# Home Health Care Nursing
## Concepts and Practice

# Home Health Care Nursing

## Concepts and Practice

**Sarah B. Keating** RN, C-PNP, EDD
Chair and Professor
Nursing Department
San Francisco State University
San Francisco, California

**Glenda B. Kelman** RNCS, OCN, MS
Doctoral Candidate, New York University
Associate Professor
Russell Sage College
Troy, New York

*J. B. LIPPINCOTT COMPANY*
*Philadelphia*
London   Mexico City   New York   St. Louis   São Paulo   Sydney

Sponsoring Editor: Patricia L. Cleary
Indexer: Ann Blum
Designer: Susan Hess Blaker
Production Supervisor: Carol A. Florence
Production Assistant: Charlene Catlett Squibb
Compositor: Maryland Composition Co. Inc.
Printer/Binder: R. R. Donnelly & Sons Company

6   5   4   3   2   1

**Library of Congress Cataloging-in-Publication Data**

Keating, Sarah B.
  Home health care nursing.

  Includes index.
  1. Home nursing.   2. Community health nursing.
I. Kelman, Glenda B.   II. Title. [DNLM:   1. Community
Health Nursing.   2. Home Care Services.   3. Nursing
Process—methods. WY 115 K25h]
RT120.H65K43   1988        610.73'43        87-2909
ISBN 0-397-54603-3

Any procedure or practice described in this book should be applied by the
health-care practitioner under appropriate supervision in accordance with
professional standards of care used with regard to the unique circumstances that
apply in each practice situation. Care has been taken to confirm the accuracy of
information presented and to describe generally accepted practices. However, the
authors, editors, and publisher cannot accept any responsibility for errors or
omissions or for consequences from application of the information in this book
and make no warranty, express or implied, with respect to the contents of the
book.
Every effort has been made to ensure drug selections and dosages are in
accordance with current recommendations and practice. Because of ongoing
research, changes in government regulations, and the constant flow of
information on drug therapy, reactions, and interactions, the reader is cautioned
to check the package insert for each drug for indications, dosages, warnings, and
precautions, particularly if the drug is new or infrequently used.

*To our husbands, Ed and Don*

# *Acknowledgments*

The authors wish to thank Karen Pardue, RNC, MS, Clinical Supervisor of Visiting Nurse Association and Home Care Inc. of Hartford, for her expert review, comments, and suggestions of the home health care principles and procedures in the text.

Chapter 8 was written by the following contributing author:

Bill Barrick, RN, MSN
Nurse Manager, Clinics
National Institute of
Allergy and Infectious Diseases
Bethesda, Maryland

# *Foreword*

Home health care is not a new nurse role. Nurses have been caring for the sick in the home since the pre-Christian era. Health promotion, as well as sick care, of persons in their homes appears in the early Roman writings so we know that home health care is not a new idea or a new role for nurses. However, home health care nursing of today is a *new* practice. Advances in technology, scientific discoveries, and the most recent changes in third party reimbursement have created a very different kind of nursing practice in the home.

Because of our ability to diagnose and treat conditions that once killed the population, coupled with the cost of that care and the need to contain that cost, patients are discharged earlier and sent to their homes in the acute phase of their recovery, often with much of the sophisticated paraphernalia still in operation to be managed by the family in the home. The high tech care of the hospital is simply transferred to the home setting. Community health nurses now find themselves functioning as acute care nurses in the home.

The home health care nurse has always devoted a major portion of time to teaching the patient and the family about how to stay well and how to manage their sicknesses. Now, however, the nurse in the home is teaching the family and the patient about high tech care. It is not uncommon to have a patient on dialysis, or on a respirator, or needing a wound or urinary catheter irrigation, or a heparinized flush of a Hickman catheter. The nurse needs to know how to care for and how to teach others to care for patients with very complex and acute health care needs.

Today home health nursing demands a different kind of nurse and one prepared with more advanced knowledge, communication, and decision-making and teaching skills—as well as psychomotor abilities—than ever before. The nursing diagnoses are more focused on acute problems, and family support is more critical. I am sure Lillian Wald, the founder of community health nursing in the early 1900s, would throw up her hands in astonishment if she could see the practice in the home today.

A major concern in these changes in home health care, and one in which I have a special interest, is how nurse educators can prepare nurses for these new roles and skills. When other roles or advances in the practice have emerged, educators have simply incorporated them into the curriculum. Resources, such as texts and research findings, were sought and experiences developed. However, there have been few resources and few experts and virtually no research, at least not until this text.

The authors of this text have accomplished a very difficult task and in a very commendable way. They have provided nurses in home health care and nurse educators with the first comprehensive home health care nursing-specific text in print. It is a text that contains information on the history and trends of home health nursing care, community diagnoses and demographics of the client population, organization and financing of home health care, specific nursing technology applied to frequently encountered nursing diagnoses, quality assurance issues, and research implications. A nurse, a student, or a faculty person would need to purchase several texts to obtain the information that is in this text. Some of the information is no other place but in this text.

As I read the manuscript in preparation for this foreword, I became very excited about how I might use it with my own community health course. I also began to see how I could provide different experiences for my students in the community setting. I believe the authors have prepared a text for a practice that is growing and changing, and that this text will help give direction and support to the way nurses are prepared for that changing practice. It is also a valuable resource for those currently practicing in the home.

Fay L. Bower, RN, DNSC, FAAN
Dean and Professor
School of Nursing
University of San Francisco

# Introduction

The book provides an overview of the expanding field of home health care nursing and a framework for nursing practice based on the caring component as the essential link between the home health care client and the nurse. The explosion in technology, including high-tech nursing procedures, coupled with early discharge from acute care settings, poses one of the greatest challenges to nurses in the delivery of care in the home. The home health care setting is rapidly becoming one of the largest practice arenas for nursing, and it is generally recognized that home health care nursing is evolving into a specialty area.

Concepts and practice in home health care nursing encompass many of the traditional nursing specialties. The nature of the practice setting and the knowledge and skills required for home health care nursing include a blending of community/public health, medical/surgical, pediatric, maternity, and mental health nursing with emphasis on community health and medical/surgical nursing. Recent debates in the profession focus on the extent to which the practitioner in home health care is a generalist or specialist and what educational and experience qualifications are necessary for practice.

It is more than likely that a master's degree in home health nursing will be required in the future. However, reality and present-day health care system needs demand nurses who can provide "high tech–high touch" services to clients requiring home health care (Backer, Frost, and Mason, 1985). Currently nurses practicing in home health care represent all specialties and levels of education, including associate degree, diploma, baccalaureate degree, and postgraduate preparation. According to Northrop (1986) home health care agencies need to test two assumptions:

> that medical-surgical nurses can go into the home health care without consideration for the difference in setting, and that public health nurses won't need medical-surgical skills for the more acutely ill patient. Employing either

assumption could raise troublesome questions about what standards of care apply. The home health care nurse should be held to the same standard as any other "home health nurse" (not hospital or public health nurse alone, but a new configuration) (p. 256).

There is a plethora of types of agencies providing home health care nursing services, including traditional visiting nurse associations, health departments, community based nursing services, hospital based home health care, nursing registries, hospices, independent professional practices, small and large for-profit agencies and corporations, specialized services agencies, and conglomerates. The type of agency in which the nurse practices home health care influences the qualifications necessary and the scope of practice.

Home health care has a long history in nursing, with its most recent history beginning with the Metropolitan Life Insurance Company's Visiting Nurses. Since the inception of the Medicare and Medicaid methods for financing health care in the 1960s and 1970s, there has been an increase in the need for providing care of the ill at home. Many of these clients are elderly and have multiple medical diagnoses with complex nursing care implications.

The federal government's plan for prospective reimbursement for hospital care has both a direct and indirect effect on home health care. Trends indicate that clients are discharged from the care-giving institution to return home at much earlier stages of their recovery and at more acute levels of illness. Long-term care in the community setting and the hospice concept of the consumer's right to die at home add other dimensions to the overall scene. This book provides the basic knowledge and techniques necessary for these types of problems.

## References

Northrop C: Home health care: Changing legal perspectives. Nursing Outlook. 34(5): 256, September/October, 1986.
Backer B, Frost AD, Mason DJ: High tech—high touch—high time. Nursing and Health Care. 6(5): 262–266, May, 1985.

# Contents

# Dimensions of Home Health Care Nursing

The first three chapters of this text present an overview of the current United States health care system as it applies to home health care nursing. The historical perspectives of home health care nursing are reviewed as they influence the present-day nursing practice and educational systems. Current trends are discussed as they influence nursing practice in the home setting.

In Chapter 2, basic concepts for assessing and diagnosing home health care needs in the community are presented. The chapter focuses on the aggregate client system, which implies nursing action on the part of the specialist or advanced nurse clinician. In home health care, the specialist or advanced nurse clinician is usually found in case management, staff supervision, consultative, and administrative roles. However, a basic knowledge of the community in which the staff home health care nurse practices is essential for identifying common problems encountered in the population served and the developing trends in the field for appropriate planning and preparation. Thus, the diagnosis of home health care needs in the community is indicated for all levels of home health care nurses.

In Chapter 3, administrative and management aspects of home health care nursing are discussed. Although the overview of financing, types of agencies, organizational structure, job qualifications and descriptions, and management principles may not apply directly to the staff nurse practicing in home health care, the knowledge base does apply to the communication and political aspects of the field. At the minimum, a brief knowledge of the financing of the system is essential for understanding client entitlement to services and the limitations within the system that prohibit the delivery of home health care nursing.

# Historical Perspectives and Current Trends

## Overview

Home health care nursing as defined by the authors is the delivery of specialized nursing care services in the home health care setting. The client system includes the person with a diagnosed health problem(s) requiring skilled nursing care and his or her family or significant others in the home setting. It requires advanced nursing knowledge and practice specific to

1. The pathophysiology and treatment of disease
2. Assessment of the person, family, and community resources
3. Nursing diagnoses appropriate to the home care setting
4. Planning and intervention
   a. Advanced communication techniques
   b. Application of high technology and advanced nursing care
   c. Teaching/education
   d. Counseling
   e. Referral
   f. Coordination of health services and personnel
   g. Application of appropriate research findings
5. Evaluation of services rendered to the person and family according to
   a. Client outcomes, including satisfaction
   b. Standards of home health care
   c. Home health care program purposes and goals

Dimensions of home health care in the health care system and their implications for nursing practice are discussed in this chapter. Historical perspectives in light of the current practice of home health care nursing are reviewed. Included in the review is a brief account of the history of the educational preparation of community/public health nurses and home health care nurses and its influence on current education for home health care nursing. Qualifications and competency expectations for the various levels of home health care nurses are also discussed.

## Historical Perspectives of Home Health Care Nursing

Home health care has a long history in nursing. Its most recent history in the United States began in the early 1900s with the advent of the visiting nurses of Metropolitan Life Insurance Company. The Medicare (federal) and Medicaid (federal and state) systems were instituted in the 1960s and resulted in increased demands for home care. The programs provided health care for Social Security beneficiaries (those 65 and older and the disabled) and other members of the population who were medically indigent (Ebersole and Hess, 1986). Because some of the benefits from Medicare and Medicaid were reimbursable to health agencies (e.g., well-baby care, skilled nursing care, and home health care), health departments, hospital-based home care units, and visiting nurse associations increased or added to their services to clients. Agencies choosing to add to or increase their services had to meet Medicare and Medicaid requirements and were certified by the federal government for Medicare and their state regulating agencies for Medicaid (Mundinger, 1983).

The current administration's prospective payment method for financing health care services and its classification of health problems into Diagnostic-Related Groupings (DRGs) have affected the home health care arena. Recent trends indicate that patients are discharged from the acute care institution to home at much earlier stages of their recovery and at more acute levels of illness. Frequently, these home health care clients are elderly and have multiple medical diagnoses with complex nursing care needs (National Center for Health Services Research and Health Care Technology Assessment, 1985). According to the National Center for Health Services Research and Health Care Technology (1985), the elderly average 22.3 home health visits annually. Long-term care in the community setting and the hospice concept of the consumer's right to die at home add other dimensions to the overall home health care scene.

### World History

From the earliest recorded times of humankind, civilizations designated certain people to visit the sick at home. The earliest nurses who visited the sick recognized the need for teaching health practices not only to cure illnesses but also to prevent them. Western Civilization tells of the Greek goddess of health, Hygiea, and Panacea, restorer of health, whose credos included health guidance as well as care of the sick. During the pre-Christian Roman era, specially prepared women were identified for visiting the sick and poor at home.

During the early Christian era, Paul's letters to the Romans (Romans 16:1-2) record the visits of Phoebe to the homes of the sick. Phoebe was the first visiting nurse identified by name (Stanhope and Lancaster, 1984). In 1617, in Europe, St. Vincent de Paul founded the Sisters of Charity whose functions were to visit the ill at home. He and a supervising nurse, Madeline Le Gras, identified additional education and professional supervision of nurses as prerequisites for providing home health care services (Clemen, Eigsti, and Mcguire, 1981).

During the Middle Ages and subsequent centuries, care of the sick and poor was considered a right of the people. The English Elizabethan Poor Law of 1601 guaranteed access to medical and nursing care for the sick and poor (Stanhope and Lancaster, 1984). Much of the care, however, was provided through charity, and, thus, quality was directly affected by the amount of available funds and numbers of qualified care providers.

Prior to the Industrial Revolution, health practices were deplorable, especially regarding sanitation of the environment. Communicable diseases were prevalent, and there were few nurses who were educated to render care and teach health behaviors. Unfortunately, nurses of those times were exemplified by Sairy Gamp of Charles Dickens' notoriety, and they did little to add to the professional image that nurses seek.

Florence Nightingale introduced the era of modern nursing in the late 19th century. It was a time of rapid explosion of scientific knowledge in the medical and health care fields. Knowledge about the causes of disease and social concerns for the plight of workers during the industrial revolution were raising the consciousness levels of the population.

In England, William Rathbone, an influential merchant and friend of Nightingale, established the first visiting nurse association. His wife had been ill at home, and the services of a nurse who came to visit at home so impressed him that he was convinced that nurses should be employed to visit the sick in their homes. He asked Nightingale to assist him in the enterprise, and, although she was unable to directly provide help, she did record her recommendations.

Based on Rathbone's notion of providing nursing for the people in the districts of Liverpool, Nightingale coined the term *District Nurses*. Nightingale believed in postgraduate education for nurses practicing in the home setting in addition to basic bedside nursing skills acquired in the hospital setting. She also recommended that nurses teach the patient and family about health care. She demonstrated her concern for the environment by recommending that District Nurses care for the sick room and home and notify health officers of any unsanitary conditions threatening the family's health (Monteiro, 1985; Smilie, 1955).

## American History

Nightingale's influence on modern American nursing is well documented. The first visiting nurses in America were termed *District Nurses*, an adoption of the English term for nurses who visited the sick and provided health teaching in the community. The first United States home visiting programs in the 1880s were under the auspices of hospital dispensaries in urban areas (e.g., the Boston Dispensary). Soon afterward in 1909, services were provided by nurses for the Metropolitan Life Insurance (MLI) Company. Lillian Wald was instrumental in establishing the latter. She and Lee Frankel of MLI were able to persuade the company that healthy workers were more efficient workers (Clemen et al., 1981). Eventually, MLI nursing activities were incorporated into visiting nurse associations or public health nursing agencies.

The first visiting nurse associations, or district nursing associations, as they were then known, were established in 1865 in Boston and Philadelphia. They were modeled after the English district nurses associations and recognized the need for health teaching of the client and family. Thus, they coined the phrase *instructive visiting nurse association*. It was also about this time that people who were interested in philanthropic causes began to establish settlement houses to help the poor and sick in urban areas (Tinkham, Voorhies, and McCarthy, 1984). They were to become the foundations for the practice of modern-day community health nursing.

In 1893, Lillian Wald and Mary Brewster established the Henry Street Settlement House in New York City to care for the sick and poor and to teach good health practices. Wald was the first to use the phrase *public health nurse* and was an early nurse activist in the political arena. Her loan of nurses to New York City schools and Health Department led to the incorporation of nurses into the public health care field (Stanhope and Lancaster, 1984).

From the early 1900s to the early 1960s, the community health care system supported basically two types of nursing service agencies. The first were the visiting nurse associations, whose primary focus was on the care of the sick at home. They were nonprofit and were supported through private funding sources such as fees for service, and community-based fund raising agencies (e.g., United Way, donations, and private foundations).

The other types of agencies with nursing services were the official health departments or public health nursing services supported by public funds. Functions of these agencies were mandated and regulated through legislation from the local, state, or regional governments. The official agencies' nursing services focused on public health activities, such as the control of communicable disease, health promotion, health maintenance, and prevention of disease. If nurses provided care for the sick at home, their function was to teach the family or other care provider how to provide care rather than to provide direct nursing care.

In some instances, visiting nurse associations and official agencies combined to form agencies supported through public and private funding sources. They shared staff and administrative functions and provided public health and bedside nursing care. These agencies were formed in the 1940s, and some continue to exist.

For at least the past four decades, community-based home health care nursing services were usually lodged in health departments, visiting nurse associations, or combined agencies. However, hospitals also provide home care for their discharged patients. With the changing health care system, additional hospital-based programs were established, and they are currently one of the major providers of home health care. Although the earliest hospital-based home care services took place in the late 1800s, one of the forerunners of today's types of services was that of the Montefiore Hospital Home Care Program in New York. The Montefiore program began in 1947 and offered comprehensive services (Stanhope and Lancaster, 1984).

There are a variety of hospital-based programs in today's home health care system. They include those who contract with established health agencies, such as visiting nurse associations, private duty registries, health departments, or entrepreneurial, for-profit agencies (e.g., those owned by pharmaceutical or medical supply companies). Based on the nature of their administrative structure, hospital-based programs may use their own nursing staff or contract for nursing services through another health agency.

## Educational Perspectives

By the turn of the 19th century, student nurses were sent by hospital-based schools to care for discharged patients at home. Nurses had to adapt what they learned from care of the sick in the hospital to the home setting, where equipment and supplies were not readily available. The situation led to ingenuity and creative approaches for providing care and the necessity to rely on other community support services. Nursing also recognized the need to teach care of the sick at home and preventive health practices to families. Based on the students' experiences, nurse educators recognized that additional education was necessary for providing nursing services in the community or home settings (Beard, 1922; Dock, 1906; Ahrens, 1905; Keith, 1905).

Stewart (1919) reiterated the need for formal preparation for public health nursing. She recommended the inclusion of content on the prevention of disease and on the family and community as clients. She recommended that schools of nursing allow students to choose the specialty of their interest during the senior year and that half of that year—not less than 4 months, preferably 8 months—be spent in public health nursing. She advised that nursing education include hygiene, sanitation, bacteriology, social sciences, psychology, teaching activities, communicable disease, and social aspects of disease. It was at that time that Teacher's College, Columbia, developed courses for application to visiting nursing. The courses included principles of public health nursing, social case work, and home economics. All these activities were in conjunction with the Henry Street Settlement under the leadership of Lillian Wald.

In 1920, the National Organization for Public Health Nursing (NOPHN) began accrediting college programs for the preparation of public health nurses. Since 1952, the National League for Nursing (NLN), the descendant of the NOPHN, has identified baccalaureate programs that receive accreditation for preparing beginning level public health nurses. The American Nurses Association stated in 1962 that public health nurses should be required to have (1) licensure, and (2) completion of a baccalaureate degree program approved by the NLN for public health preparation *or* post-baccalaureate study that includes content approved by NLN (Freeman, 1963). Although the statement was not legally binding, it signified that community health nursing content was an essential part of the baccalaureate in nursing curriculum. Community/public health nursing had come into its own. It has moved from a few days of observational home visits by students in the late 1800s to become an integral part of the baccalaureate program in the 1980s.

Today's home health care field brings yet another challenge for nurse educators in curriculum planning and development. Most experts in home health care agree that home health care nursing blends community health nursing knowledge and practice with that of acute care technology based in a home setting. The question arises concerning the placement of home health care content and clinical experiences. Is it a specialty, meriting as much attention as the other specialties, such as parent child care, gerontics, adult nursing, community/public health nursing, and psychiatric/mental health nursing? Or should it be integrated into another traditional specialty, and, if it should, which one, adult or community/public health nursing? Another problem is the clinical placement of students in home health care, where close supervision is virtually impossible yet legal liabilities for the agency and school are realities.

Schools of nursing are approaching the problem in a variety of ways. Knowledge of the health care system and its specialized programs such as home health care is usually presented in Community/Public Health Nursing or Issues in Professional Nursing courses. Because concepts and application of technical skills take place in a variety of clinical courses, some programs choose to integrate the knowledge and skills of home health care nursing into specialties such as gerontics, adult nursing, parent child nursing, and mental health nursing.

Part of the clinical experiences in these courses may include home visits to clients receiving care from those specialty units or through referral from community-based agencies. Other programs may include home health care nursing concepts and practice in community/public health nursing courses through affiliation with combined agencies (public health and home health care) or through one clinical experience in each type of agency. Clinical experiences in home health care nursing can range from 1 day of observation to an intensive clinical experience managing clients receiving home health care under the supervision of agency staff or faculty members. Many programs with a final senior year specialization track have preceptorship experiences for students in hospice nursing, home health care, or providing care for homeless people in community shelters.

History of community/public health and home health care nursing demonstrates the need for knowledge and skills beyond the level of technical nursing skills. Community health nurses diagnose complex, bio-psycho-social problems in families, teach health practices, counsel, and refer to other health care providers as necessary. These skills are in addition to the knowledge necessary for community diagnosis and planning, political action groups, and working with the multidiscipline health care team in a setting that calls for independent decision-making, collaboration, and coordination of services. Basic public health sciences, including sanitation, environmental health, statistics, and epidemiology supplement the nurses' sophisticated skills in interpersonal relationships and advanced nursing knowledge.

Acute care nurses have extensive knowledge and skills in meeting the bio-psycho-social needs of their patients. Their nursing knowledge includes a strong background in the pathophysiology of disease processes and the interventions necessary for treatment, cure, palliation, and/or rehabilitation. Acute care nurses may have specialties according to the life cycle, that is, adult, pediatric, perinatal, and gerontic nursing. Home health care nursing practice requires a blending of both of these nursing specialties and presents a challenge for nursing education and service.

The field of home health care is complex and at the present time employs nurses with both acute care and community health nursing skills. The baccalaureate-prepared nurse is a generalist. In order to keep abreast of changes in the health care system, it is recommended that students in baccalaureate programs have some exposure to home health care (including theory and clinical experience), because many may find the field attractive in the future. It is predicted that it will become a specialty, requiring post-baccalaureate preparation at a minimum.

## Current Trends

With the advent of the federal Medicare program in 1965, the numbers and services of community health nursing agencies whose focus was on care of the sick increased. It was during that period of time when the term *home health agencies* came into use to denote health care services for the sick at home. The services were reimbursable through Medicare, Medicaid, and other third-party mechanisms. Some health departments that had not previously provided bedside care assumed this dimension of nursing care to qualify themselves for Medicare and Medicaid reimbursement. The establishment of these programs marked the modern era of home health care financed by federal- and state-sponsored systems.

The Medicare system has served as the predictor of change in the health care system. Because it finances a large portion of the medical and nursing services that clients receive, changes in its thrust and implementation influence the total system. The United States' economic system was threatened by inflation in the 1980s, especially in the health care system. The federal administration initiated cost-effective programs and the Medicare and Medicaid systems were influenced. The prospective payment method of reimbursement for health care services was established to attempt to control inflation in the health care system. The program was to contain costs by paying for care estimated on the previous year's hospital budget.

In order to estimate the costs for care, the DRGs were developed. The system was created to link the necessary length of hospital care to the severity of the client's disease. The DRGs were categorized by certain medical diagnoses, the extent of the illness, the client's characteristics (age and other conditions), usual hospital length of stay for the illness, and other statistical data surrounding the diagnoses. Clients were to remain in the hospital for only the usual length of stay specified for each DRG category. Any cost exceeding that recommended for each DRG category was absorbed by the hospital.

Implementation of the DRG system resulted in shortened lengths of stay, fewer clients admitted for elective surgery, an increase in ambulatory surgery, patients in the hospital who were more acutely ill and frequently were elderly with multisystem health problems, clients discharged from the hospital at earlier stages of recovery, and patients discharged to home with problems requiring acute and intensive nursing care. The phenomenon's impact on the health care system brought the high technology of acute care into the home setting focused on the person with a diagnosed health problem and illness focused.

## Staffing Trends

### The Multidiscipline Home Health Care Team

The multidiscipline team in home health care agencies is composed of the nursing staff, various therapists, nutritionists, social workers, physicians, and other specialists. Because nursing care consumes most of the direct care time and because nurses are traditionally prepared to work with other specialists, it is logical for the nurse team member to be the coordinator of care. It is she or he who makes the initial assessment of the family and their home environment. The nurse is aware of the resources and personnel available in the community. Based on these factors, the nurse assumes leadership for the comprehensive and continuing care of the client and family. Knowledge of the other health care team members' roles and functions and their qualifications is important to the nurse. As part of the team, the nurse must have advanced interpersonal communication skills and a knowledge of group dynamics. The nurse administrator in the role of executive of the agency or director of patient care services is in charge of the administration and management of health services for all the health team members.

## Home Health Care Nurses

### Nurse Administrators, Supervisors, and Clinical Specialists

The nursing administrator needs progressive experience in staff nursing, supervision, and administration. In addition to the experience, an advanced degree, preferably in nursing, is essential. The nursing degree provides nursing theory, knowledge, a clinical base, management theory, and skills in budgeting, staff management, program planning and evaluation, research and development, management of boards of directors, legislation, and political processes.

The supervising nurse needs advanced knowledge and experience in management of patient caseloads and staff to ensure the effective functioning of her or his particular nursing service or home health care unit. It is advisable that supervising nurses have at least 2 years of progressive experience in community health nursing and advanced education. It is preferable that a master's degree in nursing be the credential for supervising nurses, with a functional area in nursing management/administration. Such an education provides the advanced nursing knowledge for delivery of nursing care and management skills, including supervision of staff, staff development, caseload management, assignments, and coordination of team efforts.

The clinical specialist in home health care usually has a master's degree in nursing in the field particularly applicable to the client population that he or she will be serving. Agencies choose to have these nurses as consultants, direct care providers, staff developers, and, in some cases, supervisors of care: for example, certified nurse midwives for high-risk pregnancy patients and clients preferring alternative birth experiences, certified family nurse practitioners who provide primary health care for families and serve the person with an illness problem, gerontologic nurse practitioners for elderly clients requiring management of chronic illnesses and health maintenance, oncology clinical specialists for home health care of cancer patients electing to have chemotherapy and other modalities of care at home, critical care nurses, and coronary care nurses for the nursing management of patients with cardiovascular problems. Close collaboration between the specialist and home health care nurses is indicated for the most effective mode of delivery of care for the client.

### Competencies and Qualifications

Knowledge about individuals, families, groups, and communities is necessary for nursing the multiple client systems in the home health care setting. Superimposed on this knowledge base are the high-tech skills necessary to care for the acutely ill person at home. The situation calls for a highly skilled nurse who has knowledge of individual bio-psycho-social health needs, application of technical skills to the home setting, family dynamics, community resources, and political climates in a milieu of complex and acute illness situations. The scenario leads to the basic question facing today's community health care system: "What qualifications must the nurse have for providing highly technical skills to a person whose needs and recovery are dependent upon the surrounding social and environmental factors?"

Agencies and communities confront this dilemma in a variety of ways. Community-based agencies may choose to educate their staffs through staff development programs providing practice for such therapies as intravenous transfusion, respiratory care, chemotherapy, and hyperalimentation. Consultants with expertise in the application of high technology to home health care are called upon to teach staff and, in some instances, to provide direct client care. Some community health agencies choose to hire clinical specialists in nursing fields such as intensive care, coronary care, and pediatric and perinatal care. Hospital-based programs may negotiate with community-based programs to rotate staff through community health nursing experiences to gain knowledge and skills in working with families, communities, and other health care agencies and personnel. Collaboration between acute care and community/public health nursing providers is indicated to integrate the highly specialized concepts and skills specific to home health care settings.

### Paraprofessionals

Simple bedside care as well as housekeeping, grocery shopping, and cooking can be provided by home health care aides or personal care aides. These paraprofessionals must be under the close supervision of the professional nurse, who conducts an initial assessment and develops a plan of care that is carried out and documented. Evaluation takes place on a planned regular basis to provide for the family's changing needs. Many agencies train their paraprofessionals or contract with other agencies for certified home health care aides. Again, federal guidelines and individual state regulations may dictate the qualifications necessary for these personnel.

## Legal Parameters

Community health agencies and other home health care agencies, such as those that are hospital based, must meet guidelines if they are to receive funding through the federally sponsored Medicare and co-sponsored state Medicaid programs. These guidelines specify the types of services that must be included, types of personnel who provide the care, qualifications of the professionals, and quality assurance programs (Ebersole and Hess, 1986).

Many states require agencies to be certified or licensed to provide home care services. Included in regulations are qualifications for staff nurses, supervising nurses, and directors of agencies. Paraprofessionals and professionals such as physical therapists, occupational therapists, speech pathologists, and nutritionists must meet certain educational, legal, and experience requirements. For example, a staff home health care nurse (RN) providing bedside skills is required to be licensed as a registered nurse; a staff community/public health nurse must have a baccalaureate degree and be licensed; a supervising home health care nurse must have a baccalaureate degree, several years of experience, and preferably a master's degree. The director of an agency or nursing service is usually required to have an advanced degree in nursing or administration. Each state's regulations vary, but most traditional agencies that include public health and/or home health care activities require similar credentials.

The entrepreneurial and for-profit agencies that have been established may or may not be regulated by government agencies. If they receive Medicare funding, they must meet federal guidelines. Otherwise, depending upon state laws, they are subject to their own quality control system. Many agencies have certain requirements for their staff based on consumer satisfaction and the legal liabilities that they may assume if unqualified people are rendering personal and/or nursing care.

## Opportunities for Nursing in Home Health Care

Proprietary agencies are competing with established community health agencies. The proprietary agencies can undercut the market through lower overhead costs and an ability to provide acute care services sooner to the client. The situation has an impact on home health care by creating a competitive market for home health clientele. Traditional agencies (visiting nurse associations and health departments) are therefore evaluating services and developing cost-effective programs. The economic influences on the system are powerful and in the end may change the system radically.

Health insurance policies may or may not include home health care nursing benefits. Beneficiaries may not be cognizant of the need for this type of coverage until the situation arises. Additionally, consumers frequently do not have the knowledge of available community resources and which of these best fits their health needs. Nursing should assume the leading advocate role by becoming knowledgeable in community resources and assisting the client to choose the highest quality, most appropriate to level of need, cost-effective, and accessible services available.

Some of the entrepreneurial agencies established to provide home health care are nurse generated and managed. Nurses who establish these services usually have business acumen, in addition to their license to practice nursing. Nurses in these roles utilize knowledge from small business experiences, accountants, lawyers, and insurance agents. Nurses in the entrepreneurial role need avanced knowledge and experience in management and business administration in addition to basic professional education and credentialing. Client care and staff management skills are essential. If business and legal skills are not part of the nurse's repertoire, consultation with experts from the business world is recommended.

## References and Selected Readings

Ahrens M: District and visiting nursing as part of training-school curriculum. American Journal of Nursing 6:817–821, 1906

Beard RO: The making of history in nursing education. American Journal of Nursing, 22:507–522, 1922

Clemen SA, Eigsti DG, McGuire SL: Comprehensive Family and Community Health Nursing. New York, McGraw-Hill, 1981

Dock LL: Training for visiting nursing. American Journal of Nursing, 7:109, 1906

Ebersole P, Hess P: Toward Healthy Aging. St Louis, Mosby, 1986

Freeman RB: Public Health Nursing Practice. Philadelphia, WB Saunders, 1963

Jamieson EM, Sewall MF: Trends in Nursing History, 4th ed. Philadelphia, WB Saunders, 1954

Keith ML: The introduction of district nursing into the training-school curriculum. American Journal of Nursing 5:599–604, 1905

Monteiro LA: Florence nightingale on public health nursing. American Journal of Public Health 75:181–185, 1985

Mundinger M: Home Care Controversy. Rockville, MD, Aspen Systems Corp, 1983

National Center for Health Services Research and Health Care Technology Assessment: Research Activities. No. 78. Rockville, MD, US Department of Health and Human Services, October 1985

Smilie WG: Public Health: Its Promise for the Future. New York, Macmillan, 1955

Spradley BW: Community Health Nursing Concepts and Practice, 2nd ed. Boston, Little, Brown and Company, 1985

Stanhope M, Lancaster J: Community Health Nursing. St. Louis, Mosby, 1984
Stewart IM: Readjustment in the training-school curriculum to meet the new demands in public health nursing. American Journal of Nursing, 20:102–109, 1919
Tinkham CW, Voorhies EF, McCarthy NC: Community Health Nursing, 3rd ed. Norwalk, CT, Appleton-Century-Crofts, 1984

# 2

# Community Diagnosis and Continuity of Care: An Aggregate Focus Applied to Home Health Care

## Overview

The unit of service in home health care nursing includes the client with a diagnosed health problem and his or her family or support systems (if any). The home health care client system differs from that of public health nursing's, which focuses on the aggregate (population at risk) and community and provides mostly primary levels of prevention. The home health care client system focus is similar to that of the community health nurse, that is, client and family, yet varies because the individual client has a diagnosed health problem mandating at least secondary levels of care and usually tertiary care. The health care needs of community health nursing clients range from primary to tertiary levels of prevention.

Primary care includes health promotion and prevention of disease activities. Secondary care is prescribed for clients with diagnosed health problems requiring activities to diagnose, cure, or prevent further illness, complications, disability, and unwarranted death. Tertiary care includes rehabilitation and palliative measures to relieve discomfort or assist the client and family toward acceptance of death and dying. Although community and home health care nurses are both involved with secondary and tertiary levels of care, home health care emphasizes tertiary levels of care.

In the hospital or acute care setting, the physician, nurse, and other care providers order the care that is provided and the rules under which the client must comply to receive care. The type of care in the acute care setting is usually tertiary and directed toward cure and rehabilitation, or palliation. The type of care is similar to that of home health care, but the ill person usually requires a higher level of short-term acute care than in the home. It is the less acute but high technology care that is brought to the home setting and that must blend with the knowledge and practice related to family care and community resources to provide today's home health care. The home health care setting creates a milieu in which the nurse is the guest of the client and family or social support system and is recognized by them as a professional expert. The situation provides the foundation for a partnership between client and nurse as contrasted to the more dependent role of the patient in the hospital setting.

The nurse administrator/manager or the professional nursing staff in home health care nursing use community diagnosis procedures to identify populations at risk for home health care and the need for specific services in the community. Community diagnosis depends upon the location of the agency, the type of agency from which services are delivered, and the nature of the population served. Types of home health care agencies include visiting nurse associations, health departments, community health nursing services, hospital-based home health care units, nurse registries, free-standing home health care agencies, corporations or conglomerates, and private practice. The following examples demonstrate how the boundaries for community home health care diagnosis are determined. Official health departments have specific geopolitical lines confining them to one location, whereas hospital-based home health care units may cross geographical lines by serving their patients and those of the physicians affiliated with the hospital.

The home health care staff nurse usually serves persons and families within a specific geographical territory and studies aggregate needs in that assigned microcosm (miniature community), such as a neighborhood or rural area. An analysis of the microcosm and its population helps to identify the most common health problems and the aggregates who are at risk for home health care services. Diagnosing aggregate health needs helps the nurse to define her or his role and functions in serving the community at large, as well as the individual client and family.

Staff home health care nurses may not have the time to diagnose in depth the neighborhood or community in which they serve the aggregate's home health care needs. However, they must have knowledge and an awareness of the community and its resources for effective coordination of care and referral of clients. Home health care administrators, managers, and clinical specialists diagnose the home health care problems of the community and its aggregate client systems, including demographic characteristics of the population served, and the sources of referrals and follow-up; this provides them with the knowledge necessary to deliver services. The diagnosis(es) assist them in developing, planning, implementing, and evaluating home health care programs.

## Demographics of the Client Population

Most specialists in home health care, acute care, and long-term care settings agree that the majority of their clients are elderly. Analysis of agency records and required reports for accrediting and regulating purposes validates this information. The National Center for Health Services Research and Health Care Technology Assessment (1985) reports that "the most intensive users of home health services are the elderly, who average 22.3 home health visits annually . . . 78% of all home health visits are received by Americans older than 65 years, even though they constitute only 43% of the user population." Hays (1986) reports that patients receiving hospice services, a specialized program within the home health care field, had a mean age of 64 years for those receiving services at home, and a mean age of 68 years for those receiving a combination of home care and inpatient services. Home health care administrators use the statistical and demographic data available as well as their personal and professional observations and judgments to project market conditions.

Although it is obvious to most providers that the majority of their clients are elderly, the other obvious dimension of home health care clientele is the increased population of clients with high-acuity health care needs, such as apnea monitoring (in infants), tracheostomy care, peritoneal dialysis, hyperalimentation, and intravenous therapy. The situation is due in large part to the impact of the prospective payment program with its related Diagnostic-Related Groupings (DRGs) on the health care system. Early discharge from the hospital and utilization of alternative methods of medical care delivery, such as surgi-centers or 24-hour surgical services, are creating population groups requiring care in the community setting rather than in hospitals. Many require high-tech nursing services at home. Advances in the application of technology to the home care setting such as home dialysis units, respirators, and other appliances have, in some instances, helped to create a younger and more acutely ill client population.

There is a dearth of current statistics reporting the demographic characteristics for home health care clientele. However, it is common knowledge that the population of the United States is aging (i.e., over 65 years of age) (almost 12% of the total population) and that the numbers of people older than 85 years of age have increased 9.1% since 1980 (Ebersole and Hess, 1985). Associated with the elderly are increased chronic disease rates requiring higher utilization of medical care, including home health care (Petrowski, 1985). Only about 5% of those people 65 years and older are under care in long-term care facilities. However, when the statistics are age-specific to people between 75 and older, the need for long-term care increases. The same situation applies to home health care. For example, Balinsky and Rehman (1984) reported that two thirds of home health care clients surveyed in 1980 in New York State were 65 years and older, and nearly 40% were 75 years of age and older.

Branch (1985) reported that 36.5% of people 75 to 84 years of age were receiving nursing home care and projected that by the year 2000, 36.8% would be in nursing homes; whereas in 2030, 38.4% would require institutional care. Branch further projected that 41.3% of people 85 years and older will require nursing home care by the year 2000, and 40% will require this type of care by 2030.

In addition to these factors, people who require home health care who are 75 years of age and older are sicker and poorer. A study by Rosenfeld (1984) comparing two states, Massachusetts and New York, demonstrated this fact; however, it must be kept in mind that the statistics for the study were based on 1976 data. It is logical to project that these numbers have increased during the past decade in accord with the increasing numbers of people in that age group.

Berk and Bernstein (1985) reported the following information related to the home health care population, based on the National Medical Care Expenditure Survey of 1977. Although the data are relatively old, the statistics from the late 1970s help to describe what is happening in the current health care system and to project for the future. Berk and Bernstein found statistically significant ($p$ = or < 0.05) differences between home health care and non–home health care populations: People older than 65 years of age had more home visits (4.4% of total population); there were more females (5.2%) than males (3.3%) older than 65 years; and more poor/near poor persons who were 65 years and over than those not poor, 5.8% compared with 3.8%.

Overall, there appear to be two basic types of home health clients; younger, acutely ill clients requiring high technology nursing care skills, and elderly clients (most of them being 75 years and older), who are ill with chronic disease and poorer than their contemporaries, with fewer resources available to them.

## Epidemiology: Common Problems Requiring Home Health Care

One of the most current studies in the literature concerning the types of health problems experienced by home health care clientele is reported by Balinsky and Rehman (1985). Their study was based on 1980 data in New York State. The primary medical diagnoses of clients, listed by percentage of the total sample of 569 were

| | |
|---|---|
| Circulatory disorders | 21.2% |
| Neoplasms | 15.2% |
| Diabetes | 18.9% |
| Accidents/musculoskeletal disorders | 20.0% |
| Other | 24.6% |

The diagnoses are consistent with the leading causes of mortality in the United States and an aging population.

Lampley and Freeman (1984) studied utilization and referral patterns of home health care clients in Mississippi in 1980. Leading health problems for their study group (N = 363) were as follows:

| | |
|---|---|
| Total bedridden or restricted activity | 88% |
| Special equipment or procedures needs | 72% |
| Assistance with activities of daily living | 80% |

Additionally, the following diseases were reported as the most common for home health clientele:

Hypertension
Diabetes
Cerebral vascular accident
Congestive heart failure
Arthritis
Arteriosclerotic heart disease
Fracture
Musculoskeletal disorders
Anemia
Urinary tract infection

The majority of hospice patients receiving care in Hays' (1986) study were diagnosed with cancer—lung cancer being the most predominant. When comparing the home care hospice clients with those receiving a combination of home care and inpatient services, Hays found that home care hospice clients had fewer symptoms (pain, nausea/vomiting, respiratory distress, elimination problems, nutritional deficit, and mental status deficit) than those patients receiving care at home and in the acute care setting. Their families exhibited less anxiety and fatigue during the last 6 days of their lives compared to the families of patients in the combined home care/ inpatient care program.

Dalton (1985) identified cardiac output, alteration in: decreased, as a major nursing diagnosis found in the discharge records of a visiting nurse association. The alteration in cardiac output diagnosis and the medical diagnoses previously listed are consistent with common problems identified by nurses involved in home health care services for the northeastern region of New York State in 1983–1985 and northern California in 1986 (see Chapter 12, Table 12-2). In the latter studies, nurses identified the following nursing diagnoses, which correlate with the medical diagnoses previously listed:

Activity intolerance
Alterations in cardiac output
Alterations in comfort
Impaired physical mobility

Included in the list of nursing diagnoses are those that have an impact on the family of the ill person such as coping, ineffective: family, and alterations in family processes related to an ill family member.

## Community Diagnosis

### Assessment of Home Health Care Needs

Home health care administrators and staff nurses delivering services to clients need a knowledge of their community and its services relating to home care. A home health care needs assessment verifies the existence of a client population for the agency. It also identifies the market prospects for delivering home health care and can be driven by monetary motivation to either support continuation of the agency or create a profit-making enterprise.

The needs assessment projects future needs of the community for home health care services, including staffing, agency housing, and special services needs. It identifies existing services in the community to

1. Avoid duplication of services
2. Identify existing resources
3. Provide a base for referral and collaboration among agencies and health care providers

The process of diagnosing a community helps to identify the community support and interest of people in the services. Client participation and volunteer services for care of the ill at home are crucial to the success of the home care enterprise. Community diagnosis identifies such community support systems, informal and formal, and the financial resources available for home health care services.

Conducting a community needs assessment becomes efficient and thorough if it is a group effort and includes community leaders, community residents, and members of the health care team representing the various health disciplines. Home health care assumes that clients need at least the secondary level of care (diagnosed illness) and that most clients are in tertiary stages of need (complex illness). The latter groups require rehabilitation, alleviation of discomfort from chronic disease, and/or a comfortable death at home. Data collection focuses on information describing the characteristics of the population, its health status, resources existing in the community for health care, and major sources of financing health care.

Warren's (1978) description of the horizontal and vertical patterns of community organization serves as a model for collecting data for home health care. The horizontal pattern in the community as defined by Warren is, "the structural and functional relation of its various social units and subsystems to each other" (p 164). Figure 2-1 illustrates the adaptation of Warren's model to a community diagnosis for home health care needs.

When assessing for home health care needs, horizontal patterns include specific health-related social institutions within the community. Institutions within the community such as religion, education, commerce, industry, transportation, communication, government, and recreation are listed. Data pertaining to institutions having a direct bearing on home health care needs are collected.

### Example

*Religion:* What religious services are available for members confined to their homes? Are there friendly visitor programs?

*Education:* Are there home health care continuing education programs for clients and their families? What continuing education programs exist for professionals?

*Commerce:* Are there commercial vendors or loan closets for home care equipment and supplies?

*Industry:* What role do major employers in the community take in providing employees with home care services?

*Transportation:* What services are there for transfer of clients from one health care delivery scene to another?

*Communication:* Do emergency call systems exist, such as home phone emergency call buttons? How is new knowledge in the field disseminated?

*Government:* What government programs on the local level are available to clients and families?

*Recreation:* What support systems exist in the community for rest and relaxation for clients and care providers (e.g., YM/WCA, cardiac rehabilitation programs)?

Family as an institution is considered a part of the needs assessment. It includes an analysis of family characteristics such as structure; religious

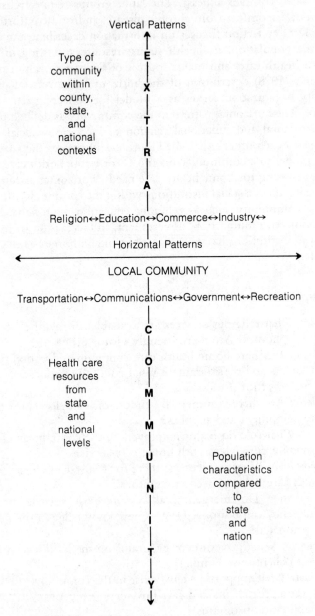

Figure 2-1. Adaptation of Warren's (1978) Patterns of Community Organization to Community Diagnosis for Home Health Care Needs.

support; average family age and size; and support systems. Health care institutions having a direct bearing on home health care needs include acute care institutions (hospitals, emergency centers, surgical centers), ambulatory care centers, clinics, physicians' offices, pharmacies, health care equipment vendors, health maintenance organizations, nursing homes, health-related facilities, homes for the aged, senior citizens' centers, health departments, visiting nurse associations, and other voluntary or official community health agencies.

Health statistics, including population base, age groups, socioeconomic status, census track characteristics, morbidity, and mortality rates, help to reveal existing and potential health problems. Sources of data can come from the U.S. Census Bureau, surveys conducted by the National Center for Health Statistics, Centers for Disease Control, state and local health departments, and health agency records.

Health agency records assist in the data collection by reporting the acuity level of the clients it serves, unmet needs, major diagnoses or health problems treated, the sources of financing for the health care provided, methods of referral, and to whom clients are referred for continuity of care.

The vertical pattern for community organization as defined by Warren is "the structural and functional relation of its various social units and subsystems to extra-community systems" (p 163). The vertical pattern relating to home health care is the means by which the community meets its needs through secondary and indirect sources. For example, local health departments are regulated by state health department activities and the laws of the state. In turn, the federal government has certain programs and legislation that regulate the state agencies. The Older Americans Act is an example of how the federal government provides certain programs that interface with local levels and provide direct care (Kaye, 1984).

The Medicare and Medicaid programs have federal, state, and local impact on implementation of services and quality of care. Medicare is regulated by the federal government, whereas federal, state, and local interpretations influence the Medicaid program. Other sources of health care financing come from private insurance and other health plans, many of which are large corporations and include, on a national level, the main corporation, politicians, and influential lobbying and professional groups such as the American Nurse's Association, American Medical Association, Joint Commission for the Accreditation of Hospitals, and the National Home Care Association.

Data collection for a needs assessment begins with information concerning the horizontal strands in the community. Each portion of the horizontal pattern is traced through its vertical pattern to identify possible resources or barriers to care outside the community.

A thorough community diagnosis is time-consuming and can itself become a barrier to delivery of care. Those wishing to conduct a brief needs assessment for program development can use certain indices in the community that provide accessible and critical information describing the community. The recommended indices are

1. Population size and age
2. Existing agencies providing care
3. Leading morbidity and mortality rates
4. Financial support systems

Appendix A outlines a community assessment model for identifying home health care needs.

### Sources of Data for Assessing and Diagnosing Levels of Home Health Care Needs in the Population and in Data Analysis

The outline in Appendix A serves as a tool for collecting and analyzing data to formulate tentative diagnoses of home health care problems in the community. Analysis will indicate the need for services, the target population group(s), types of problems, and financial support systems. The following outline and discussion provides possible sources of data for each item in the Appendix and suggested analyses for formulating diagnoses and making decisions.

### Horizontal Patterns

I. Community geopolitical boundaries
   A. Sources
      1. Maps
      2. Political subdivisions
      3. Health systems agencies
   B. Analysis
      Initial decisions are made at this point, and the diagnosticians delineate the parameters of health care needs that they wish to identify. Decisions depend upon the population group they wish to serve, the geographic practicalities, the governmental and political boundaries that specify legal limitations, the financial eligibility of clients for programs of health services, and the previously agreed upon boundaries of services for provision of care by existing agencies.
      The area is defined and surveyed according to the aforementioned considerations. The process of data collection helps to inform the people of the community of the needs assessment and may stimulate their interest in program development. It

provides a format for their perceptions of health care needs and can provide initial qualitative data that assist in diagnostic activities. Samples of communities could include a city, an incorporated village, a small rural county, a school district, a township, a neighborhood, or a census tract.

II.  Population Characteristics
 A.  Sources
   1.  Vital statistics from city, county, state, or town clerk records
   2.  Demographics from the latest census
   3.  Health statistics from health departments, community agencies, long-term facilities, hospital records, and random sample interviews of health personnel and the general population
   4.  Information regarding financial support systems from insurance agents and companies, health and human services agencies
 B.  Analysis
   Review of the data will indicate leading diseases, vulnerable population groups (aged, sick, poor), and financial gaps or possible support systems for provision of health care services.

III.  Community Resources
 A.  Sources
   1.  Health systems agencies
   2.  Local health departments
   3.  Registries
   4.  Professional organizations
   5.  Telephone book
 B.  Analysis
   A comprehensive list of all agencies, numbers of personnel in private practice, and personnel employed in agencies is developed. Analysis of the list indicates numbers of private for-profit health care agencies and public or private nonprofit services. The list of agencies, personnel, and services is compared with the previously identified health care needs derived from the population characteristics to judge adequacy of services within the community.

## Vertical Patterns

I.  Community Characteristics
 A.  Sources
   1.  Maps
   2.  Political subdivisions on local, state, and national levels
   3.  Government publications

B.  Analysis

Maps are studied, and the local community is surveyed to identify its location in comparison to county, state, and national political and geographic boundaries. For example, a community defined by school district borders can cross county and town lines, which, in turn, could influence government health care services.

II.  Population Characteristics
A.  Sources
1.  National health survey
2.  Health and human services publications on health statistics
3.  U.S. Census
4.  Home health care publications, such as the journal *Caring*
B.  Analysis

Population groups are compared with the larger communities' trends in population groups, which are identified according to age, socioeconomic levels, education, and cultural values, and major health problems (morbidity and mortality rates) are compared and projected for future needs. High-risk groups are identified.

III.  Health Care Resources from State and National Levels
A.  Sources
1.  Government publications
2.  Professional organizations' publications
3.  Health service agencies' directories
4.  Telephone listings under local, regional, and national categories
5.  Catalogs
6.  Advertisements
7.  Insurance brochures
B.  Analysis

Each local agency's organization and financial structure is examined and analyzed for its parent organization's influence; legal regulations and professional standards relevant to home health care are examined on the local, regional, and national levels for their impact on local programs.

## Diagnosis of Home Health Care Needs in the Community

Diagnosis of health problems for the community as the client is comparable to the nursing process applied to the individual or to the family as client.

Diagnosing home health care needs in a community is based on a needs assessment. Analyses of the community's home health care needs provide the documentation for services within the community. Nursing diagnosis problems are those within the legal definition of practice and amenable to nursing care. Most diagnoses on the community level imply collaborative problems, because they require the efforts of the population, health care providers, and various representatives of community institutions and organizations.

## Sample Health Care Needs

A frail elderly population (75 years and older with chronic disease or the potential for debilitating conditions) indicates a need for support systems providing continuity of care. A large elderly population, age-specific to the 65- to 75-year-old range, implies future health care needs for an at-risk client group in another decade of time. Increased morbidity and mortality rates for chronic disease such as heart disease, cancer, and cerebral vascular accidents indicate the need for specific nursing services that provide rehabilitation at home. High rates of accidents and arthritis indicate the need for musculoskeletal rehabilitation programs, including physical therapy. A low socioeconomic status for specific population groups, or for the community as a whole, as in an economically depressed area, implies vertical patterns of care for financial support. Samples of community diagnoses based on these hypothetical needs for home health care services are presented in the next section.

## Sample Diagnoses

*Diagnosis 1:* Activities of daily living support for frail elderly in their homes related to the aging process and chronic disease complications and disabilities.

*Diagnosis 2:* Potential need for home health care services for clients experiencing chronic debilitating diseases related to increased heart, cancer, and cerebral vascular accident morbidity and mortality rates in the community.

*Diagnosis 3:* Community health services dysfunction related to lack of adequate rehabilitation services for clients with musculoskeletal disorders as demonstrated by high morbidity rates within the general population.

*Diagnosis 4:* Lack of local financial support systems for home health care services to a community at high risk for acute care and chronic disease problems.

## Planning for Home Health Care in the Community

### Formulation of Long-Term and Short-Term Goals

The health care team reviews the list of diagnoses identifying home health care needs in the community. Priorities of needs are agreed upon, and the realities for support of programs by the community are reviewed. The changing home health care market makes it difficult to predict trends and outcomes. Medicare and Medicaid programs that could be relied upon in the past are no longer secure. Many health insurance plans do not carry home health care benefits. Although it has been demonstrated that home health care is more cost-effective than long-term facility expenses, there are no firm financial support systems in place to support home care programs. For example, not every health insurance plan contains a benefit for home health care. Medicare will provide services for only 90 days, Medicaid home health care services vary from state to state, and private fees for long-term home health care services can prove to be prohibitive to all but the wealthy. It thus becomes difficult to develop long-term and short-term goals that are dependent upon the method of financing for program planning purposes.

The health care team must take all these facts into consideration and develop long-term goals that are subject to revision as time passes and the health care system changes. Short-term goals are usually developed within 6-month frameworks, and the expectations for what will be accomplished and when are established. These become the process evaluation standards that lead toward the final outcome and meeting of the long-term goals. Plans, including periodic review, allow for the formation of new goals or for abandonment of original goals. See Chapter 11 for discussion of program evaluation and quality assurance.

Examples of long-term goals and related objectives for the four diagnoses listed in the previous discussion follow. Each diagnosis can have more than one long-term goal. Several short-term goals (objectives) are necessary for each long-term goal as the processes, or steps, for reaching the long-term goal(s). The examples list a few goals for each of the diagnoses to illustrate format (several more goals for each diagnosis are usually necessary).

### Examples

*Diagnosis 1:* Activities of daily living support for frail elderly in their homes related to the aging process and chronic disease complications and disabilities.

*Long-Term Goal:* Within 5 years, the frail elderly (population 75 years of age and older, and ill) will be supported in their homes as demonstrated by a 75% rate residing at home.

*Short-Term Goal (Objective):* Within 6 months of the implementation of home care activities of daily living program, admission rates to hospitals, long-term care facilities, and health-related facilities will remain stable or decrease.

*Diagnosis 2:* Potential need for home health care services for clients experiencing chronic debilitating diseases related to increased heart, cancer, and cerebrovascular morbidity and mortality rates in the community.

*Long-Term Goal:* Within 1 year, referral rates to home health care agencies will increase twofold over present rates for clients experiencing chronic debilitating diseases related to heart, cancer, and cerebrovascular accidents.

*Short-Term Goal (Objective):* By the end of 3 months, all community acute care hospitals and health care provider offices will receive information about home care rehabilitation services available to clients with heart, cancer, or cerebrovascular accident health problems.

*Diagnosis 3:* Community health services dysfunction related to lack of adequate rehabilitation services for clients with musculoskeletal disorders as demonstrated by high morbidity rates within the general population.

*Long-Term Goal:* Within 1 year, 90% of clients experiencing rehabilitation needs related to musculoskeletal problems will demonstrate optimal levels of functioning.

*Short-Term Goal (Objective):* Community health agencies will increase their services for rehabilitation by increasing referrals, adding staff, and increasing the number of visits to clients with musculoskeletal disorders.

*Diagnosis 4:* Lack of local financial support systems for home health care services to a community at high risk for acute care and chronic disease problems.

*Long-Term Goal:* Within 10 years, the community will have cost-effective and self-supporting financial support systems for home health care services for populations at risk for acute care and chronic disease problems.

*Short-Term Goal (Objective):* By the end of 1 year, several grants or projects for seed money to financially support home health care services will be completed and submitted to potential funding agencies.

A review of the community diagnoses and goals assists the community in deciding the priority of problems. In the aforementioned hypothetical situations, it is obvious that lack of financial resources for home health care services becomes the most crucial. In order to develop programs targeted for the at-risk aggregate (the frail elderly), financial resources must be found to support the programs. The health care team, in collaboration with the community, would develop programs targeted toward that specific problem in order to influence positive outcomes for the other diagnoses. Since the community and its at-risk population has limited financial resources, external funding sources (vertical patterns of organization) are sought.

Federal grants to support innovative programs meeting the needs of the elderly are available. The team must write a grant proposal to obtain the necessary funds. It must be kept in mind that grants are "soft" money and will only last for short periods of time; thus, the proposal must include plans for how the community will become self-sufficient in financing the home health care needs it wishes to provide. For example, the grant may be used to establish home health care services, hire staff, and create a demonstration model of providing services that includes a sliding scale fee for helping to support costs. Other funding agencies within the community should be explored, such as gaining financial support from volunteer organizations focused on helping the poor or patients with specific diseases (e.g., United Way, American Red Cross, Salvation Army, American Cancer Society, American Heart Association).

## Program Development

Planning for care on the community level involves program development. The health care provider reviews existing home health care programs to identify services that exist. These services and agencies may be used by the new agency in the future for collaboration, coordination of community services, and referral of clients. This type of action prevents duplication of services and indicates gaps in services that could be integrated into the program. It also identifies lack of services and the need for new programs.

Each diagnosis and its related long-term goals and short-term objectives serve as guidelines for program development. Based on the review of existing programs, decisions are made to either supplement existing programs or create new ones. The opportunity for networking with other agencies and personnel is reviewed and instituted as appropriate to the program.

If the home health care program is a new one, organization and staffing patterns are developed. Financial organization and budget systems are set up. An administrative head, board of directors, or advisory board is established. Various policies and procedures to initiate the program are developed. The health planners review the goals and set specific time frames for meeting them. From these time frames, people who will accomplish the goals and objectives are identified. Plans for filling the positions with existing personnel or recruitment plans for additional staff are formulated.

Once the personnel are in place with specified job expectations, plans for their activities are developed. Team conferences and staff meetings are frequently held in the beginning and at regular intervals thereafter in order to evaluate the progress of the program toward its goals. Eventually, according to the pre-set objectives or short-term goals, clients are admitted into the program for direct services. Admissions must be on an orderly basis. Goals and objectives are reviewed to evaluate whether they should be changed to meet client needs without jeopardizing the organization as a result of inadequate staff or too few clients to make the program economically feasible.

Integration of new home health care services into existing programs follows the same steps as previously outlined for new programs with the exception of establishing a new organization and administration. Staffing patterns are reviewed, and new positions are added or old positions are changed according to needs within the existing program and projected needs for the new program. Formative evaluation of the progress toward goals and objectives remain the same as those for new programs (see Chapter 12).

## Implementation of Home Health Care in the Community

### Continuity of Care

Implementation of home health care occurs after programs have been established and care is being delivered to the clientele. Home health care relies upon the concept of continuity of health care. Continuity of care is defined as the planned delivery of health care services, in a variety of settings, for clients experiencing health problems requiring various levels of care throughout the continuation of the problem—to recovery, to rehabilitation, or to death.

A client's entry into the health care system occurs through a variety of circumstances. An acute illness can bring a client to a hospital emergency room, where, depending upon the diagnosis, the client may be admitted or referred to a primary care provider. Other clients enter the system through self-referrals or through case-finding activities on the part of health care providers in the community. For example, a home health care nurse on a routine home visit may find a client with problems requiring hospitalization, ambulatory care, or long-term care.

When a client enters the system, an initial assessment is conducted to predict the potential for recovery. The information projects health care needs and the probable length of time for recovery. Information includes the client's financial resources, family and friends' support, employment status, implications for return to daily activities, types and levels of care usual for the medical diagnosis and nursing diagnoses, and the resources available to the client as care progresses.

Planning for continuity of care occurs upon entry into the system and requires assessment of the client for future services. If the client requires long-term care, the client and family are informed and referred to appropriate agencies. The discharge planner in the acute care setting and community agencies work with the client and family to coordinate transfer from one facility to another. For the patient in the hospital, plans for home care are included in the initial interview for preliminary identification of agencies serving the client's home community, for agency planning, prior assignment of staff, and review of eligibility requirements. The family and client are referred to the admissions coordinator of the agency, and mutual plans are made between the care giving agency and the future care providers.

## *Referral*

Referral is the process through which continuity of care is planned and initial contact is made for providing services. Referral is carried out by health personnel and clients or by consumers. All health team members are eligible to refer; however, it is usually the primary care provider who has the major responsibility. The latter types of personnel include nurses, physicians, social workers, and discharge planners (usually nurses) in the acute care setting.

The client and family must be involved in the process of referral for a satisfactory outcome. If the client and family are not involved in the planning and implementation, they are less committed to the process and its eventual outcome. Therefore, it is recommended that the client participate in the referrral process with the health care provider's guidance, if necessary. When the client initiates the referral, he or she is demonstrating interest and commitment to continuity of care. Additionally, when the client arranges the referral, a third party is eliminated, preventing inconvenient appointment times and confusion. If the health care provider believes that the client may have difficulty making the contact, it is permissible to make arrangements.

Referrals can be initiated by a single person or by multiple parties. They can be formal, usually written and documenting the reason for referral and the recommendations for continuity of care. Referrals can also be informal, usually on a verbal basis through telephone arrangements or person-to-person contact. Informal referral takes little time and is especially effective in times of emergency or at a time when the client is motivated and indicates a willingness to receive services. Informal referral does not have the advantage of a formal written referral, which provides documentation of plans for care. Written referral has the latter advantage and also requires explicit information that is helpful for planning of care. Most agencies and private practitioners use formal referral forms to ensure continuity of care for the client and to document action. When informal contacts or referrals occur, agencies or personnel usually follow up the action with written documentation for quality assurance and documentation of care purposes.

### Follow-Up

It is not unusual for the formal referral process to cease when the client enters a new health care setting or receives the new health care provider's services. Most agencies and health care personnel do not have the time or the awareness of the value for providing follow-up information to the referring agency. This is unfortunate, because follow-up of every referral is critical to the future needs of the client, in the event that he or she must return to the initiator(s) of care. Follow-up communications to the referring agency or person provide for documentation of services. They also provide the health care worker with a knowledge of the success of the referral and the need for future improvement in the referral process. It leads to closer collaboration between the health care team and agencies and provides a potential data base for program planning, evaluation, and research.

## Documenting Care

### Recordkeeping and Evaluation

Agencies and health care providers need to keep records of the care and services provided to the consumer. In Chapter 4, recordkeeping for the individual client and family receiving home health care is described. The present discussion is confined to record systems applying to the community as client.

The needs assessment to demonstrate home health care adequacies within the community serves as the baseline for creating services and programs. It should be organized logically and in certain categories. The outline in Appendix A serves as the format for recording the baseline data. The purposes for keeping these data are (1) to use as a needs assessment, (2) to formulate nursing diagnoses or health problem lists, (3) to provide a history of activities, (4) to predict trends, (5) to serve as a baseline to update information, (6) to provide data for funding and regulating agencies, and (7) to document activities relating to the provision of care based on need and resources within the community.

Records of the diagnoses or problem list and their associated goals and objectives serve as guidelines for program development and evaluation. They document the progress of the services toward solution of problems for the community. A record of the implementation activities demonstrates health care providers' accountability to the community. Types of records that demonstrate services include minutes of meetings and conferences; copies of bylaws, and the constitution if indicated; policies and procedures; staffing positions and their role expectations; staffing patterns; staff files, including qualifications; inventories of agency equipment and supplies; statistics concerning numbers of visits, types of services provided, major health problems encountered, and population groups served.

## Computer Technology

Each home health care agency can incorporate recordkeeping activities into computerized systems. Computerized record systems can be established through a system that feeds into a main frame (centralized system) with computer terminals in suboffices or personal computers within each subsystem of the agency. The records mentioned in the previous section could be entered into a computerized system. Examples include

1.  Data-based systems for needs assessment information
2.  File systems for recording statistics and staffing patterns
3.  Statistical packages for analyzing health statistics, including morbidity and mortality rates, population groups served, numbers and types of home visits
4.  Spread sheets for financial accounting systems

Agencies can take the state of the art of computer technology into account and incorporate it into recordkeeping and accounting activities. Many computer companies have developed programs and systems specific to home health care administrative needs. Even though establishing the system may be time-consuming, computerized systems speed the process of preparing reports, record analyses, and evaluation of programs. Computer technology supplies statistical analyses in a few short hours that previously took years of time. It enhances evaluation and research activities that are critical to program planning for the future and for demonstrating accountability to the consumer.

## Conclusion

Community diagnosis for home health care needs is a function of the administrative/management staff of home health care agencies. Staff nurses providing home health care services in a specific neighborhood or community use diagnostic information for identifying resources in the community, coordinating care for their clients and families, and referring clients to appropriate services.

Community diagnosis for home health care is a nursing process and includes a needs assessment for home health care problems and services, diagnosis of community-based problems specific to home health care and nursing action, development of long-term goals and related short-term goals or objectives, planning for care through program development, implementation through direct and indirect care for clients, and evaluation based on the outcomes of program services and client and families' improved health status and satisfaction.

# References and Selected Readings

Balinsky W, Rehman S: Home health care: A comparative analysis of hospital-based and community-based agency patients. Home Health Care Services Quarterly 5(1):45–60, 1984

Berk ML, Bernstein A: Use of home health services: Some findings from the national medical care expenditure survey. Home Health Care Services Quarterly 6(1):13–24, 1985

Branch LG: Home care is the answer: What is the question? Home Health Care Services Quarterly 6(1):3–12, 1985

Dalton J: A descriptive study: Defining characteristics of the nursing diagnosis cardiac output, alterations in: Decreased. Image: The Journal of Nursing Scholarship 17(4):113–117, 1985

Ebersole P, Hess P: Towards Healthy Aging, 2nd ed. St Louis, Mosby, 1985

Hays JC: Hospice policy and patterns of care. Image 18(3):92–97, 1986

Higgs ZR, Gustafson DD: Community as a Client: Assessment and Diagnosis. Philadelphia, F.A. Davis, 1985

Kaye LW: The adequacy of the Older Americans Act home care mandate: A front line view from three programs. Home Health Care Services Quarterly 5(1):75–88, 1984

Lampley P, Freeman R: Utilization and referral patterns for home health services: A data base for needs determination. Home Health Care Services Quarterly 5(1):89–106, 1984

National Center for Health Services Research and Health Care Technology Assessment. Research Activities. No. 78, Rockville, MD: US Department of Health and Human Services, October 1985

Petrowski DD: Handbook of Community Health Nursing. Essentials for Clinical Practice. New York, Springer Publishing Company, 1985

Rosenfeld AS: Home health services and long term care: A two-state comparison. Home Health Care Services Quarterly 5(1):5–34, 1984

Warren RL: The Community in Action, 3rd ed. Chicago, Rand McNally, 1978

Watson NM: Community as client. In Sullivan JA: Directions in Community Health Nursing, Chapter 3. Boston, Blackwell Scientific Publications, Inc, 1984

# Administration and Management of Home Health Care Agencies

## Introduction

Chapter 3 reviews common types of home health care agencies and their organizational patterns. Included are traditional agencies that have provided home health care services over the past century and the newer types of agencies that are providing services today in the changing, high technology, multicorporate health care market. The administrative structure of various home health care agencies and the roles and functions of personnel, including the board of directors, chief executive, management/supervisory staff, professional, and paraprofessional health care provider staff, are discussed.

The financing and budgeting of agencies are reviewed, with an overview of the marketing aspects in today's health care system and its relationship to home health care. The legal and political climate for home health care is examined, and program development and evaluation are briefly discussed in relation to the changing health care system, needs assessment of the community in which the agency operates, and standards of care for evaluation purposes. The chapter concludes with a brief discussion of change theory and its application to program development and evaluation in home health care.

## Organizational Patterns: Types of Organizations

### Visiting Nurse Associations

From the early 1900s until the 1960s when Medicare and Medicaid programs were instituted, Visiting Nurse Associations (VNAs) provided most of the home health care or bedside nursing care services in the community. These agencies were also leaders in providing preventive health care services. For example, they established prenatal classes, provided health supervision of infants and children, and conducted school health visits. As time progressed in the early 1900s, official agencies under the mandate of state or local public health laws assumed the disease prevention and health promotion activities while visiting nurse associations focused on bedside nursing in the home. The VNAs were among the first in the 1960s to become eligible for Medicare home health care reimbursement programs and currently depend upon Medicare and Medicaid, other third-party payments, fees for service, and charity or endowments as sources of income.

Some VNAs are having financial difficulties as federal and state funds decrease, client eligibility requirements become more stringent, the caseload of patients with higher acuity levels of need increase, and new companies enter the home health care industry (Mershon and Weslowski, 1985). Other problems facing the agencies are the increased demand for services from multiproblem patients with high technology needs and from a growing population of frail elderly whose delivery of services contribute to high overhead costs for the agencies. Many VNAs are currently engaged in or considering collaboration, merger, and diversification of services with other health care agencies such as hospitals, health departments, long-term care facilities, and private health care agencies (Caring, 1985).

## Health Department Nursing Services

The other traditional type of health care agency in the community exists within the public sector and is created by local, regional, and state legislative acts. The original focus of services for these types of official agencies was on health promotion and prevention of disease through public health activities. When the Medicare and Medicaid programs were instituted in the 1960s, some of the agencies became interested in providing services to vulnerable population groups within their communities and in the potential revenues for their programs. Many health department nursing divisions created home care services and, in accordance with regulations for reimbursement eligibility, included skilled nursing care and at least one therapy such as occupational therapy, physical therapy, speech therapy, or medical social worker consultation in their services.

To meet the needs of this new cadre of clients, community/public health nurses needed to add technical home health care skills to their repertoire of health teaching, counseling, and coordination of care activities. Examples of the technical skills include administration of medications, activities of daily living support, dressing changes, monitoring of health status, and catheterization. The skills were provided from the agencies by community health nurses, registered nurses, practical nurses, or home health aides and were under the supervision of the community/public health nurses or their administrative staff.

Adding home health care services to the official agency's programs resulted in the sacrifice of some of the health promotion and health supervision activities of community/public health nurses. Agencies came to depend upon the revenue home health care visits generated through Medicare, Medicaid, and other third-party reimbursement programs and placed priority on these types of services, with wellness programs frequently taking second place. Health departments that chose not to assume home health care services decreased in size owing to their dependence upon general revenues from government-sponsored programs and the de-emphasis on health in a disease-focused, acute care–driven health care system.

## Proprietary Agencies

As the need for home care increased, entrepreneurial health professionals, agencies, and businesses recognized the financial opportunities for providing services. Entrepreneurial agencies provide an array of services and, in some instances, operate at lower overhead costs than the established VNAs and health department nursing services. In the recent decade, there has been a tremendous increase of proprietary (for profit) agencies in the health care system (Janz and Burgess, 1985). Some agencies are sponsored by pharmaceutical companies or other health care equipment suppliers such as suppliers of respiratory care, orthopaedic devices, and hospital equipment. As the home care industry grew, these supplier agencies began to add nurses and other providers to their staff. Most of them delivered services through technical personnel who were usually under the supervision of registered nurses. These agencies either charge fees for services or are reimbursed under insurance plans or other third-party systems.

There are also specialty organizations that provide home health care personnel such as home health aides, homemakers, and other technicians. These agencies usually operate through contracts with existing agencies, including VNAs, hospitals, and health departments. Training and nursing supervision of the paraprofessional personnel are part of the agreement and can be provided by either agency.

## Hospital-Based Home Care Services

Prior to the early 1980s' prospective payment method for financing health care, a few hospitals with a focus on service to the community established home health care services for their discharged patients. However, most hospitals referred patients who required nursing care to existing community-based agencies such as VNAs or health departments. The prospective payment method and its use of the Diagnostic-Related Grouping (DRGs) categories resulted in decreased lengths of stay for clients in the hospital. As acute care delivery needs decreased and hospital units closed, hospitals looked for alternate models of delivery of health care within their own organizational structure for financial recovery or stabilization. Hospital-based home health care programs provided one of the models they were seeking. In the current health care market, hospital-based home health care services have become one of the major providers within the community (Janz and Burgess, 1985).

## Private Practice

Another type of home health care model is private practice. Services are provided by professionals and others interested in the entrepreneurial aspects of the changes in the health care system. Professionals include nurses, therapists, pharmacists, and durable medical equipment distributors. Physicians have indicated an interest in entering home health care, as demonstrated by a survey conducted by *Home Care Market Outlook '85*. Of the physicians surveyed, 78% indicated interest in education concerning high-tech home health care compared with 47% demonstrating an interest in learning about investment opportunities (Louden, 1985).

Few professional nurse practices or corporations are established as for-profit enterprises; however, the rapidly expanding field of home care creates independent for-profit nursing practice possibilities. An advantage of private practice and corporations, compared with large non-profit organizations, is their potential for low overhead costs, which are cost-effective for the client and profitable for nurses.

## Nurse-Managed Home Health Care Services

Shelton, in 1985, stated, "The nursing profession will offer many other exciting opportunities for nurses over the next several years. Midwives, nurse practitioners, and nurse-managed alternative delivery systems such as birthing centers, hospice care, and home health care, all have come to the forefront of new nursing opportunities. . . . Because nurses are the most visible, available, and continuous care providers, they can serve as vital links between quality and cost" (p 253).

Shelton's statements point out the opportunities for nurses to enter the health care market and to offer cost-effective, quality nursing care services. There are many nurses who have succeeded in establishing and maintaining their own health care business. There are two major methods for establishing an independent nursing service business: (1) private practice through solo practice or partnership and (2) professional corporations. It is also possible to establish one's own home health care agency; however, it is usually subject to licensure or certification procedures according to state or federal regulations.

The private practice model offers the opportunity for nurses to start an independent business. They must follow the laws of the state relating to the legal practice of nursing and those regulating professional corporations. Third-party reimbursement for nurses depends upon the specific state laws that allow payment for professional services rendered. A few states, for example, California, New York, and Maryland, have legislation that specifies reimbursement for nursing services; however, the extent and type of services provided and nurse provider qualifications for providing services vary. It is too early to read the impact of these programs on the potential for financial support of the private practice of nursing. Nurse-managed agencies that are certified or licensed by state government regulating bodies and meet state and federal guidelines are usually eligible for reimbursement for services.

Nurses in private practice or private nursing corporations charge fees for services, and it has been demonstrated that clients are willing to pay for these services. In many cases, groups of clients such as senior citizens and those in industry and church groups are willing to contract with nurses for services to their group members. This model serves as a cost-effective way for delivering services and providing profit for nurses while, at the same time, delivering quality care for clients who otherwise could not afford services individually.

## Summary of Types of Home Health Care Organizations

According to Janz and Burgess (1985), the numbers of home health care agencies in California increased in the 1-year period from September 1984 to August 1985. The percentage of types of home health care agencies providing services included:

| | |
|---|---|
| Visiting nurse associations (VNAs): | 0.2% |
| Rehabilitation-based: | 26.0% |
| Hospital-based: | 49.0% |
| Proprietary: | 35.0% |
| Private, nonprofit: | 9.6% |

Types of agencies that decreased in numbers included:

| | |
|---|---|
| Official (government-based): | −2.0% |
| Combination (VNAs and health departments): | −2.0% |
| Skilled nursing facilities: | −15.0% |
| Unidentified (other): | −74.0% |

In 1985, there was a total of 5698 home health care agencies, compared with

4847 in 1984. The three major types of agencies (more than 1100) were official agencies, hospital-based, and proprietary.

## Organizational Structure: Informal and Formal Patterns

### Informal Patterns

The formal structure of agencies provides the official channels of communication in the agency and can take the form of hierarchic, democratic, or flat lines of functioning. Formal lines set the purposes, philosophy, goals, and organizational lines for functioning. They provide the legal basis for providing services to clients and delineate the financial structure and staffing patterns of the agency. Informal structure provides the channels of communication for accomplishing goals and emphasizes the human interactions within the organization. Informal communication provides the staff members the ability to interact with each other, their clients, supervisors, administration, and the governing board.

Informal communication creates the milieu and work environment for the staff. Effective administrators create an informal, yet professional, warm, and supportive environment in which staff can communicate freely. The milieu promotes the sharing of problems, the opportunity for praise and constructive criticism in a nonjudgmental atmosphere, and the development of personal and professional relationships. Positive informal networks are essential to job satisfaction and the mental health of the personnel in health agencies. Negative networks with their gossip, negative criticism, and destructive behaviors lead to a demoralizing situation affecting the quality of care provided to the consumers of services. The administrator needs open communication channels to informal levels in order to monitor for problems and to intervene if necessary.

### Formal Patterns

Within the health care system, formal patterns of home health care agencies fall under two major categories of financing, proprietary and nonproprietary. Proprietary agencies and professional practices are within the private sector of the health care system and operate for profit. Examples of these types of agencies include some hospital-based programs, health agencies developed by drug companies, durable medical equipment suppliers, and entrepreneurial interests, including private practice and corporations. The latter groups include nurse-owned and -operated agencies as well as those owned by other health care providers, including physicians, physical therapists, and some non–health care professionals such as business people and lawyers. Some nonprofit agencies have considered converting to for-profit based on the changing health care system and its competitive market.

Flanagan (1985) discusses some of the legal and practical considerations for changing a home health care agency from nonprofit to profit. He points out that this strategy may not solve financial stress. Agencies changing to a for-profit basis need to consider many factors, including tax-exempt status, laws and regulations, needs of clients, and financial benefits.

Proprietary agencies are usually run within a corporate structure and have a board of directors. Members of the boards may be stockholders or act as advisors for the agency. In the case of proprietary agencies, the board members are usually stockholders and serve as the officers of the corporation. They choose the administrative staff of the agency. As members of the board, they are responsible for legal matters, finances, and policies regarding the types of services that the agency will provide. If the home care services are part of another larger, for-profit corporation, such as a hospital or long-term care facility, its structure is subsumed under the parent institution. Figures 3-1 and 3-2 illustrate sample organizational charts for the two types of agency structures (proprietary home care agency and hospital-based home care services).

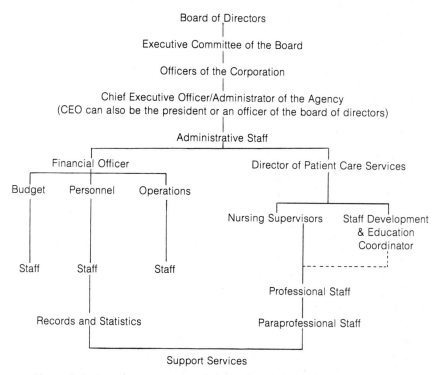

Figure 3-1. Sample organizational chart of proprietary home care agency.

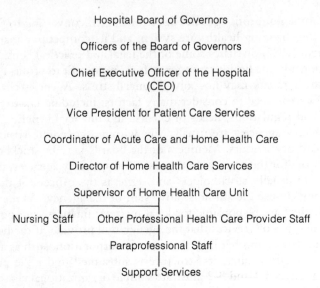

Figure 3-2. Sample of hospital-based home care services organizational chart.

There are nonproprietary (nonprofit) agencies within both the public and private sectors of the health care system. Examples of these agencies include VNAs and other agencies in home care that do not operate for-profit, some hospices, home health aide agencies such as those sponsored under United Way, and private health care provider practices and corporations that choose to operate under nonprofit auspices and pay themselves salaries from the organization's income.

Similar to some hospital-based home health care units, a few VNAs and other home health care agencies have chosen to diversify their corporate structure by combining with other health care provider organizations. These multicorporations share financial resources, organizational structures, office facilities, and personnel resources to continue to offer their services and yet become more cost-effective in a climate of fiscal constraint (MacKenzie, 1985). Administrative and personnel management issues, including fringe benefits for employees and delineation of roles and functions, are negotiated. Many of these agencies are new on the health care scene, and their effect on staffing patterns, services rendered, and client outcomes must be studied.

Official agencies that are governed and supported through general revenues, such as health departments and social services, belong to the public sector. With the advent of the Medicare and Medicaid financing programs, many of these agencies chose to meet certification requirements as home care providers. Figure 3-3 illustrates the organizational structure of a typical official agency with home health care services. Organizational charts of an agency providing home health care services indicate the lines of authority and power of the administrative staff and personnel within the agency. Examination of the sample charts reveals the potential power of nursing within home health care agencies. Nurses placed in positions of higher lines of authority and power such as Director of the Agency, Director of Patient Care Services, and member of the board of directors are going to have more influence on the policies of the agency and quality of home health care services provided to the consumer of services.

Many more complex organizational structures occur when existing home health care agencies such as VNAs and hospital-based home care units or official and private agencies merge their services. Some agencies choose to do this in order to restructure their financial organization to become cost-effective and to provide additional comprehensive services (Mershon and Weslowski, 1985). Diversification helps to eliminate competition for the market and yet opens additional market opportunities for the agencies involved. A classic example of such a merger is the combining of health departments and VNAs.

In today's health care system, it is more frequent for health product suppliers, hospitals, and visiting nurse services to combine. Such mergers have many advantages in addition to financial gain; these include personnel expertise, combined resources for the supply of equipment, a community-based home health staff, and acute care hospital-based personnel. Merger offers each agency experienced personnel for operating services within the community and acute care settings. Mergers are complex, and there are

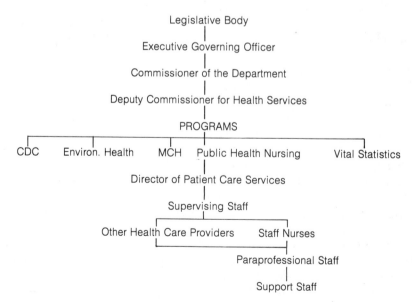

Figure 3-3. Sample official agency organizational chart.

many organizational models of administration. Because of their complex nature, it is not unusual for initial negotiations to work out administrative details to continue over long periods of time. Each merger is unique; therefore it is difficult to portray them schematically.

## Boards of Directors and Advisory Boards

Agency boards of directors and advisory boards serve two distinct purposes. The board of directors, members of which own stock in the corporation or agency, assumes financial responsibilities as well as legal liabilities for the agency. This is the governing and policymaking body. The board of directors can choose to delegate responsibilities to the executive committee of the board, the executive officers, or the administrator, or the members may choose to keep operations under their direct control. Advisory boards are established for both proprietary and nonproprietary agencies. The boards offer professional expertise and represent the various functions, interests, and responsibilities of the agency.

For example, a board may have a lawyer to offer legal advice, an accountant for financial consultation, a businessman to advise about marketing conditions and projections for the future, advertising people to develop public relations, and professionals to offer health expertise for client services. Their combined expert knowledge and services are essential to the running of both types of agencies, with advisory boards particularly applicable to the nonprofit agencies.

The type of relationship that the staff and administrators of the agency have is established by the purposes and functions of the boards of directors. The administrators and staff may act as employees of the board and are responsible for client services according to the policies and procedures formulated by the board. If the board of directors acts in an advisory capacity, the administrator and staff consult board members for advice and professional counsel.

Both types of boards usually meet monthly. As is true of all groups, the boards vary according to individual and combined personalities and defined roles and functions. Some boards are puppets to the chief executive officer and serve to give their seal of approval to executive decisions. Others operate democratically under parliamentary procedure and act on problems through multiple channels of decision-making such as special task groups, needs assessment surveys, committee meetings, and advice and counseling from others.

It is important for the administrator(s) and staff of the agency to recognize the type of role that the board plays, to communicate often and effectively with the board, to recognize its power, and to use it in the best way for providing services to the client population. As vacancies occur on boards of directors, new people are selected based on criteria set by the board, administrators, and staff of the agency. The criteria are set according to the philosophy and goals of the agency and the specific needs for expertise and power from the community. There should be a mechanism for representation of the agency's administration and staff on the board to enhance relationships. This type of structure opens channels of communication to the board and leads to understanding among the groups rather than creation of adversary situations.

## Administration

Administration of the agency consists of an appointed chief executive officer. The officer can be the president of the board of directors of the agency or corporation, or a person hired by the governing board. The administrator meets criteria set by the governing body and accrediting organizations such as state regulating agencies, the Joint Commission on Accreditation of Hospitals, and the National League for Nursing/American Public Health Association.

It is recommended that the administrator have advanced education in administration and progressive experience in the field. Although it is not necessary that the person be a health professional such as a nurse, physician, or therapist, it is essential for the person to have a knowledge of the types of client health problems and the services provided by the agency. If the administrator is not a health professional, a nursing position equal to that administrative line is created to manage client care services. The chief nursing administrator meets education and experience criteria for the position. Quality of services can be compromised if a person's position is influenced by the politics of the moment; therefore, the position should have tenure assurances based on performance and the meeting of agency goals.

The administrator represents the agency and is responsible for enhancing the image of the agency. The person represents the agency in public relations, in political action and representation to governing bodies, and in networking within the community. Because of the complexity of the position, the major responsibilities delegated to the administrator, and the expertise required, it is expected that the position will provide economic incentives as well as opportunities for personal and professional development. An excellent reference for administrators of home health care is the *Administrator's Handbook for Community Health and Home Care Services* by Fish (1984).

## Staffing

Staffing the agency is based on a needs assessment. The major client health problems determine the numbers and types of personnel necessary. For example, if there are many clients with high-tech acute care needs, skilled nurse clinicians are indicated; if the agency also provides care to a substantial number of chronically ill clients with less-skilled nursing care needs, home health care aides under the supervision of nurses constitute a large part of the staff. A large population requiring rehabilitation indicates the need for professional therapists and technicians to carry out plans of care in collaboration with the nursing staff.

The community's home health care needs are compared with costs for implementing services. For example, home health care aides may be indicated for clients with long-term needs, compared with experienced professional nursing staff needed to provide high-tech skills for clients with acute care needs. Using professional staff helps to prevent complications and disabilities that could result in clients requiring additional long-term care. Appropriate levels of care based on client need and financial support systems are examined in relation to intermittent home health care (periodic care over a limited time), 24-hour home care, respite care to provide the family care provider with rest and relaxation, day care to which the client is transported, and hospice models of care, including in-home and hospital care.

Patient education and agency staff development needs are identified to promote the effective use of personnel and to ensure participation of the client and family in their own care. Support staff supplement the services of the professional staff and are cost-effective to the extent that they relieve professional staff from recordkeeping and other nonprofessional, time-consuming activities.

## Staff Management

**Lines of Authority.**    The organizational structure of the agency determines the lines of authority for staffing. The executive director delegates patient care services to the appropriate director or supervisor of that program. In home health care agencies, that person is usually a nurse with advanced education in nursing administration and experience in the delivery of patient care services. The director has a staff of nursing supervisors who manage special programs within the patient care services or supervise teams of nursing staff and other health personnel who deliver care to specified client populations or geographic regions. Examples of specific programs that might require such supervisors are hospices, home health aide training, and rehabilitation services. Examples of health care teams who deliver services to specific client populations and might require this type of supervision are parent–child services and oncology services. Examples of health care teams in geographic locations are those located in districts or satellite offices.

Usually, the hierarchy of the agency is such that the director of patient care services is responsible to the executive director, the supervising nurses to the director of patient care services, and the staff to their supervisors. Informal communication systems can circumvent the formal organizational lines and can be positive or negative.

***Position Titles, Qualifications, and Descriptions of Duties.*** Each position within the agency has a job description. It includes a list of the functions within the job that define the legal or mandatory requirements of the job, role expectations, qualifications, and experience necessary for filling the position. It is expected that the chief nursing administrator has advanced education and progressive experience in the field, including supervisory and fiscal management experience. Supervising nurses, or nurse supervisors, usually have advanced education and experience (at least 2 years) as home health care nurses. Nurse clinicians have advanced education in their field of expertise and at least 2 years of experience in clinical practice. See Chapter 1 for a discussion of the recommended educational qualifications of nurses in home health care.

In home settings, nurses make independent judgments since other members of the health care team are not easily accessible for consultation; therefore, it is essential for home health care nurses to have advanced preparation and experience. Beginning-level professional nurses must have at least a bachelor of science degree in nursing. Associate degree- and diploma-prepared registered nurses practice in-home health care, usually under the supervision of the community health nurse and the supervising nurses. Paraprofessionals such as home health aides, attendants, and homemakers are under the supervision of professional nursing staff and should be graduates of certified training programs.

The Director of Nursing/Patient Care Services is the chief administrator of the agency's nursing services. He or she is ultimately responsible for the quality of nursing services provided to clients and may choose to delegate certain authority and responsibilities to other members of the administrative staff. Depending upon the size and type of the agency, the director may be in charge of the agency's fiscal management; development of policies and procedures and their implementation; recruitment, hiring, retention, and promotion of employees; and contract negotiations with the employee union or other representative groups. In some instances, he or she may direct supervision of services and staff members.

The director is responsible for program planning and evaluation and conducts periodic needs assessments for future program changes. He or she acts as liaison between the agency and the community and as advocate for home care services to the community at large, including politicians and regulating agencies. Through public relations, the director represents the agency and nursing services to the public.

Supervising nurses give direction and consultation to the staff who provide the direct services defined by the agency. The goals and objectives of the agency's programs provide guidelines to the supervisors and staff for the delivery of care. Supervisors are quality control agents. They promote the personal and professional development of the staff to ensure quality of services and staff job satisfaction, and they act as advocates for the staff to the administration as the need arises. Supervisors represent the staff and the agency to the community and are active in public relations.

Supervisors are essential to the recruitment, hiring, promotion, and retention of personnel. They are responsible for orientation of staff, implementation of personnel policies, maintenance of personnel records, and direct and indirect supervision of staff through periodic performance evaluations. Supervisors provide guidance, support, and expert consultation to the professional staff who are responsible for implementing specific programs and services and for the training and supervision of paraprofessional staff such as home health aides and homemakers. Fish (1984) discusses in detail the role of the supervising nurse and includes examples of various levels of staff performance appraisal forms.

Supervising nurses have a dual role: staff development and staff evaluation. Staff development activities include diagnosing the learning needs of staff, keeping abreast of changes in the field and sharing them with staff, and providing an environment that is stimulating and promotes professional growth. Supervisors provide support to staff by creating a milieu in the work environment that facilitates open discussion of the problems confronting staff as they deliver services to clients. Genuine concern for the staff's personal and professional needs is part of the function of the supervising nurse. He or she is an interested listener and counsels staff regarding their professional needs and personal problems that may interfere with job performance. If indicated, the staff are provided with the time to solve personal problems according to personnel policies and are referred to appropriate resources as necessary. As middle managers, supervisors need the support of the administration and staff in defining and implementing the two basic functions of the role (staff development and evaluation).

Professional nursing staff consist of persons who are self-directing and who are responsible for the direct care of clients and the supervision of paraprofessional staff. These front-line personnel deliver care, teach, and also supervise the delivery of care. Qualifications include at least one year professional clinical nursing experience. If they have not had experience, they should be under the mentorship of experienced staff members and supervisors. Paraprofessional staff are responsible to professional staff and the client. Their activities are carefully monitored, and plans of client care are developed by their supervisors (professional staff). The plans must be specific and are evaluated periodically by the paraprofessionals providing client care and their supervisors to ensure quality care.

The number and types of personnel vary from less than half a dozen in a small agency to several hundred in large metropolitan agencies. The greater the number of staff, the more complex the system of staff management. Large numbers of staff contribute to greater overhead costs of the agency. Thus, the structure of the agency is evaluated in terms of income and outlay, including staffing, cost of maintenance, and recordkeeping expenditures to determine cost-effectiveness. The evaluation can lead to structural decisions for the agency, for example, to remain as a large health agency, become a corporation, diversify and offer multiple services, merge with other agencies, or contract for services from other agencies.

## Financing and Budgeting

The market for home health care services has changed dramatically with the implementation of the prospective system of payment and the emphasis on cost containment. Home health care needs are increasing for patients who are discharged earlier from the hospital and for an aging population with chronic diseases requiring supportive services; however, the financial base for supporting these services is in a constant state of flux. It was initially anticipated that Medicare would help to support the elderly and others eligible for funds in the home care setting. Although the Medicare and Medicaid programs provide the major source of funding for many home health programs (Knollmueller, 1984), funds for these programs are decreasing with recent federal budget cuts. Insurance companies are providing some limited home health care benefits for their participants; however, they follow Medicare and Medicaid patterns and their percentage of financial support has, for the most part, not increased (Knollmueller, 1984).

Balinsky (1986) reported that approximately $300 million (6%) of the total Medicaid budget went to home health services in 1981 in New York state. Medicare reimbursement in New York in 1979 was about 10% of the total federal Medicare budget. In his survey, 85% of the patients reported that these two systems were their primary sources of payment for services. However, Wood (1984) reported that with the Omnibus Reconciliation Act of 1980, Medicare home health programs were cut. For example, the 100-visit limitation was eliminated, eligibility requirements mandated that clients must have been in the hospital 3 days prior to home health care, and $60 of the home health care cost became deductible under Part B. Balinsky reported that Medicare and Medicaid reimbursement for services seems to target medically related services, whereas reimbursement for social support services such as homemaker and transportation services has been decreased or eliminated.

Knollmueller (1985) reported that the current emphasis is to cut home care expenditures rather than to view home care as a program in its own right. Expenditures for home care reimbursement from Medicare and Medicaid programs represented about 5% of the total expenditures for all health services; yet, the two programs were the major sources of financial support for home health care agencies.

### Cost Containment Programs

The Medicare and Medicaid systems are short-term and do not cover the long-term needs of many chronically ill clients. Medicaid funds and other governmental support systems are at risk. Many local and state governments are operating with deficit budgets, and the total health care financial structure is in peril, especially with costs continuing to soar.

Private pay clients exist and help to support the cost of agency services. However, agencies with large overhead costs must at times charge prohibitive fees, which can eliminate many clients from services. In order to maintain services, agencies are examining cost containment programs, projecting needs for the future, and identifying methods for decelerating the cost of providing care.

Cost containment measures include appropriate use of personnel for each situation. Examples include:

1. Acute care on a short-term basis provided by specialists who refer continuing lower level care to less expensive health care providers under the specialists' supervision
2. Teaching certain skills to clients and family members rather than continuing to provide services that are costly and could be provided by nonprofessionals.

Other cost containment measures include using equipment and supplies that can be recycled, establishing efficient record systems that cut personnel time and office supplies, and consolidating travel expenses through staffing plans that take into account travel time and distances.

### Cost-Effective Programs

According to Shelton (1985), the health care system business "accounted for nearly 11 percent of the nation's Gross National Product" (p 251). It costs the United States nearly $1 billion per day and employs nearly 8 million people. Shelton predicts that industry and businesses will be financing more of the health care benefits and care for their employees in the near future. The change is due in large part to the new prospective payment system to contain costs. Employers are reconsidering the benefits of preferred provider organizations, and nurses are among the professionals who can establish this type of model for delivery of health care.

Many established home health care agencies that have depended upon third-party reimbursement are concerned about the present financial picture in the health care field and recognize the changing market in the health care system. The hospital system's change from the retrospective method of reimbursement to the prospective payment method has demonstrated the possibilities for creating cost-effective program incentives. This type of model is sure to spill over into the home care scene (Knollmueller, 1984).

The journal *Caring*, July 1985, was devoted to the problem of cost-effectiveness in home health care and gave examples of agencies who have confronted the problem and developed methods for cost-effective programming. Examples include diversification of programs, corporate restructuring, and reorganization of the agency. The point was made that such restructuring must be based on a needs assessment that includes patient perspectives (Shaw, 1985).

The diversification model consists of agencies that approach others to contract for the provision of additional services or providers for their clients. Corporate reorganization or restructuring involves several agencies agreeing to merge by combining their organizational management and financial support systems. They include both for-profit and nonprofit models (Daniels, 1985). Many of the corporate structures have become enormous and operate according to a "supermarket" concept, offering a comprehensive selection of goods and services to the client. Smaller independent agencies become the "neighborhood grocery" by meeting the special needs of consumers and neighbors.

### Agency Funding

Sources of revenue for agencies include insurance benefits, fees for service, endowments and foundations, contributions, government support programs, Medicaid, and Medicare. A cost analysis of the services provided by the agency is important. Analysis helps to identify the source of income for the services, how much of the income will be realized, what the cash flow will be per annum or fiscal year, and how the provided services match clients' needs, that is, supply and demand. If the agency exists in a fairly high-income community, if it has the support of the local industrial complex, if clients are enrolled in health care benefit programs, and if clients are eligible for federal programs, the financial outlook is promising. If the agency is not located in such an atmosphere, it must search for other methods of support.

Alternate sources of income include separate insurance plan benefits, grants from foundations and official agencies, veterans' benefits, private donations, and support from community coordinating agencies such as United Way, Salvation Army, American Cancer Society, and the American Red Cross. Although it is difficult to predict financial outlook in these times of change, it is vital to an agency to have a 5-year financial plan with a forecast for the future. The plan includes contingency funds and methods for cutting back services without jeopardizing client, staff, and agency safety. Agencies considering diversification and joint ventures with other health care–providing agencies or personnel are directed to the series of articles previously mentioned in *Caring* (DeVita and Elwell, 1985; Lorenz, 1985; Simione and Elwell, 1985).

The agency budget is planned for a fiscal year. The fiscal year can coincide with federal funding time periods such as July 1 to June 30. Other fiscal years may coincide with the founding date of the agency or with the new year, that is, January 1 to December 31. For new agencies, initial budgets include seed money for conducting needs assessments and advertising services. Included in the seed money are the costs of a survey (e.g., mailings, forms, typing) and the salary for the staff conducting the needs assessment.

After the agency is established, the budget includes agency building funds or rental of space, operating expenses (heat, light, other utilities), salaries of personnel, fringe benefits, unemployment insurance, disability insurance, liability and malpractice insurance for staff and the agency, car and travel expenses, phones, paper, typewriter or word processor, record-keeping utilities, legal consultation, equipment, supplies for providing care, and so on.

Recordkeeping activities include an inventory of the agency equipment and supplies, personnel records, expenditures for maintaining service to clients, overhead costs, and records of income and outgo. The records are maintained by an accountant and are audited periodically. The executive director or the administrator of the program are kept appraised of the financial condition of the agency to support those programs responsive to client needs and to adjust programs that are not cost-effective. Decisions are made according to the debit and credit balance of the budget.

### The Home Care Market

According to Louden (1985) "high-tech" home care includes services for home infusion/nutrition therapies such as home parenteral and enteral nutrition therapy and antibiotic and chemotherapy treatments. Louden recognized that while these are the major treatments currently classified under the high-tech rubric, other treatment modalities will be added as the experience grows. In a home care marketing survey, Louden reported the following: Twenty-nine percent of hospitals surveyed were involved in high-tech home care, another 36% were entering the field, and 62% of home care agencies surveyed were involved in the delivery of high-tech services or goods.

Louden pointed out that the continued growth of the industry will greatly depend upon the reimbursement system. Only recently have the Medicare and Medicaid programs begun to address this issue and develop financial plans for support of the programs in home care. Under Medicare, parenteral nutrition therapies are allowed for the following conditions: short bowel syndrome, intestinal obstruction from carcinomatosis, inflammatory bowel syndrome, motility disorder, radiation enteritis, mesenteric infarction, and massive bowel resection (Louden, 1985). Louden advises that agencies and health care providers move cautiously in the market of home health care. The system appears to be moving toward disorganization and fragmentation. It reflects many of the existing problems in the American health care system with no organized approach to planning and evaluation of services.

Louden (1985) reported the Health Care Financing Administration's (HCFA) prediction that by 1990 high-technology care (parenteral and enteral) will increase in the home setting by 30%. In the 1985 Home Care Market Outlook Survey, 61% of home care agencies were providing high-tech services to their clients. Based on similar market projections, many varieties of health care agencies were established. Instead of consolidating services, the home care market became fragmented. Although home care saves in the cost of delivery of care, Louden stated, "However, at the present time, existing and prospective providers should proceed cautiously given the potential reimbursement pitfalls and increased competition. . . . Agencies have a variety of choices to make regarding high tech home care: provide specialized nursing care, provide equipment/supplies, handle billing, or handle it at all. Whatever the approach, it is critical to understand the reimbursement aspects and target marketing efforts to hospitals, high tech product companies, HMOs and perhaps, more important, physicians" (p 25).

According to Cabin (1985), "the basic reason for diversification is to put the entity in a better market position by expanding its range of services and sources of revenues" (p 6). Windley (1985) reported that diversification opportunities exist within the health care system for various models of home care. He gave an example of a pharmacy and its services as part of the health care delivery for clients receiving home care. Benefits in insurance plans are beginning to include private duty nursing services. Durable medical equipment supply can be a joint venture between the health care agency and the distributors. Physical therapy services can be diversified through therapy clinics or as part of the comprehensive services offered through outpatient clinics.

Millman (1985) discussed legal concerns facing home health care agencies by introducing high-technology care to the home setting. Her discussion includes Medicare reimbursement, certificate of need issues, product liability, and malpractice and informed consent issues. Home health care agencies providing high-technology services to clients need to consider these legal and ethical parameters of practice.

Health maintenance organizations (HMOs) and preferred provider organizations (PPOs) are starting to provide home health care services through their existing agency structures or through joint ventures with other agencies. Hospital joint ventures with home care agencies are becoming more common, and both provide the combined professional expertise of acute and community health nursing skills necessary for the delivery of high-tech services. High-tech services such as respiratory services are well suited for merging with hospital programs and often affiliate with community home-based agencies. Community-wide emergency systems provide an arena for coordinating care and for referral to the acute care of community-based agency.

## Marketing Services

*Marketing* is defined as a systematic process of identifying the needs and wants of customers/clients and developing services to meet these needs. Marketing focuses on the customer, with the basic belief that satisfied customers' payment for services produces the profit (for proprietary agencies) or surplus for the nonprofit agencies to support the financial base of the organization (Drucker, 1974; Wilkins, 1986). There are four components to the marketing process:

1. *Market research.* A needs assessment to survey and interview the population, identify the potential customers/clients, and their needs and wants.
2. *Program development.* Based on the needs and wants of the consumer population, an existing program may be repackaged to meet the customers' needs, an existing program from another community agency may be purchased and become part of the total package offered to clients, or the agency may choose to diversify and combine its services with other agencies.
3. *Market planning.* Setting the goals, objectives, and strategies for implementation of the new program or product.
4. *Market communication.* The advertising phase for promoting the program and entering into sales contracts with customers.

Advertising techniques are based on the motivations of the target consumer population. What they consider as quality services, such as a clean, modern, and attractive physical facility and a service personnel staff who care, are emphasized. The management of the organization is concerned about client satisfaction and will develop quality assurance measures such as utilization review and peer review indices.

Hiring professional advertising agencies or consultants assists in increasing the public's awareness of services; however, it is costly if consultation is long-term. It may be advantageous for large agencies to have their own marketing services to identify the consumer population and to develop and maintain strategically planned advertising campaigns. It is essential that an adequate consumer market exist to support initial start-up expenses. An agency may wish to establish itself by providing limited services with plans for future expansion as demands increase. The strategy is financially less risky if the expected caseload is not realized and the agency must be discontinued.

The agency philosophy and goals serve as a foundation for the image it wishes to project to the community. Advertising campaigns are directed toward the potential consumer/client population, with an emphasis on the specific services to be provided. Serving a few clients well with high-quality services is one of the best public relations mechanisms. Word of mouth spreads, and a sense of trust in the agency, its services, and its personnel develops. A new agency that is part of an established reputable institution in the community has the advantage of being associated with a proven record of excellence.

An effective means for publicizing services is to build a network of other health care providers with similar services, especially those who refer clients to the new agency. It is also advantageous to have a person on staff with a wide network of contacts and an established reputation in the community. The person is employed by the agency to make personal visits to key people in the community in order to gain support for the agency and to publicize its services. Display 3-1 lists potential home health care markets for agencies, corporations, and private practices who may be seeking a consumer/client population.

Attractive, to the point, professional, and informative brochures help to advertise. They can be distributed by hand or through the mail. Distributing brochures to agencies frequented by clients, such as hospitals, nursing homes, clinics, and health care providers' offices, is another method for raising public awareness. The extent of advertising depends upon the budget and the benefits of the advertising campaign over time. The initial campaign influences the success or failure of the agency, and is deserving of careful planning on the part of the founders. A well-supported and professional campaign has potential for early utilization of services by clients and a financially sound base.

---

*Display 3-1*
**List of Major Consumer/Client Markets
for Home Health Care**

Hospitals
Other health care agencies
Physicians, nurses, and other health care providers
Past clients
Insurers and other third-party payors
Senior citizens organizations
Employees
Durable medical equipment vendors
Business and industry
The public

## Consultation Services

Much of the previous discussion about starting an agency, marketing services, organizational structure, and management indicates the types of consultants useful to an agency. Even a small proprietary, professional practice or corporation consisting of several people is wise to invest in the services of experts. Examples of experts who are valuable to home care agencies include:

Accountants for business decisions and accounting procedures.
Lawyers for advice about local and regional laws, legal liabilities, malpractice matters, corporation taxing concerns, staffing concerns, and so on.
Insurance brokers for liability coverage, malpractice, employee benefits, and so on.
Public relations and advertising firms for marketing home care services.
Professional clinical experts for types of services and the personnel needed.
Health care suppliers to explain products for client or agency purchase or rental.
Real estate agents to discuss building needs.
Politicians to advise on the political and governmental climate.
Consultants from regulating agencies to advise about laws and regulations regarding the establishment of home health care agencies and the standards of care expected.
Other health care agency administrators to share their experiences and advise on effective methods of practice.

## Legal and Political Climate

The changes in the current health care system are a result of governmental legislation activities. Historically, the first major impact on the system occurred with the amending of the Social Security Act in the 1960s. The advent of the Medicare and Medicaid programs and the accompanying legislation creating regional health planning agencies and quality assurance programs such as utilization review committees helped to set the stage for future legislation and changes. Although these legislated programs applied only to hospitals and long-term care facilities where patients were recipients of Medicare and Medicaid benefits, they had an impact on home health care agencies.

Medicare and Medicaid and some private insurance companies recognized the need for support of home care services and provided for benefits during specified amounts of time after discharge from the hospital. The length of coverage for home care was 90 days and required certain diagnoses and provision of "skilled nursing care." Definitions of skilled nursing care were, at times, controversial, for example, early definitions did not include patient teaching.

The Medicare portion of the Social Security Act (Title XVIII) is administered by the HCFA. Currently, Medicare provides home health care for people 65 years and older if prescribed by a physician. The services must include care by registered nurses and at least one of the following: therapists (speech, occupational, or physical) social workers, or home health aides. Some supplies, equipment, and appliances are allowed. For example, oxygen therapy is allowed under Medicare for the following diagnoses (COPD; restrictive lung disease; pulmonary hypertension, with hypoxemia; significant or severe hypoxemia; cystic fibrosis; bronchiectasis; and widespread pulmonary neoplasm). Medicare does not provide reimbursement for angina pectoris in the absence of hypoxemia, shortness of breath without congestive heart failure or hypoxemia, or terminal diseases that do not affect the lungs. Intravenous therapy provided by hospital outpatient services is not allowed under Medicare but is included in home health benefits, that is, it can be provided through certified home care agencies. Medicaid (Title XIX) provides services for low-income people and, in some states, provides nonskilled services (homemaker) if the agency has these types of programs.

Title XX of the Social Security Act allowed for block grants to states for homemaker, chore, and companion services. The grants are based on a competitive basis among states and are based on population statistics. The 1978 amendment (Title III) of the Older Americans Act consolidates services for the elderly, including nutrition and social services, in an effort to provide coordinated and comprehensive services (Knollmueller, 1984).

The implementation of the prospective method of payment for Medicare patients in the hospital created shorter lengths of stay and earlier discharge. Patients are leaving hospitals with acute care needs and require nursing services at home. Because the system is recent and constantly changing, it is difficult to document: (1) who provides services for the clients, (2) if clients receive care, (3) to what extent clients are recovering, and (4) who is paying for services.

Many studies have demonstrated that home care is less costly than institutional care. Most of the studies were conducted prior to the impact of the DRGs and the prospective payment method of financing. Studies are needed to analyze how the health care system has changed during the last 5 years. Planned health care support is indicated with programs that are cost-effective yet provide the appropriate type of care at the correct time in the illness episode.

The Older Americans Act amendment of 1978 helped to demonstrate the effectiveness of coordination of activities for directing clients to appropriate care. Coordination of care allows the system to provide quality care that is cost-effective. For example, expensive programs delivering unnecessary services are eliminated, and savings are invested in programs that promote quality of life. Hospitalizing the terminally ill and providing heroic measures of care to maintain nonquality life are examples of the need for ethical considerations when viewed from the perspective of their tremendous costs to an overburdened health care system.

Health care providers need to have facts in order to take issues of concern to the community and politicians. Raising the public's awareness about the costs of health care services, the waste, the inappropriate expenditures of monies for care that is unnecessary, and the lack of services to promote health and rehabilitation and to provide supportive services for those dying at home is part of the activities of the health care worker. Information is presented to government leaders and legislators who can create changes in the laws and health care system.

Health care workers bring about change through membership in professional organizations that in turn send lobbyists to the government. Lobbyists for health care and professional organizations influence politicians and help to explain issues to the legislators and their aides. They help to campaign and point out the value of voting for candidates who represent the public's health interests. Politically savvy health professionals provide expert knowledge to those in power and may occupy political positions themselves in order to directly affect the system. Political awareness and participation in government are part of the professional role in today's health care system if the health care team is to effect change.

## Overview: Program Development and Evaluation

Chapter 2, Diagnosis of the Community for Home Health Care Needs, describes in detail the assessment process for diagnosis. Program development based on the identified needs includes a philosophy, purpose of the program, formation of agency goals, and specification of the objectives to meet goals. If it is a new agency as well as a program, the philosophy of the agency and its goals of services are developed. Within these broad goals are the specific programs of services and their objectives for delivery of care.

In a multiservice agency, there may be specific programs for cancer patients, individuals dying at home (hospice concept), rehabilitation programs for those with conditions whose recovery is essential to therapy programs, support services for the frail elderly. Each of the programs has an overall purpose. Long-term goals and short-term objectives for reaching the goals are set. Time frames are defined, whether it is a term program (ending by a specific date) or a continuing program based on need. In all cases, an evaluation plan is built into the program to judge its progress and the outcomes of its services. Evaluation leads to decisions to change the program, continue it, or discontinue services.

Chapter 11 describes in detail the concepts of program evaluation, an essential part of the provision of services based on quality of care and community need. Agencies are directed to the National League for Nursing Publication: *Criteria and Standards Manual for NLN/APHA Accreditation of Home Health Agencies and Community Nursing Services* (1980) for a listing of the 28 criteria that agencies must meet for accreditation. These same criteria serve as standards for agencies in evaluating their programs.

## Change Theory Applied to Home Health Care

Program planning, development, and evaluation operate within the conceptual framework of change theory. Change is the driving force of viable health programs. Change can be planned or unplanned. Leddy and Pepper (1985) defined *planned change* as involving "a deliberate process that has direction. The purpose is the improved functioning of the system" (p 266). For program planning, change occurs through a projection of needs for the future and the resulting responsive changes in the program.

Change can also occur as a result of situations arising in the environment that are out of the control of the health care provider. According to Leddy and Pepper (1985), there are three major types of unplanned change: (1) haphazard, which is random and unpredictable; (2) spontaneous, occurring in response to a natural uncontrollable event; and (3) developmental, in which one phase leads to the next in a progressive fashion (pp 266–267). For these latter types of change, the health care worker usually must react to the situation rather than having the advantage of thoughtful, purposive preplanning.

In those situations, it is best, if there is time, for the health care workers to meet as a group of providers and consumers to make decisions. One person is not as apt to consider all variables operating in the situation and alternatives for action. Emergency situations do arise, however, and there are times when the administrator must respond immediately. Staff in the agency need to know on whom they may call in case of emergency and the need for speedy decisions. When change is occurring and health care workers are aware of the situation, they can use the unplanned occurrence of change to make positive changes prior to reverting back to the usual ways.

Lewin (1951) and Schein (1969) developed theories of change as they relate to planned change. The three major steps in the process of change are unfreezing, changing, and freezing. A knowledge of the change process assists administrators and staff in program development, planning, implementation, and evaluation. By recognizing when change is occurring or by initiating change through raising the awareness of those involved that a problem or situation exists that needs attention, the program developer can take advantage of an unfreezing of status quo. It is at this time, when the situation is fluid, that change can be instituted.

In the case of anticipated change, the purpose for change, goals and intended outcomes, impact on the existing system, and benefits should be well thought out in advance and presented to the power group for action. Persuasion and the willingness to compromise are two key concepts for creating healthy change. When a situation becomes stable, freezing takes place by the system's return to its previous state or by the implementation of a new system or program. The successful institutionalization of a new system or program is measured by its official standing within the agency; that is, it has a title, staff, funding, and provides services to clients.

The current health care system is in a state of unfreezing, and home health care personnel can use change theory to respond to this rapidly changing arena of care. Needs assessment for home health care and the identification of long-term goals assist in targeting appropriate responses to changes in the health care system. Alternative strategies for program implementation are developed in collaboration with the client system. The selected strategies are then ready for action when the time for implementation is appropriate. Prior planning during the unfreezing stage helps to institutionalize new programs in the future and to create an improved system of care to meet client needs.

## References and Selected Readings

American Nurses' Association: A Guide for Community Based Nursing Services. Kansas City, American Nurses' Association, Ch-12, 2.5 M, 8/85, 1985

Balinsky WB: A comparative analysis of agencies providing home health services. Home Health Care Services Quarterly 6(1):45–64, 1986

Byers M, Jones B, Al-Sarraf E et al: On the scene: Corporate nursing and consulting. Nursing Administration Quarterly 10(4):25–57, 1986

Cabin W: Corporate reorganization overview. Caring 4(7):4–7, 1985

Caring, Washington, DC, National Association for Home Care, July 1985

Daniels K: Hospital home health care agency of California. Caring 4:16–19, 1985

DeVita, R, Elwell D: Corporate restructuring. Caring 4(7):60–61, 1985

Drucker PF: Management: Tasks, Responsibilities, Practice. New York, Harper & Row, 1974

Fagin C: Opening the door on nursing's cost advantage. Nursing and Health Care 7(7):353–357, 1986

Fish CW: Administrator's Handbook for Community Health and Home Care Services. New York, National League for Nursing Pub No 21-1943, 1984

Flanagan M: Conversion from nonprofit to profit; Legal and practical considerations. Caring 4(7):52–55, 1985

Janz K, Burgess B: Home health care. Stanford Nurse 7(3):6–9, 1985

Knollmueller RN: Funding home care in a climate of cost containment. Public Health Nursing 1:16–23, 1984

Knollmueller RN: The growth and development of homecare: From no-tech to high tech. Caring 4:3–8, 1985

Leddy S, Pepper JM: Conceptual Bases of Professional Nursing. Philadelphia, JB Lippincott, 1985

Lewin K: Field Theory in Social Science. New York, Harper & Row, 1951

Lorenz B: Corporate reorganization: The accounting perspective. Caring 4(7):62–66, 1985

Lorenz B: More sophisticated cost finding. Caring 4(7):75–79, 1985

Louden TL: Planning your niche in the "high tech" home care market. Caring 4:21, 1985

MacKenzie JA: Order out of chaos: Changes in community health and home care. Nursing Outlook 6(1):37–38, 1985

Mershon K, Weslowski M: Strategic planning for the business of community and home health care. Nursing and Health Care 6(1):33–36, 1985

Millman DS: Advances in medical technology: Legal problems and approaches. Caring 4:11–18, 1985

Mundinger M: Home Care Controversy. Too Little, Too Late, Too Costly. Rockville, New York, Aspen, 1984

National League for Nursing: Criteria and Standards Manual for NLN.APHA Accreditation of Home Health Agencies and Community Nursing Services. 2nd printing. New York, National League for Nursing, Pub No 21-1306, 1980

Schein EH: The mechanisms of change. In Bennis WG, Benne KD, Chin R (eds): The Planning of Change, 2nd ed. New York, Holt, Rinehart, and Winston, 1969

Shaw S: Market and program changes for the traditional intermittent provider. Caring 4:8–10, 1985

Shelton J: Cutting health care's bottom line. Nursing and Health Care 6:250–254, 1985

Simione WJ, Elwell D: Cost allocation: The problem and the solutions. Caring 4(7):67–71, 1985

Tulga G: Ethical and business decisions for home I.V. programs. Caring 4:19–20, 1985

Wilkins S: Marketing of health care services: Presentation at Looking Ahead Health Care 1990's. Sponsored by AORN California, San Jose Chapter of Association of Operating Nurses, 1986

Windley R: Diversification opportunities in the 1980s and beyond. Caring 4(7):10–12, 1985

Wood JB: Public policy and current effect on home health agencies. Home Health Care Services Quarterly 5(2):75–86, 1984

# Nursing Diagnostic Clusters and the Nursing Process in Home Health Care

Part II of this text is organized according to commonly encountered medical and nursing diagnoses in home health care. The authors propose a conceptual model for clustering nursing diagnoses appropriate to the practice of home health care. The model is based on an exploratory research study conducted on the east and west coasts from 1983 to 1986. One of the purposes of the research was to investigate the fit of nursing diagnosis classification systems to home health care and to medical diagnoses (DRGs). Another purpose was to develop a tool to audit client records and measure client outcomes, also linked to nursing diagnoses and their related client-centered goals.

The authors recognize that the proposed model for home health care nursing practice is limited because of the small size of records in the sample studies, the need for further research, and the nature of the evolving specialty of home health care nursing. The proposed model is an attempt to begin to classify nursing diagnoses appropriate to the field and to use it as a model for conducting further research. It is not the authors' intent to include every nursing diagnosis and related interventions, but rather to present a sample of those that represent

1. Major health problems commonly encountered in home health care
2. Selected nursing strategies consistent with interventions that relate to the problems

The model is discussed in detail in Chapter 4 and is described according to the four domains of nursing (nursing, person, health, and environment) and their interrelationships in the home care setting. The conceptual base for nursing diagnosis classification systems is reviewed, and several systems are discussed according to current nursing practice and the home health care setting. The authors develop *Nursing Diagnostic Clusters* within functional health patterns, which are relevant to home health care practice as contrasted to the acute care setting. The diagnostic clusters are further classified into two of the domains of nursing practice that the authors identify as crucial to client care in the home setting: *person* and *environment*.

The concept of caring as the essential link between nurse and client, family, and social support systems is proposed, with the notion that caring creates the working relationship to promote the client's recovery, maintain the family's health, and develop client and family self-care strategies. The ultimate goal of the nursing process is the client and family's improved health status and their ability to function independently or interdependently to meet their health needs. The authors recognize that the specialty of home health care nursing is evolving and acknowledge that the rapid changes also affect practice. The nursing process chapters attempt to meet the practical needs of present-day home health care clients and their primary care providers.

The description of the conceptual model is followed by a review of the fundamental steps of the nursing process as adapted to the home health care setting. Nursing assessment, diagnosis, contracting with the client, planning and implementation, monitoring of client status, and evaluation are reviewed. The Problem-Oriented Record System is presented as an efficient method for recording the home health care nursing process. An example of the application of the nursing process in the home health care setting is illustrated in tabular form.

The remaining chapters of Part II are presented according to the conceptual model of Home Health Care Nursing Diagnostic Clusters. Each chapter is organized around a diagnostic cluster and its list of nursing diagnoses. Frequently, encountered diagnoses and possible related diagnoses are selected from the cluster. The etiology and defining characteristics of the selected diagnoses are discussed, and a focus for nursing care is identified. The outcome criteria for the focus of nursing care are listed and serve as guides for the nursing care plan and standards of client care. The nursing process follows with assessment of the client, planning and implementation, and monitoring of client status. To complete the nursing process cycle, evaluation takes place by measuring client outcomes against the preformulated outcome criteria.

Chapters according to diagnostic clusters and the concepts of person or environment are listed below.

## Concept: *Person*

Chapter 5
>   *Diagnostic Cluster:*
>   Cognitive, sensory-perceptual patterns
>   *Selected Diagnoses:*
>   Knowledge deficit; educational needs for home health care providers; learning needs and teaching strategies for home health care clients
>   *Focus of Nursing Care:*
>   Teaching plan
>   *Selected Diagnosis:*
>   Comfort, alterations in
>   *Focus of Nursing Care:*
>   Noninvasive pain intervention strategies; invasive pain intervention strategies

Chapter 6
>   *Diagnostic Cluster:*
>   Circulatory and ventilatory patterns
>   *Selected Diagnosis:*
>   Respiratory function, alterations in
>   *Focus of Nursing Care:*
>   Airway and ventilation therapy and equipment; home apnea monitoring
>   *Selected Diagnosis:*
>   Cardiac output, alterations in: decreased; tissue perfusion, alterations in
>   *Focus of Nursing Care:*
>   Cardiac rehabilitation; pacemaker monitoring; stroke rehabilitation

Chapter 7
>   *Diagnostic Cluster:*
>   Fluid, nutrition, and elimination patterns
>   *Selected Diagnosis:*
>   Fluid volume deficit
>   *Focus of Nursing Care:*
>   Intravenous therapy in the home
>   *Selected Diagnosis:*
>   Fluid volume excess
>   *Focus of Nursing Care:*
>   Continuous abdominal peritoneal dialysis (CAPD)
>   *Selected Diagnoses:*
>   Skin integrity, impairment: related to stoma problems; knowledge deficit: related to stoma management

Chapter 8
    *Diagnostic Cluster:*
        Activity patterns: self-care, integument, exercise, mobility, sleep,
        sex
    *Selected Diagnoses:*
        Infection, potential for; oral mucous membranes, alterations in; sex-
        ual dysfunction
    *Focus of Nursing Care:*
        Nursing process for the homosexual client with AIDS
    *Selected Diagnoses:*
        Diversional activities deficit; infection, potential for; skin integrity,
        impairment
    *Focus of Nursing Care:*
        Nursing process for the intravenous drug user client with AIDS

## Concept: Environment

Chapter 9
    *Diagnostic Cluster:*
        Interaction and communication patterns
    *Selected Diagnoses:*
        Coping, ineffective; grieving; self-concept, disturbance in
    *Focus of Nursing Care:*
        Coping strategies for clients and families experiencing chronic and
        terminal illnesses

Chapter 10
    *Diagnostic Cluster:*
        Health promotion and maintenance/management: safety patterns
    *Health Promotion and Maintenance/Management Patterns in the Home
    Environment*
    *Selected Diagnoses:*
        Coping, ineffective; family processes, alterations in; health main-
        tenance management, alterations in; home maintenance man-
        agement, impaired; knowledge deficit; self-care deficit
    *Focus of Nursing Care:*
        Counseling, consultation, and referral
    *Safety Patterns:*
        Prevention of injury
    *Selected Diagnoses:*
        Family processes, alterations in; health maintenance management,
        alterations in; home maintenance management, impaired; injury,
        potential for; knowledge deficit; mobility, impaired; self-care
        deficit

*Focus of Nursing Care:*
Creation of a safe physical environment
*Safety Patterns:*
Control of infection
*Selected Diagnoses:*
Family processes, alterations in; health maintenance management, alterations in; home maintenance management, impaired; infection, potential for; knowledge deficit
*Focus of Nursing Care:*
Aseptic technique through the application of "bag technique"

# 4

# *Nursing Process in Home Health Care*

## *Nursing Diagnosis*

Nursing diagnosis provides a framework for organizing patient assessment and data collection. Shoemaker, in Kim, McFarland, and McLane (1984), stated at the Fifth National Conference for Classification of Nursing Diagnosis:

> Nursing Diagnosis is a clinical judgment about an individual, family, or community which is derived through a deliberate, systematic process of data collection and analysis. It provides the basis for prescriptions for definitive therapy for which the nurse is accountable. It is expressed concisely and it includes the etiology of the condition when known. (p 94)

Currently, there are 72 nursing diagnostic categories accepted by the North American Nursing Diagnosis Association (NANDA, 1986). These diagnoses have been categorized by several nurses in an attempt to standardize data collection. Gordon (1982) developed a framework for organizing nursing diagnoses based on 11 functional health patterns:

1. Health Perception–Health Management
2. Nutritional–Metabolic
3. Elimination
4. Activity–Exercise
5. Sleep–Rest
6. Cognitive–Perceptual
7. Self-Perception
8. Role–Relationship
9. Sexuality–Reproductive

*10.* Coping–Stress Intolerance
*11.* Value–Belief

The current diagnostic categories accepted by NANDA, 1986, are grouped under Gordon's 11 functional health patterns and are listed in Appendix B.

Doenges and Moorhouse (1985) developed 12 diagnostic categories to assist the nurse in the collection and standardization of data. The categories are alphabetized for ease of use, yet the authors emphasize that the diagnostic categories can also be prioritized and individualized to meet individual patient needs. Diagnostic divisions include:

*1.* Activity/Rest
*2.* Circulation
*3.* Elimination
*4.* Emotional Reactions
*5.* Family Pattern Alterations
*6.* Food/Fluid
*7.* Hygiene
*8.* Neurologic
*9.* Pain
*10.* Safety
*11.* Teaching/Learning
*12.* Ventilation

The diagnostic divisions and nursing diagnoses as developed by Doenges and Moorhouse are listed in Appendix C.

Carpenito (1983), in her text *Nursing Diagnosis Application to Clinical Practice*, states that "this standardization of data should not interfere with the nurse's theoretical or philosophical beliefs. It directs the nurse to the data that should be collected, not to the approach that should be used in interpreting the data or determining the intervention" (p 12). These divisions only serve as a *structure* for data collection, not as a conceptual model or theoretical framework.

One nursing diagnosis classification system particularly applicable to community/public health nursing is that developed by the Visiting Nurse Association of Omaha, Nebraska (Omaha, VNA), *A Classification Scheme for Client Problems in Community Health Nursing* (Simmons, 1980). The uniqueness of this classification system is that it is data based. The client problems were derived from a review of representative client records of the Visiting Nurse Association starting with a pilot study in 1976. The system identified four major domains of client problems:

*1.* Environmental—focus on problems external to the client affecting health
*2.* Psychosocial—refer to patterns of behavior, communication, relationship, and development

*3.* Physiologic—refer to the functional status of life maintenance processes

*4.* Health Behavior—refer to activities to maintain wellness or to promote recovery and rehabilitation (p 8).

Many of the client problems from the Omaha VNA scheme, such as those relating to the environmental domain, apply specifically to community/public health nursing clients. However, there are client problems that are very similar or identical to the NANDA's classification system and also apply to home health clientele. Examples of similarity are as follows:

Anxiety (identical)
Human sexuality: impairment (similar)
Bowel function: impairment, constipation (similar)
Therapeutic regime: noncompliance (similar).

Appendix D lists the Omaha VNA Classification Scheme for Client Problems in Community Health Nursing.

Part of the project by the Omaha VNA included identification of expected outcomes for each of the problems and criterion measures to increase specificity of and measurement potential of the expected outcome (Simmons, 1980, p 17). These client-centered problems and their related outcomes are relevant to home health care and community-based agencies that have chosen this scheme for the home health care population.

## Conceptual Framework and Nursing Diagnostic Clusters

Current nursing theories and nursing models provide nurses with several views of nursing, yet most theorists identify four concepts central to the domain of nursing, which include person (client), health, environment, and nursing (interaction, process, and therapeutics). Meleis (1985) states that the domain of nursing involves persons who are in constant interaction with their environment, who have unmet needs or are not able to care for themselves, or who are not adapting to the environment because of interruptions or potential interruptions to health. Nursing, with its caring approach, focuses on health promotion and interventions to enhance self-care abilities and to assist those persons or their social support systems unable to care for themselves. The nurse practicing in home health care is in collaboration with the client and family. Together, they identify unmet needs and build on the client and family strengths to move toward an improved health status.

The authors of this text used a deductive approach to develop a conceptual model of home health diagnoses by recognizing that clients enter the home health care system with a prediagnosed health problem. The model is congruent with the notion of the interaction of two of the central concepts in the domain of nursing: nursing care and the person's health status. The model identifies client home health care problems as within the domain of nursing, and it specifically addresses frequently encountered nursing diagnoses of the client in the home environment as differentiated from diagnoses found in the acute care and community health settings. The nursing diagnoses common to the home health care setting are grouped into six *nursing diagnostic clusters* that address the concepts of person and environment and prioritize the needs of the client and family in the home environment.

## Caring: The Humanistic Approach to Home Health Care

The nursing concept of caring is based on Leininger's theory (1978) and is identified as the central and unifying link between nursing, the dynamic state of health and illness, and the client and family/support systems. Professional caring emphasizes helpful, enabling activities, including nursing behaviors, techniques, processes, and patterns that improve or maintain health conditions.

As early as 1860, Florence Nightingale charged nurses to care for patients as whole persons. Today, the concept of caring remains a somewhat elusive phenomenon and is a neglected area of nursing theory and research. Recent work by Watson, Roy, Travelbee, Bevis, and Leininger and the National Caring Conferences within the last 10 years has begun to explore caring behaviors, characteristics, processes, and their cultural implications (Leininger, 1980).

Leininger defines caring as "those human acts and processes which provide assistance to another individual or groups based on an interest in or concern for that human being, or to meet an expressed, obvious, or anticipated need" (1980). Leininger describes the link between curing (which is the major focus of health care) and caring. She contends that there can be no curing without caring, but that there can be caring without curing. She also proposes that more emphasis be given to caring. She estimates that three fourths of health services represent caring and that only one fourth represents curing.

The conceptual model developed by the authors identifies home health care nursing and its caring nature as the linkage for bringing the client (person) within the home environment to an improved health status. Styles (1982) states:

> Nursing is "caring": both the attitude and the activity. Nursing is caring by promoting health and self-reliance for all. Nursing is caring for those who need to be nurtured in relation to their health status, wherever, as long, and as frequently as they need it, until that need is removed or revised by recovery, independence or death. (pp 230–231)

In the home setting, the nurse brings caring to the client with a health problem and the client's family or significant others. It is the caring nature of the nurse that generates trust and collaboration in the care of the ill client and the maintenance of health of the other family members. The nurse's genuine concern and care for these client systems is the foundation for building a trust relationship, contractual agreements, delivery of care, client and family compliance with medical orders, participation in the nursing prescription, and the eventual assumption of self-care.

Caring implies a moral and ethical commitment on the part of the nurse. It mandates a nursing care plan guided by client-centered goals that move the client and family toward an improved health status. Health status is recognized as a dynamic state, everchanging, and thus requiring a flexible plan of care that adjusts to the physiologic changes in the health condition as well as the wishes of the client and family.

The nurse's support and advocacy for the right to die at home and for the client and family's wishes to be carried out is an example of caring in its ultimate form. Continuing to care for the family of the deceased client, to provide grief therapy, demonstrates the hospice and home health care nurse's role in caring. Finding alternate ways to provide support and health counseling through referral to other community resources demonstrates care when health care system funding ceases or the initial health problem has been resolved.

High-tech care in home health care calls for emphasis on the nurse's human touch as a method for communicating with the client. This form of communication represents an activation of the caring process (Hudak, 1986). It becomes a very important component of practice for the home health care nurse. With the increase in complex procedures and the use of specialized equipment in the home care setting, caring becomes depersonalized. Human touch may be lost to the technology of manipulation, adjustment, and monitoring of *equipment*, instead of focusing on tactile contact and meaningful conversation and interactions with the client and family.

Caring for the client and family in their own home environment calls for an awareness and respect for the environment that is inseparable from the people. The nurse assesses the environment for physical safety factors as well as a therapeutic milieu that supports the recovery of the ill client and a healthy environment for the family. The nurse will not impose personal and professional values on the family that conflict with cultural practices and lifestyle. Home health care nurses must learn about clients' cultural practices and avoid ethnocentrism (the nurse's belief that her or his way is the best; Shubia, 1980). When conflict is identified, the nurse and family will discuss together the issues in the environment or health practices on the part of the family that are of concern to the nurse.

Health care practices that are at variance between the nurse and the family are sorted out, and those identified as neutral (neither positive nor negative effects) or beneficial (having positive effects on health) will remain

(Stanhope and Lancaster, 1984). Those issues that are harmful to the family are openly discussed, and ways to resolve the issues are formulated. If the family and nurse remain at odds over these issues, some conclusion must occur, such as a plan for change, termination of visits by the nurse, or reports to authorities in the case of illegal behaviors, such as abuse of a family member.

Leininger (1980) states that the majority of the behaviors of nurses take place in the caring mode compared with the curing mode. In the home setting, caring must take place in order for cure or improved health status to occur. The nurse is on the turf of the client and family, who have the right to accept or reject services. It is through the caring nature of the nurse that she or he is accepted by the client and family. Caring by the nurse helps to accomplish cure, rehabilitation, a peaceful death, acceptance of loss, and/or self-care and family health promotion activities. As illustrated in the Keating and Kelman conceptual model for home health care, it is the link between the person and environment and health.

## Development of Conceptual Model

Figures 4-1 and 4-2 represent the acute and home health care models according to the four major concepts within the nursing domain: nursing, person, health, and environment. Although the catalyst for the person's entry into both the acute and home health care settings is referral for a

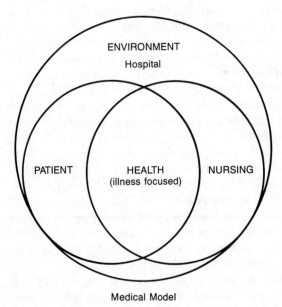

Figure 4-1. Traditional health care conceptual model.

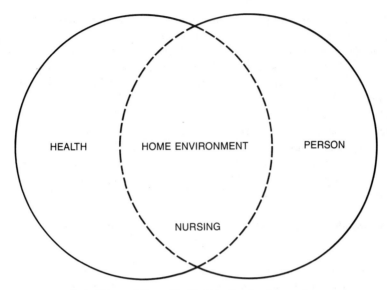

Early Stages of Home Health Care Nursing Interventions

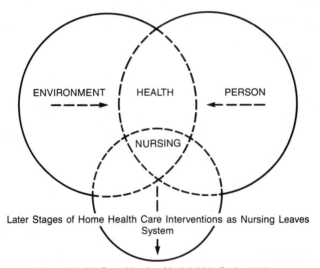

Later Stages of Home Health Care Interventions as Nursing Leaves System

Home Health Care Nursing Model With Caring Linkage

Figure 4-2. Keating and Kelman's home care conceptual model.

diagnosed health problem, there are major differences in the environment, client system, and nursing care. Acute care is dominated by the institutional setting, with its bureaucratic constraints that focus on illness and interventions within the institutional setting. In contrast, the home health care setting is in the client's familiar environment and allows for maximal control by the client, family, and significant others who actively participate in the formulation of goals and implementation of the care plan.

The Keating and Kelman home health care conceptual model of nursing diagnostic clusters is based on health problems and nursing diagnoses frequently recorded in home health care agency client records and identified as problems by experts in the field of home health care (see Chapter 12). Synthesis of the functional patterns of Gordon (1987), the diagnostic divisions of Doenges and Moorhouse (1985), the National American Nursing Diagnosis Association (NANDA, 1986), the Omaha VNA's (1980) four domains of client problems, and the frequently encountered nursing diagnoses in home health care led to the development of the diagnostic clusters that pertain to home health care. Table 4-1 lists the six diagnostic clusters and their nursing diagnoses.

Although the same nursing diagnoses can repeat within clusters, the

**Table 4-1.** *Nursing Diagnostic Clusters According to the Concepts of Person and Environment and Listing of Nursing Diagnoses Developed by Keating and Kelman for the Home Care Setting*

| Nursing Diagnostic Cluster | Nursing Diagnosis |
| --- | --- |
| *Concept:* **Person (Client)** | |
| 1. Cognitive, Sensory-perceptual patterns | Comfort, alterations in, pain |
| | Coping ineffective: |
| |    Individual |
| |    Family |
| | Health maintenance, alterations in |
| | Home maintenance management, impaired |
| | Knowledge deficit |
| | Noncompliance |
| | Sensory-perceptual alterations: |
| |    Self-concept, disturbance |
| |    Sexual dysfunction |
| |    Thought processes, alterations in |
| 2. Tissue perfusion and respiratory function patterns | Activity intolerance |
| | Cardiac output, alterations in |
| Circulatory and ventilatory patterns | Comfort, alterations in |
| | Communication, impaired |
| | Home maintenance management, impaired |
| | Knowledge deficit |
| | Mobility, impaired |
| | Respiratory function, alterations in |
| | Self-care deficit |
| | Sexual dysfunction |
| | Tissue perfusion, alterations in |

**Table 4-1.** *Nursing Diagnostic Clusters According to the Concepts of Person and Environment and Listing of Nursing Diagnoses Developed by Keating and Kelman for the Home Care Setting (Continued)*

| Nursing Diagnostic Cluster | Nursing Diagnosis |
|---|---|
| 3. Nutrition, fluid, and elimination patterns | Bowel elimination, alterations in<br>Fluid volume deficit<br>Fluid volume excess<br>Infection, potential for<br>Knowledge deficit<br>Nutrition, alterations in<br>Skin integrity, impairment of<br>Sexual dysfunction<br>Urinary elimination, alterations in |
| 4. Activity patterns (self-care, integument, exercise, mobility, sleep, sex) | Activity intolerance<br>Diversional activity deficit<br>Family patterns, alterations in<br>Infection, potential for<br>Knowledge deficit<br>Mobility impaired,<br>Oral mucous membrane, alteration in<br>Self-care deficit<br>Sexual dysfunction<br>Skin integrity, impairment of<br>Sleep pattern disturbance |

*Concept:* **Environment**

| | |
|---|---|
| 1. Interaction and communication patterns | Anxiety<br>Communication, impaired<br>Coping, ineffective:<br>  Individual<br>  Family<br>Family processes, alterations in<br>Grieving<br>Knowledge deficit<br>Powerlessness<br>Self-concept, disturbance in<br>Social interactions, impaired<br>Social isolation<br>Spiritual distress |
| 2. Health promotion, maintenance, and management patterns<br>Safety patterns | Coping, ineffective family<br>Family processes, alterations in<br>Health maintenance alterations in<br>Home maintenance management, impaired<br>Infection, potential for<br>Injury, potential for<br>Knowledge deficit<br>Mobility, impaired, physical<br>Self-care deficit |

81

DECISION GUIDE
STEPS FOR DETERMINING NURSING DIAGNOSES FOR HOME HEALTH CARE CLIENTS

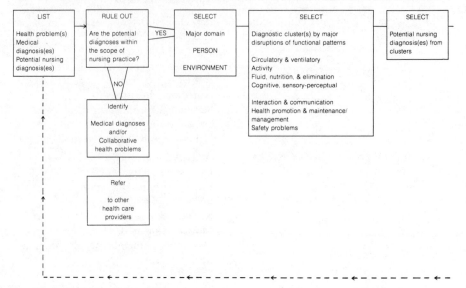

Figure 4-3. Decision guide for selecting home health care nursing diagnoses.

model presents and emphasizes those that occur most frequently within a given cluster. For example, knowledge deficit related to self or family care of the ill client is encountered more frequently in the cognitive, sensory-perceptual patterns, yet it may also apply to the safety, health promotion, maintenance, and other patterns.

Figure 4-1 represents the traditional structure of client care in the health care system. Health is illness-based, with a disease or system focus with very little emphasis on the individual as a holistic being. The institution (environment) defines the parameters of care and becomes the controlling agent for health–illness dynamics, nursing, and the patient. The artificial limitations imposed by the hospital environment on the patient and family hinder independence and health-promoting behaviors. The patient becomes entrapped within the bureaucratic structure of the health care system, has little control over his or her care and the environment, and thus becomes dependent upon the health care provider to meet basic needs.

Figure 4-2 represents the conceptual model developed by Keating and Kelman. The individual is a unique, holistic being, greater than the sum of his parts. Health is wellness-focused. The home health care client and family coexist with the environment. Health can occur without nursing input. The person is viewed as a consumer and an independent or interdependent agent with unique problems. Nursing interacts collaboratively with the client, family, and social system to implement a plan of care. The person and home environment are critical to the effectiveness of care and set the limits with

AND FAMILIES

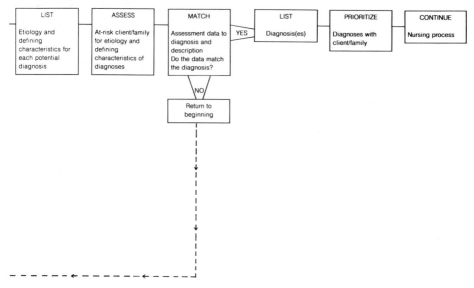

which nursing and members of the health care team operate to bring about changes in the health–illness dynamic state. To assist the nurse and client to formulate a realistic individualized plan of care, the nursing process is modified and revised for home health care. As the client and family move toward wellness and use health promoting behaviors, interactions with the nurse decreases.

Based on the home health care nursing conceptual model in Figure 4-2 and the findings from two pilot studies to review client records in home health care agencies, the nursing diagnoses in this text are grouped into diagnostic clusters. The clusters are organized around the nursing domain concepts of person, environment, dynamic state of health–illness, and nursing, with caring being the link between nurse, client, environment, and health status. Medical diagnoses and other health problems contribute to the etiology and defining characteristics of the nursing diagnoses.

Home health care nurses who choose to use the Keating and Kelman diagnostic clusters conceptual model may wish to use a decision guide for identifying those health problems that belong to the nursing domain, medical practice, or collaborative problems indicating the participation of other health care team members. McKnight (1985) and Carpenito (1984) present such decision trees for distinguishing between health problems and relegating them to domains of nursing. Keating and Kelman offer a decision guide (Fig. 4-3) for determining nursing diagnoses of concern to the home health care client and family from the diagnostic cluster model.

Home health care nurses may also wish to use a series of critical questions to identify nursing diagnoses related to the client and family's medical/health problems. Additional questions are posed as they relate to nursing intervention and the client and family's responses and outcomes. The critical questions are as follows:*

1.  What is/are the medical/health problems of the client and family?
2.  What is the current and prescribed medical therapy for the client at home?
3.  What are the possible negative outcomes that could occur as they relate to the medical/health problem(s) of the client and family?
4.  What do the nurse, client, and family need to know in order to monitor and assess for early signs of negative outcomes?
5.  How will the nurse, client, and family recognize adverse responses?
6.  Can the nurse, client, and family intervene/act to prevent the negative outcomes?
7.  How will the nurse, client, and family know if the patient is responding?

## Nursing Process Applied to Home Health Care

The nursing process applied to home health care includes assessment, diagnosis, planning for care, intervention, and evaluation. Even though the steps of the process are the same as those in hospitals and long-term care facilities, they are often more complex owing to the nature of the setting, the additional variables influencing the client and family, and the need for integration of community health nursing concepts. Figure 4-4 illustrates the nursing process applied to home health care.

Clients are referred to home care agencies by other community health care agencies, hospitals, long-term care facilities, health care providers, and community organizations and through case finding activities on the part of nurses. Referrals for home care clients usually contain medical diagnoses and related nursing diagnoses. Thus, the approach to the nursing process becomes a deductive one, leading from the referring diagnoses, to diagnostic clusters, to assessment, and, finally, to refinement of specific nursing diagnoses unique to the client in the home setting.

### Overview

During the initial assessment of the client and family, the nurse lists all health problems in the family record. Health problems are categorized into

* Adapted from lecture by Keenan, 1985.

three types:

1. Problems indicating collaboration with other professionals or referral to other health care providers
2. Medical diagnoses
3. Nursing diagnostic clusters

Frequently, the problem list is long and consists of multiple problems. The nurse, client, and family review the list and set priorities according to needs and family preference. Usually, the basic physiologic needs of the ill family member are of primary concern to the client, family or significant others, and the care providers.

After assessing the individual client, family, social support systems, and the environment and identifying health-related problems and formulating diagnostic clusters, the nurse, with the client and family, develops client-centered long-term goals that define the desired outcomes of care. The long-term goals are "ends standards." They serve to list the final expected outcomes of care and are used as criteria against which to measure the success of nursing intervention.

Throughout the process, the nurse and client add to the data base and refine the diagnoses to reformulate related goals. Short-term goals (objectives) based on the long-term goals are listed. These objectives provide the steps that the nurse and client take to reach the long-term goals and serve as an outline for developing the nursing care plan. They are the "means standards" to measure the client's progress toward an improved health status.

The nurse, client, and family develop a plan that specifies what will be done, by whom, when and how often, where, the method, and the recording or documentation of the care received. Implementation of the plan can involve the following people:

Home health care nurse (baccalaureate-prepared)
Other members of the nursing staff such as:
    Registered nurses (associate degree or diploma)
    Licensed practical or vocational nurses
    Home health aides
Other professionals such as
    Physical therapists
    Occupational therapists
    Speech therapists
    Physicians
    Nutritionists
    Social workers
    Client
    Family or significant others

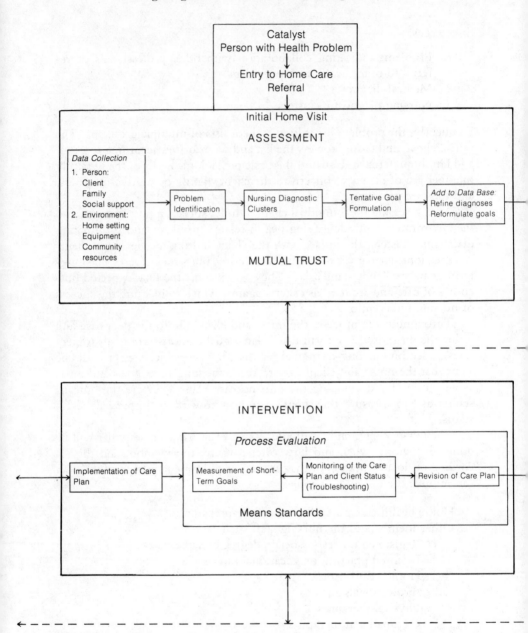

Figure 4-4.  Nursing process for home health care.

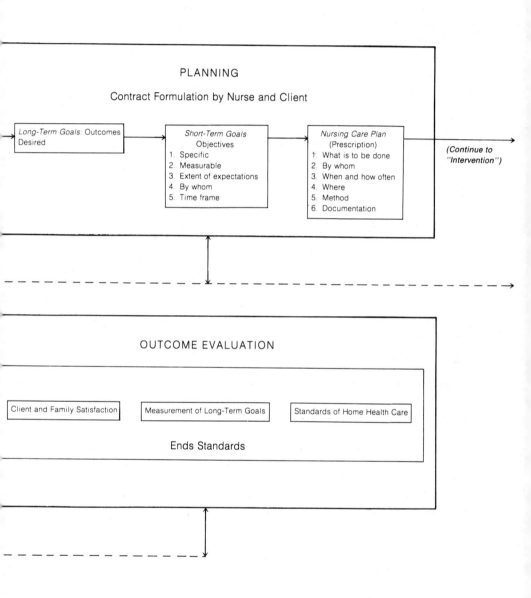

PLANNING

Contract Formulation by Nurse and Client

| *Long-Term Goals:* Outcomes Desired |
|---|

| *Short-Term Goals* Objectives |
|---|
| 1. Specific |
| 2. Measurable |
| 3. Extent of expectations |
| 4. By whom |
| 5. Time frame |

| *Nursing Care Plan* (Prescription) |
|---|
| 1. What is to be done |
| 2. By whom |
| 3. When and how often |
| 4. Where |
| 5. Method |
| 6. Documentation |

*(Continue to "Intervention")*

OUTCOME EVALUATION

| Client and Family Satisfaction | Measurement of Long-Term Goals | Standards of Home Health Care |
|---|---|---|

Ends Standards

Neighbors and friends
Vendors of durable medical equipment and supplies

The nursing care plan contains process evaluation techniques for measuring the client's progress toward the final outcome. Process evaluation is conducted through the assessment of the client's progress toward reaching the short-term goals (objectives or means standards) and monitoring activities on the part of the nurse. Ends standards are the measures for meeting long-term goals, client and family satisfaction, and established standards of home health care. There are two major long-term goals for clients receiving home health care:

1.  To improve the individual client's health status
2.  To maintain the family's health during the client's illness.

## Assessment

Assessment of the home health care client consists of collecting data specific to the client's health needs, including information about the home environment, client's family and other support systems, care provider(s), and actual or potential community resources. The data are collected systematically on an initial assessment tool. The tool organizes the information into subjective and objective categories. Subjective data contain information gathered from an interview of the client and family. The objective data include observations and examination of the client and family by the nurse, laboratory reports, and observation of the home environment. Commonly used health history and physical examination forms, family profiles, and referral formats serve as data-gathering tools for assessment.

### Individual Client Assessment

Current nursing texts on health assessment contain suggested outlines for collecting individual client health data. Because the home health care client usually carries one or more major medical diagnoses, the analysis of a symptom or chief complaint portion of the health history becomes extremely important for formulation of nursing diagnoses and the progress of care. Sources of data for the initial assessment include:

Referral form
Referring agency
Health care provider
Health history and physical assessment of the client
Interview of the family and/or significant others

Home health care nursing diagnostic clusters are identified, and preliminary nursing diagnoses specific to the client, family, and situation are formulated. The existing client health problems listed on the referral form and the new data gathered during the initial home visit serve as resources for formulating diagnoses and planning care.

## Family Assessment

The initial assessment of the family and/or significant others living at home with the client includes a description of the family cluster. Social support systems include extended family members, friends, and neighbors who serve as actual or potential care providers. For ease of reading, the terms *significant others* and *social support systems* are subsumed under the term *family* for the remainder of the text.

Each family member living in the home is listed by name, role, age, and general health status. Role in the family includes that of dependent, major income provider, nurturer, care provider, and/or counselor. Included in the description is how the various members' roles will be influenced by the presence of an ill member in the family. The tasks each member will assume in the care of the client, if any, are reviewed and discussed for planning purposes.

Major cultural, religious, and language factors are identified as they influence the family's health care practices, beliefs, and values. The nurse discusses these with the family to clarify any potential professional values and health behavior conflicts that might arise.

The nurse observes the family dynamics, and, eventually, as a trust relationship is developed, these interrelationships are discussed with the family. It is important to identify the member(s) of the family who will be providing care for the client in order to institute teaching–learning strategies for the management of nursing care. Additionally, it is important to know which member of the family is the sustainer or provider of basic necessities to ensure maintenance of basic human needs for the family.

Usual decision-making processes within the family are reviewed by the nurse to implement care and develop changes that promote the health of the family. The primary communicator or spokesperson for the family serves as the contact person or coordinator of communications between the health care provider(s) and the client and family. A profile of the essential data to collect from families with a member receiving home health care is outlined in Appendix E: Assessment Guidelines for Family Profile of Home Health Clients.

The family economic resources for basic necessities and coverage for health care are listed. In case of need, resources outside the family, including extended family, friends, neighbors, and social agencies are identified as potential sources of assistance to the family. Included in the socioeconomic assessment are the major expenditures facing the family, such as housing, utilities, food, clothing, home maintenance expenses, educational expenses, leisure time activities, health care, and equipment or assistive devices necessary to the care of the ill family member. The following discussion relates to the assessment and evaluation of durable medical equipment indicated for the home health care setting.

## Assessment of Home Health Care Supplies, Equipment, and Vendors

Major categories of home health care products follow, with a few examples for each:

1. Patient's room furniture (e.g., bed, table, safety devices, traction equipment, chair, transfer items, commodes)
2. Medical equipment (e.g., thermometers, sphygmomanometers, biologic testing meters and supplies, humidifiers, vaporizers, oxygen therapy, cold and heat therapy items, massagers, infusion pumps, suction machines, respirators)
3. Physical therapy equipment (e.g., appliances, supports, prostheses, walkers, wheelchairs, safety devices such as grab bars, ramps, shower benches, and raised toilet seats, whirlpool baths, shower hoses)
4. Occupational therapy equipment (e.g., reaching aids, utensils, flexors)
5. Ostomy and urologic supplies (e.g., tubing, syringes, catheters, pastes and powders, drainage bags, personal care items)
6. Surgical and first aid supplies (e.g., dressings, tapes, pads, gauze)

Home care agencies, their staff, and clients make decisions regarding the provision of necessary equipment, devices, medical supplies, and appliances for care. Prior to the current increase in the delivery of acute care in the home setting, clients discharged from the hospital and needing equipment for continuity of care at home were referred to hospital social workers, therapists, or discharge planners. These specialists referred clients to dealers in the community or supply houses where equipment could be purchased or rented. The therapists (physical, occupational, and respiratory) knew which products were best for clients' needs. Social workers and discharge planners were familiar with resources in the community and referred clients to community health agencies with loan closets or stores where items could be purchased or rented.

With the changes in the health care system, enterprising stores, pharmacies, and distributors experienced an increase in the demands for equipment for patients at home. They established warehouse supply stores and/or retail stores. Some of the stores expanded rapidly and became large supermarkets of medical supplies. As demand grew, they began to add services such as special therapists and nurses who provided care and taught clients how to use the equipment. Thus, companies and suppliers began to provide the care and education necessary for maintenance of the client at home, and, eventually, they became home health agencies in their own right.

Some hospitals, realizing the potential market for supplying medical equipment from discharged clients, established home care supply centers. Nonprofit hospitals established holding companies for distributing equipment. Profit from renting or selling products to clients is returned to the hospital through the holding companies. The income generated from the holding company helps to defray the loss of revenues by the hospitals from the declining client population.

In the current home health care system, home care agencies, their staff, and clients have the following three basic choices for supplying clients with durable medical equipment and other supplies:

1. To establish an agency supply station with
   a. A dispensary for renting or selling equipment and supplies to clients; or
   b. A loan closet for borrowing equipment and supplies; or
   c. A holding company that sells or rents items to clients
2. To contract with a dealer to supply the agency, which, in turn, supplies the client
3. To refer clients to wholesale or retail dealers

While health care providers can present choices to their clients for access to products, they also have a responsibility to provide safe and reliable equipment and supplies. There are a myriad of products and suppliers from which to choose. Providers who enter home health care without experience in this aspect of care should refer clients to established resources in the community. If the provider or agency finds that it must obtain equipment, the guidelines listed here are offered.

### Guidelines

*Geographic Location/Accessibility:* How far is the distributor from the home? Is the vendor or distributor accessible if the client or health care provider must return or pick up any additional supplies or equipment? If a service call is indicated, how long will it take, especially in an emergency situation?

*Operating Hours:* Consider the availability of the vendor and the services offered. What are the normal operating hours? Are services provided evenings, weekends, and holidays? Will house calls be made to deliver repair equipment if needed outside of business hours? Is there an answering service? Is the answering service local or regional?

*Set-Up and Delivery:* Does the vendor make an initial hospital visit to review equipment and supply needs? Is there a charge for delivery and set-up?

*Financing Billing/Charging:* Consider the assignment of benefits. Can bills be submitted directly to insurance companies, Medicare, Medicaid? If not, what is the procedure? Is billing by the month with an itemized printout? It is essential that the client determine whether he or she has coverage for supplies and home therapy.

*Maintenance and Repair of Equipment:* Does the client contract with the company for repairs? Is there an additional fee? Is the equipment routinely cleaned and repaired when returned to the vendor?

*Back-Up System for Equipment and Spare Parts:* Is there a back-up system for equipment that may break down or malfunction? How does the back-up system operate? Some companies have a computer system that assists in tracking inventory.

*Compatibility of Equipment:* If more than one vendor is to be used, it is important to determine whether the equipment is compatible and interchangeable with other equipment that may need to be used.

*Inventory and Condition of Equipment:* Consider the availability and selection of equipment offered by the vendor. Is the equipment new and in good condition? If the client has extra supplies and equipment no longer needed, can these items be returned or will the client receive credit?

*Nurse's Role in the Vendor's Company:* Consider the role of the nurse. Does the nurse have an active role in regard to home health care management, including instruction and validation on the use of equipment?

*Comparative Costs vs Other Vendors and Distributors:* Consider the cost of the vendor's equipment and services and compare it with that of other companies.

*Total Services Offered vs Other Vendors and Distributors:* Consider the total services that each vendor offers and determine which best meets the needs of the client.

*Communication:* Consider how the people employed by the vendor interact with the client, family, and health care team. Are they encouraging and supportive? Do they consider health teaching and instruction regarding equipment and use of supplies to be a priority?

Appendix F contains a checklist for the selection of vendors that nurses and their clients may find useful as a guideline.

Equipment should be durable and safe. If the agency plans to loan or rent equipment to clients, it is best to purchase quality medical equipment with a known reputation. Even though the equipment is more expensive than less well known products, the life of the product and ease in cleaning and maintaining will prove to be cost-effective over time. As items become outdated, they may still have a useful purpose for some clients to whom the equipment can be sold for a reasonable price, saving the client considerable expense for new equipment and allowing the agency to profit to some extent from the loss of outdated inventory.

Some home health agencies have little expertise with high-technology products. If, for example, intravenous therapy is to be one of the services, clinical nurse specialists and staff nurses in hospitals are the best advisors for types of supplies necessary for the patient. They know which brands are of the best quality, "nurse and patient proof," and least expensive, and those that provide ease of administration.

The various therapists are the experts to consult for orthopaedic appliances, bedside care furniture, therapy aids, transfer devices, and mobility appliances. The therapists may be employed by the agency or can be consulted in hospitals, clinics, or private practice.

## Home Environment Assessment

An assessment of the home environment is included in the physical and sociologic data collection. In Chapter 9, home environment aspects are discussed as they relate to the diagnostic cluster: "Environment: Safety Patterns." Appendix G contains a Home Environment Assessment Guide. The guide collects data describing how the family provides home health care and helps to identify possible etiologic or contributing factors to the aforementioned nursing diagnoses.

The home environment assessment provides the nurse and family with information about the facilities and equipment readily accessible in the home for client care and for the additional materials that need to be procured. A neighborhood and community assessment provides information about resources and locations for obtaining necessary articles. The review of the clients' economic status guides the nurse and family to appropriate agencies and reimbursement systems that help supply the articles of care through loan, rent, or purchase.

Assessment and diagnosis of the home environment lead to the listing of the supplies and equipment specific to the clients' needs for health restoration and/or comfort measures. The list is comprehensive and is reviewed by both client and health care provider to identify those items that are in the home or that may be substituted with home equipment. The review helps to avoid unnecessary cost and expense in equipment and supplies.

Examples of items on the list include bowls and pans that can substitute for basins; food and canning tongs for forceps; roasting basters for large irrigating syringes; empty jars and cans for solutions or dry materials; white rags for large nonsterile dressings and bedding materials; newspaper pads covered in old pillow slips for bed pads; old towels and blankets for positioning patients; blocks to raise beds to a comfortable care-providing height; and sturdy metal or wood chairs for bathing and showering purposes.

All equipment is cleaned, and some items can be sterilized by boiling or baking. Because equipment is used only for the client in his or her home environment, the danger of cross-infection is decreased. Using home supplies and equipment can greatly decrease the cost of care and the negative impact of disposable supplies and equipment on the community's environment. Specific equipment needs for each nursing diagnostic cluster are included in the following chapters.

A review of the routine schedules of family members and the client helps to identify gaps in the care giving regimen and the need to plan for continuity of care. Part of the plan must include respite for the primary care giver in the home to prevent burnout and to maintain individual and family health.

## Nursing Diagnosis and Tentative Goal Formulation

Nursing diagnostic clusters are identified according to person (client and family) and environment. Tentative nursing diagnoses and their related goals are formulated. As the planning and contract phases of the nursing process develop and assessment continues, certain of the diagnoses are eliminated, and specific diagnoses are identified and prioritized for intervention. Increasing numbers of community and home health care nursing agencies are using classification systems for nursing diagnoses. The major systems are the Classification Scheme for Client Problems in Community Health Nursing (Simmons, 1980) and the National Group for Classification of Nursing Diagnosis (Kim et al, 1984).

Many agencies use the International Classification of Diseases or the Diagnostic Related Groupings (DRGs) (Shaffer, 1983) as guides for documenting the care requested and provided. The latter method (use of DRGs) relates to the prospective payment of medical care instituted in the U.S. health care system in the early 1980s. It is possible to articulate these medically oriented diagnoses within the framework of the nursing classification system. The nursing classification system helps to identify the human responses to medical diagnoses or other health problems, yet it is specific to nursing intervention.

## Planning With Family, Community, and Support Systems

### Mutual Trust

Home health nurses use the knowledge and skills of communication theories, family dynamics, and community or aggregate health diagnoses in providing home health nursing care. These knowledge bases and skills are essential to the delivery of care. Freeman (1970) emphasized initial building of trust between the nurse and client in the home setting as imperative for satisfactory interpersonal relationships.

The first client contact with the care provider creates an initial impression and is comparable to the bonding process that occurs between mother and infant or significant other. It is therefore essential that during the first visits, the primary nurse conducts the initial assessment, diagnoses the nursing problem, and plans for the nursing care. The main care provider in the home and members of the family and/or significant others should be present during the first visit. Adequate time for the visit provides time to build trust, conduct the initial assessment, develop a plan of care with short- and long-term goals, and draw up a contract of agreement for care among all interested parties.

The trust-building process involves a genuine interest by the nurse in the client and family, with a display of warmth and empathy and a willingness to interact with them. The home environment of the client creates the milieu in which the nurse must function and adapt nursing knowledge, practice, and professional values to the delivery of care. Frequently, the nurse finds that personal and cultural beliefs vary from those of the client and/or his or her family. Knowledge and acceptance of cross-cultural values and behaviors are important for the nurse to facilitate communication, acceptance of differences, and collaboration with the client and family in order to restore the person to optimal health or level of functioning.

### Refining Diagnoses and Reformulating Goals

The process of collection of data for assessment of the client, family, significant others, and the community helps to create a mutual understanding of health needs. Identifying the specific nursing diagnoses from the nursing diagnostic clusters and referring non-nursing diagnoses to appropriate resources with the client and family helps to set priorities and begin the planning phase. If a nursing diagnosis exists only in the mind of the referring agent or the nurse, planning and implementing care will probably not succeed owing to the lack of client involvement.

## Contract Formulation

Having a contractual system for providing care between the nurse, client, and family helps to validate diagnoses, set priorities and goals, and plan for the actual care. Steckel (1982) and many basic community health nursing texts provide the theory for contracts between nurse and clients and present samples of contracts.

The essential ingredients included in a contract are

Mutually agreed upon diagnoses (problems)
Priority of problems
Major long-term goals or outcomes of care
Short-term goals (objectives) or steps leading to achievement of the outcome, including a time frame and estimated number of visits
List of all the health care providers (including the client and family or significant others) and their functions
Specific tasks for all those providing and receiving care.

The contract is in nontechnical language and at a level at which the client and/or family can understand. Goals, objectives, and specific tasks are stated in behavioral terms, with time parameters and level of competency specified to measure the final outcomes of care (see section discussing evaluation).

## Nursing Care Plan

The nursing care plan (prescription) is drawn up and specifies the type of care necessary, who will provide it and when, and a method for recording the care. The care plan is posted in the home, and a flow sheet (see sample in Figure 4-7) is kept in the home and in the agency to record activities of care and the client's progress. The care is implemented, and all participants evaluate the care given, the client's progress toward improvement in health status, and the client's and family's satisfaction with the care provided.

## Intervention and Evaluation of Home Health Care

### Process Evaluation

The nursing care plan is implemented according to its prescription. The care provided is evaluated from the time of initial implementation through the final outcome or discharge of the client and family from service. Although process evaluation includes all phases of nursing care—assessment, diagnosing, planning, implementing, and evaluation—it is especially relevant to the implementation stage of the nursing process. Short-term goals (objectives) serve as process criteria and are included in the care plan. They direct the nurse, client, and family toward the prevention or alleviation of the altered state of wellness. Process criteria can focus on three major areas to assist the client to

> Use his or her resources more effectively to facilitate an optimal level of coping
> Seek other resources to facilitate an optimal level of coping
> Modify his or her activities of daily living and usual lifestyle when resources are diminished or inadequate (Carpenito, 1983, p 41).

The written nursing care plan with its specific nursing diagnoses, client goals, operational objectives, plans for nursing care, and health care provider objectives provides the criteria for measuring the effectiveness of process measures. Thus, it is important to state nursing and client goals and objectives in measurable terms. Objectives must specify who is involved and include action verbs, what is expected, the measure of success, and the time parameter involved. The data from the nurse's troubleshooting activities and subsequent revision of the care plan provide additional criteria for process evaluation.

Monitoring of the client's health status by the nurse minimizes and/or reduces the risk of failure. It also identifies potential problems that may jeopardize the client's recovery. Problems can include client illness and recovery factors, family coping abilities and resources, and environmental limitations. Monitoring activities include the assessment of equipment and assistive devices used by the client with input by the nurse regarding their usefulness and appropriateness to the care setting. After problems are identified and resolved, the care plan is revised and implemented while process evaluation in terms of meeting the objectives and monitoring activities continue.

## Outcome Evaluation

Outcome evaluation refers to the long-term client-centered goals. For home health care clientele, the outcome is twofold: the improved health status of the ill person, and the maintenance of the family's health. Evaluation of the quality of care delivered to the individual client and/or family is measured by the extent to which the predefined goals and outcomes of care are met. Carpenito's text lists outcomes for each of the nursing diagnoses listed in her text (1983). Carpenito defines outcome criteria as "the expected change in the status of the client after he has received care" (p 41). Examples of process and outcome goals for selected hypothetical diagnoses follow.

## Examples

*Nursing diagnosis:* Potential for infection related to surgical incision postmastectomy.

*Outcome (long-term goal):* By the end of 1 month, the nurse will care for the client's surgical incision, which will be healed with no evidence of inflammation or infection.

*Who is involved:* The nurse and client

*Action verb:* Will care for

*What is expected:* Surgical incision will be healed

*Measure of success:* No evidence of infection or inflammation

*Time parameter:* At the end of 1 month

*Process (short-term goal):* By the end of 1 week, the nurse will observe that the client's incision is healing, because it will be well approximated, dry, and free of purulent exudate, and there will be less inflammation.

*Who is involved:* The nurse and client

*Action verb:* Will observe

*What is expected:* Incision is healing

*Measure of success:* Well approximated, dry, no purulent exudate, less inflammation, absence of fever

*Time parameter:* By the end of 1 week

The long-term goals serve as one set of criteria for outcome evaluation. Other criteria are client and family satisfaction with the services provided, and standards of home health care. Setting standards of care for the agency and health care providers is prerequisite to evaluation of nursing services. Sources for standards of care can come from professional organizations such as the American Nurses Association, National Home Care Association, American Public Health Association, Oncology Nursing Society, State Health Department regulations, Medicare and Medicaid guidelines, and accreditation agencies such as the National League for Nursing or Joint Commission on Accreditation of Hospitals. Evaluation is part of quality control systems within agencies or private practice and demonstrates professional accountability to the consumer. See Chapter 11 for further discussion of quality assurance.

## Documentation of Care

### Client and Family Records

Community and home health care nurses agree that recordkeeping activities consume a large part of their work time. Home health care nurses can make as many as six or seven visits per day, all of which must be recorded to document care and in the type of language that qualifies the agency for financial reimbursement for services. Recordkeeping activities are one of the greatest sources of stress to nurses in the community (Sevee, 1984). Nurses, health care agencies, professional organizations, and regulatory agencies need to make a concerted effort to ease the problem and streamline the health care system. Supervising nurses and staff development personnel can assist nurses by reviewing their recordkeeping activities, identifying problem areas and techniques of recordkeeping that are more efficient, and holding workshops to teach newer and more effective recordkeeping methods.

Dictating notes by dictaphone or telecommunications are examples of speedy and efficient strategies used by nurses. Office staff assume the recording activities in these instances with a method of quality control built in by periodic review of records by the nurses and management. With computerized systems available, nursing services have the opportunity to interface with the systems to keep records, document care, and evaluate services and staff. The systems will provide a data bank with fertile ground for research in clinical nursing and health care management that will lead to improved client care.

Documentation of care through recordkeeping is an essential part of nursing and its accountability to the consumer. At the same time, however, the amount of time spent in recordkeeping by professionals is costly and takes time away from direct client care. Record systems must be as concise as possible and must, at the same time, substantiate the provision of care.

Nurses practicing in the community setting define their unit of service as the family, whereas acute care nurses define their unit of care as the patient or individual. In many instances, the home health care nurse will visit a home with only one resident, but, like the community health nurse, it is more usual to visit families with one or two members experiencing health problems amenable to nursing care. The problems have an impact on the family system; thus, the nurse must take into account family dynamics and other related factors while caring for specific persons.

In many instances, the family as a unit is experiencing a problem such as home maintenance problems, potential for violence, or parenting problems. Because of the focus on family in community and home health nursing, records for families and the individuals within them are complex. Complicating the picture even further are regulations imposed upon health care providers that require separate records for each person. It is this confusion in recordkeeping that causes redundance, large amounts of paper work, and volumes of records.

The nature of the community, its demographic characteristics, and the health statistics of its population influence the style of nursing service and recordkeeping. Agencies' utilization of one of the nursing classification systems of client problems and adaptation of a system such as the problem-oriented medical record (POMR) system (Weed, 1969) can assist in recordkeeping.

The ideal record system consists of one family record (cross-referenced if surnames are different), with the baseline information contained on a form similar to the one outlined in Appendix E. Each member of the family, regardless of that person's health status, that is, health supervision or home health care problem, should have a baseline health assessment, identification of nursing diagnostic clusters, nursing diagnoses, related goals (outcomes), and progress notes to document the care given for the area of concern during each visit. According to the financial structure of the agency and the type of services provided, the records may need to be kept in subfiles of the family file in order to demonstrate care provided for third-party payors.

Flow sheets (see Fig. 4-7) correlated with the diagnoses, patient outcomes or goals, and objectives related to plans of care serve to document care and the client's progress toward the goal. Flow sheets are more than check lists; they include evaluation statements that describe the amount of progress achieved. If they document the extent of progress or deterioration of the situation, lengthy progress notes (narrative notes) are not necessary. Flow sheets are particularly appropriate to the high-technology procedures related to the current home health care scene.

Figure 4-5 illustrates the recommended organization for client records. Records include the family file with identifying data and a suggested form for the nursing diagnosis list. Figure 4-6 presents a sample outline for recording family progress notes.

## Individual Records

Each folder includes subfiles for individual family members. The subfiles are organized as follows:

1. Baseline Health Assessment: Includes initial referral and its follow-up reply.
2. Nursing Diagnostic Cluster: Person and/or environment; nursing diagnoses and related goals (Outcomes) list. Where appropriate, these diagnoses are related to medical diagnoses for financial systems analysis.
3. Progress Notes (most recent first) in the following SOAPE format:
   (S)ubjective—data collected from client report, interviews, and health history
   (O)bjective—data collected from actual observations, physical assessment, and documented facts
   (A)ssessment—impressions and problems, nursing diagnosis, and current status of problem: i.e., improved, same, deteriorated (complications disabilities, unwarranted death), or new diagnosis

(P)lan—client-centered long-range goal or outcome of care, objectives for accomplishing goal, method of care, care provider, time parameters, reports

(E)valuation—measurement of outcomes of care using prestated goals (outcomes) and objectives as criteria. Includes client care providers' satisfaction.

(*Text continues on p. 105*)

**Family Nursing**        **Diagnosis List**

Diagnostic Cluster: (Check all those that apply)

Environment:
Safety patterns ✓
Health promotion and maintenance/management patterns ____

Rule out:
Family processes, alterations in ✓
Home maintenance management, impaired ✓
Infection, potential for ____
Injury, potential for ____
Mobility, impaired, physical ____
Self-care deficit, total or partial ____

| Date Admitted | Diagnosis: # and Title | Goal: # and Title | Date Discharged |
|---|---|---|---|
| 2/20 | 1. Alterations in family processes related to ill family member | 1.1 Verbalize feelings 1.2 Participate in care of ill member 1.3 Maintain basic needs for members | |
| 2/20 | 2. Impaired home maintenance management related to principal family member's illness | 2.1 Seek outside resources 2.2 Delegate functions to other members | |

Diagnostic Cluster: (check all those that apply)

Person:
Circulatory and ventilatory patterns ____
Activity patterns ✓
Fluid, nutrition, and elimination patterns ____
Cognitive, sensory-perceptual patterns ✓

Rule out:
Self care, deficit, Total ✓ Partial ____
Skin integrity, impairment ____
Oral mucous membrane, alteration in ____
Infection, potential for ____

Figure 4-5. Sample of recommended organization chart for family records.

Activity intolerance ____
Diversional activity deficit ____
Mobility, impaired, deficit ____
Sleep pattern disturbance ____
Sexual dysfunction ____
Rape trauma syndrome ____
Self-concept disturbance ____
Thought processes, alterations in ____
Coping, ineffective, individual ____
Coping, ineffective, family ____
Comfort, alteration in, pain ____
Sensory perceptual alterations ____
Knowledge deficit ____

## Individual Family Member's Nursing Diagnosis List

| Name | Date Admitted | Nursing Diagnosis: # and Title | Goal: # and Title | Date Discharged |
|------|--------------|-------------------------------|-------------------|-----------------|
| Mary | 2/20 | 1. Self-care deficit related to inability to carry out activities of daily living | 1.1 Assist care taker in ADL 1.2 Express satisfaction with hygiene | |
| | | 2. Alterations in comfort related to acute pain from pathologic rib fracture | 2.1 Receive empathy for discomfort 2.2 Express improved status in comfort | |
| ____ | ____ | ____ | ____ | ____ |
| ____ | ____ | ____ | ____ | ____ |

## Identifying Data and Baseline Assessment for Family

*Name:* Smith/ Jones

*Address:* 416 Main Street
Lima, CE 003249

*Phone:* 000-678-3244

*Directions:* Single-family home on Main Street, 8th house on the right coming from the south. House is a two-story blue frame with white trim.

*Family Members:*   Husband: John Smith
Birthdate: 5/6/53    Health Status: excellent

Wife: Mary nee: Lane, (Jones, 1st marriage) Smith
Birthdate: 11/2/58    Health Status: Metastatic breast cancer

Children:
Louise Smith
Birthdate: 4/3/77    Health status: hayfever, no other problems

Jacob Jones
Birthdate: 7/14/82    Health status: excellent

Melanie Smith
Birthdate: 2/28/84    Health status: excellent

Figure 4-5. (continued)

## Family Progress Notes

*Family Member(s):* Mary     *Date:* 2/20

*Individual Diagnosis #:* 2.   *Diagnosis Title:* Alterations in comfort related to acute pain
from pathologic rib fracture from metastatic breast cancer

See referral form: Medical Diagnosis: Metastatic breast cancer

*Subjective data:* Client reports generalized acute pain, weakness, inability to carry out
ADL; says she is "depressed."

*Objective data:* Vital Signs: B/P: 100/70, P:96, R:32; T: 97
Skin: jaundiced, diaphoretic, restless

*Assessment:* Generalized debilitated state

*Evaluation:* Condition deteriorating

*Plan:*  1. Provide comfort measures: positioning, relaxation/visualization techniques,
medication
2. Encourage client to verbalize

*Family Member(s):* John Smith, Louise Smith, Jacob Jones, Melanie Smith

*Family Diagnosis #* 1.  *Title:* Alterations in family processes related to ill family member

*Subjective data:* Family members are angry and frustrated with Mary's condition; express
need to discuss her condition with physician; Melanie is unkempt, cries frequently; indicates hunger.

*Objective data:* All members are home; house is in disarray.

*Assessment:* Family unable to meet basic necessities; exhibit grieving process at anger
stage.

*Evaluation:* Dysfunctioning family unit

*Plan:*  1. Allow family to express anger
2. Assist members in organizing activities to maintain basic necessities
3. Refer to community resources for home care, i.e., home health aide; American
Cancer Society; counseling services.

Re-visit 2/21.

*N.Taylor, RN*

## Client Record

*Client and I.D. #:* Mary Doe   000-00-000

*Date of Initial Diagnosis:* 5/6/86

*Nursing Diagnosis:* # 1. Potential for infection related to surgical incision postmastectomy.

*Goal:* By the end of 1 month, the nurse will care for the client's surgical incision, which
will be healed with no evidence of inflammation or infection.

*Objectives:*

Week 1:  By the end of 1 week, the nurse will observe that the client's incision is healing,
because it will be well approximated, dry, exhibit no purulent exudate, and exhibit no accumulation or fluid under incision located near axilla, and there will
be less inflammation. No fever present.

Week 2:  By the end of the week, the incision will be dry with no exudate and resolving
inflammation.

Week 3:  By the end of 2 weeks, the incision will be healed.

Figure 4-6. Sample family progress notes (see also Fig. 4-5).

## Nursing Care Plan

Week 1: The nurse will change the mastectomy dressing using sterile technique q.i.d.
The nurse will observe the incision for complications q.i.d.
The nurse will encourage patient to view the incision while changing the dressing.
The nurse will report complications to the physician for follow-up p.r.n.

Week 2: The nurse will make two visits during the week to monitor progress.
Visit 1:
The client will assist the nurse to change the dressing.
The nurse will refer client to physician and readjust plan; if complications occur.
Visit 2:
The client will change the dressing.
The nurse will reassess the client and make recommendations for continued rehabilitation.

Week 3: If the incision has healed and there are no complications, the problem is resolved and the diagnosis is closed.

Figure 4-6. (continued).

## Flow Sheet

**Week 1:**

| Visit | Day 1 | Day 2 | Day 3 |
|---|---|---|---|
| *Time of Visit* | 10:00 A.M. | 10:30 A.M. | 10:00 A.M. |
| *Incision condition*:* | * | * | * |
| *Action:* | Scanty exudate, cleaned with sterile saline, xeroform gauze dressing | Same | Intact dressing D.S. dressing |
| *Initials:* | SK, RN | SK, RN | SK, RN |

|  | Day 4 | Day 7 |
|---|---|---|
| *Time of visit:* | 10:15 A.M. | 10:00 A.M. |
| *Incision condition:** | Intact | Intact |
| *Action:* | Call MD, d/c dressings | Diagnosis resolved |
| *Initials:* | SK, RN | JS, RN |

* Describe if other than dry:

**Week 1:**
Day 1: Small amount of serous exudate, no odor, slight inflammation, cleaned with sterile saline, client observed dressing
Day 2: Less amount of serous exudate, no odor or inflammation, cleansed with sterile saline, dry sterile dressing applied.
Day 3: Clean and dry, no inflammation, client assisted with dressing, client is viewing incision
Day 4: Incision is closed, no exudate, referred to Reach for Recovery visit in 3 days
Day 7: Incision edges well approximated, no inflammation, client reports no problems, phone call to MD, d/c dressings, client is in contact with Reach for Recovery, nursing diagnosis resolved

**Week 2:**
Follow-up visit. No evidence of inflammation or infection of incision, client continues rehabilitation program. Will contact agency as necessary.

Figure 4-7. Sample flow sheet for postmastectomy patient with potential for infection related to surgical incision.

Laboratory reports, interagency information sheets, and interdisciplinary communications are included in the progress notes and are placed with subjective or objective data as appropriate.

4. Flow sheets (most recent first)

Related to nursing diagnosis, client outcome, and objectives/plan of care (see Fig. 4-7).

Using a system such as the Problem-Oriented Medical Record (POMR) will help to eliminate unnecessary recording. Only essential information is recorded in the progress notes and flow sheets. Narrative notes are unnecessary. Reports include the care provided, current assessments of the client's progress, and evaluation of the nursing care plan's implementation within the nursing diagnosis classification and its related goal(s).

The POMR and the nursing classification systems lend themselves to quantitative recording, computerization, and analysis. As more agencies and providers of care in the health care system use these systems, and, as the financial system mandates cost-effectiveness, information systems will improve. There will be a sharing of information, and systems will refine recordkeeping for more accurate documentation of care and research activities. The resulting efficiency of recordkeeping will provide relief for nurses from the stress of paperwork and the time consumed for these activities. Additionally, valuable retrievable data, easily accessible for nursing research, will become available.

## References

Carpenito LJ: Nursing Diagnosis Application to Clinical Practice. Philadelphia, JB Lippincott, 1983

Carpenito LJ: Is the problem a nursing diagnosis? AJN 11:1418–1419, 1984

Doenges M, Moorhouse M: Nurse's Pocket Guide: Nursing Diagnoses With Interventions. Philadelphia, FA Davis, 1985

Freeman R: Community Health Nursing Practice. Philadelphia, WB Saunders, 1970

Gordon M: Manual of Nursing Diagnosis. New York, McGraw-Hill, 1983

Hudak C, Gallo B, Lohr T: Critical Care Nursing, pp 33–43. Philadelphia, JB Lippincott, 1986

Keenan, M: Lecture. Albany, New York, 1985

Kim MJ, et al: Classification of the Nursing Diagnoses: Proceedings of the Fifth National Conference. St Louis, Mosby, 1984

Leininger M: Transcultural Nursing: Concepts, Theory and Practices. New York, John Wiley & Sons, 1978

Leininger M: Caring: A central focus of nursing and health care services. Nursing and Health Care 1(10):135–143, 1980

McKnight PM: Decision tree for distinguishing nursing diagnosis, clinical nursing problems, and clinical medical problems and relegation to relevant domains of nursing. Nursing Diagnosis Newsletter 11(4):1985

Meleis A: Theoretical Nursing Development and Progress. Philadelphia, JB Lippincott, 1985

NANDA: New diagnoses accepted. Nursing Diagnosis Newsletter 13(1):1986

Sevee AD: Work Stressors of Community Health Nurses. Unpublished master's project. Troy, NY, Russell Sage College, 1984

Shaffer FA: DRG's: History and overview. Nursing and Health Care 4(7):383–396, 1983

Shubia S: Nursing patients from different cultures. Nursing '80 10(7):78–81, 1980

Simmons DA: A Classification Scheme for Client problems in Community Health Nursing. Hyattsvile, MD, U.S.D.H.E.W., No HRA 80–16, 1980

Stanhope M, Lancaster L: Community Health Nursing: Process and Practice for Promoting Health. St. Louis, CV Mosby, 1984

Steckel SB: Patient Contracting. Norwalk, CT, Appleton-Century-Crofts, 1982

Styles M: On Nursing: Toward a New Endowment. St. Louis, CV Mosby, 1984

Weed L: Medical records that guide and teach. N Engl J Med 278:593, 1969

# 5

# Diagnostic Cluster: Cognitive and Sensory-Perceptual Patterns

The nursing diagnoses listed in the cluster of cognitive, sensory-perceptual patterns are related to numerous medical and health problems encountered by nurses providing home health care to clients and their families. All the diagnoses are potential health problems and are identified according to etiologic and defining characteristics and priority of client need. Although most of these diagnoses are interrelated, the authors chose to discuss two of them because of their frequency reported in client records and because they are diagnoses that override many other diagnoses and client conditions. The two selected diagnoses discussed in this chapter are knowledge deficit and comfort, alterations in: related to pain. Included with the pain discussion are the related diagnoses of knowledge deficit, sensory-perceptual alterations, and sexual dysfunction.

## Nursing Diagnoses

Nursing diagnoses related to this cluster and frequently encountered in the home health care setting are

Comfort, alterations in, related to pain
Coping, ineffective, family
Coping, ineffective, individual
Health maintenance, alterations in
Home maintenance management, impaired
Knowledge deficit
Noncompliance
Self-concept disturbance
Sensory-perceptual alterations

Sexual dysfunction
Thought processes, alterations in.

## Selected Diagnoses From Cognitive Patterns: Knowledge Deficit

### Learning Needs and Educational Strategies for Home Health Care Providers

The home health care field is changing rapidly and affecting nursing services in acute care and community health nursing agencies. Traditional home health care agencies and health departments are expanding their nursing services to include care for the acutely ill at home and the terminally ill who choose to die at home. With shortened lengths of stay in the hospital, hospitals are closing acute care units and entering the home care business with their own nursing staff and support services. Nontraditional agencies and entrepreneurs are also entering the home health care field.

Educational needs abound in the current health care system, and there is a demand for preparing community/public health nurses and acute care nurses for home health care. Collaboration between the two groups of nurses is indicated. Acute care nurses can provide training for community health nurses in such techniques as venipuncture, medication administration, transfer techniques, activities of daily living for clients confined to bed, physical therapy, feeding techniques, and dressing changes. Additionally, home health care nursing practice includes high-technology skills such as ostomy care, wound care, catheterizations, intravenous therapy, hyperalimentation, total parenteral nutrition, respirator care and oxygen therapy, and medication and other palliative measures for intractable pain.

Acute care nurses who plan to practice in the home setting need to acquire community health nursing knowledge and skills, including the referral process, coordination of care among health care providers, financial recordkeeping systems, environmental assessment for safety factors, application of legal parameters of practice care to the home setting, community assessment for resource and system support, and family assessment and care. Community health nurse colleagues can share their expertise in these skills with acute care nurses.

Nurses who provide care for clients in the home setting demonstrate the usual needs of adult learners. For principles guiding the educational needs of adult learners, the reader is referred to Knowles (1980), who has studied the many variables affecting adult learners. Professional qualifications and characteristics vary greatly between the types of nurses involved in home health care.

Community health nurses are usually required by agency and governing body regulations to have at least a baccalaureate level of nursing preparation. The credentials of nursing personnel employed by nontraditional agencies, hospital-based programs, or entrepreneurial nurses involved in home health care may vary from associate degrees to doctoral degrees. Credentials of acute care nurses practicing in the home setting also vary, although clinical specialists usually have advanced knowledge and skills in their specialty of nursing, with a minimum of a master's degree.

The home health care field is composed of a paraprofessional nursing staff who also have teaching–learning needs. Included in this cadre of health care providers are licensed practical or vocational nurses, home health care aides, housekeepers, and outreach workers. Their educational backgrounds range from less than a high-school education to highly educated people. Adding to the characteristics of all learners are their multivariate life experiences.

## Etiology and Defining Characteristics

The selected nursing diagnosis from the diagnostic cluster's cognitive patterns is knowledge deficit and relates to the learning needs and educational strategies for

1. Health care providers in the home setting
2. The client and family and/or significant others

Knowledge deficit as defined by Carpenito (1983) is "the state in which the individual experiences a deficit in cognitive knowledge or psychomotor skills that alters or may alter health maintenance" (p 254).

The nursing diagnosis of knowledge deficit for home health clientele carries numerous defining characteristics and etiologies. Primary to the diagnosis are the health problems or medical diagnoses that cause the client to require home health care services. Thus, etiologic factors include the pathophysiology and other variables that cause or contribute to the medically diagnosed condition and the related therapeutic regimens that are prescribed for cure, rehabilitation, or palliation. The related stresses, including the high anxiety levels and grieving processes that occur as a result of the illness, are also etiologic factors and add to the complexity of the learning needs of the client and family. Knowledge of the health resources and community support systems presents other parameters of learning needs for clientele in their ability to cope with the crisis situation, adjust to new lifestyles, and learn to use systems available to them.

Defining characteristics of knowledge deficit in the home care setting include the existence of a new health condition or situation that has not been encountered previously, the need for the client and family to understand the cause of the condition, the pathology involved, and the therapeutic measures needed for improvement of the condition; there is also the need for motivation on the part of the clients to learn and achieve the knowledge and skills necessary for improvement in health status.

The home health care system provides a temporary, episodic interlude of care for clients. The financial support for home care is limited to a prescribed number of visits for various health conditions and is usually confined to "skilled" nursing care and other professional therapies. The situation leads to the need for the client, family, or support system to assume the care of the ill client at home. Although it is not necessarily supported financially, the home health care nurse becomes responsible for the future needs of the client by teaching the client and family the assessment and home care interventions that will improve and maintain the client's health.

## Focus of Nursing Care

The teaching plan serves as the selected focus of nursing care for the home health client and family as they learn about the problems they are facing and the health care strategies they will need to assimilate. Teaching–learning strategies are synthesized to simultaneously meet the needs of the home health care personnel, individual clients, and their family or significant others. The situation calls for highly skilled nurse educators and clinicians who can assess learning needs and develop appropriate teaching plans. The plans must be specific to the characteristics of the learner, commonly encountered health problems, specialized nursing techniques, and the home setting. The teaching plan is discussed in detail later in this chapter as it applies to the home health care client and family, with a sample case study at the end of this section.

## Outcome Criteria

The following outcome criteria are listed by Carpenito (1983):

The person will
actively participate in the health behaviors prescribed or desired
experience less anxiety, related to fear of the unknown, fear of loss of
    control, misconceptions, or previously given misinformation
describe the disease process, causes, and factors contributing to symp-
    toms, and the procedure(s) for disease or symptom control (p 260)
perform techniques of care for the maintenance of the ill client at home
    (author's addition).

While these criteria appear to be client and family-centered, they also apply to health care personnel.

## Application of the Nursing Process to the Learning Needs and Educational Strategies for Home Health Care Providers

### Assessment

The complexity of the system and the diversity of its practitioners require an assessment and diagnostic approach to the teaching–learning needs of health care providers. The situation calls for close collaboration among the clinical specialists in the acute care setting, community health care nurses in the field, and nursing educators in institutions. Educators include those who are involved with staff development in the health agencies, private nursing education services, and faculty in formal academic settings.

Each agency examines its needs for staff education. The following cost-effective questions are posed:

1. Is it more effective to re-tool all staff or selected members of the staff, or hire specialists to serve in the agency?
2. What types of nursing services best meet the needs of the agency's clients?
3. Should community health nurses be placed in acute care settings, or are acute care clinical specialists in the community agency best suited to the needs of the program?

### Planning and Implementation

Planning for teaching–learning needs is identical for all nursing care plans. After the assessment of the learner(s) takes place and the diagnosis of knowledge deficit is reached, client-centered (home health care provider) goals are developed. Objectives are formulated and provide the process for achieving the goal. The usual rules governing statements of objectives apply; that is, verbs are behaviorally stated, what is to be done is included and by whom, to what extent success is to be measured, and when the goal is to be completed. Based on the objectives, the content and teaching strategies are developed.

The present financial structure of the health care system with its emphasis on cost-effectiveness does not provide for adequate financial support of educational programs. Because of this situation, many nursing service administrators and nurse educators have developed innovative programs. For example, two large metropolitan health departments use the local university's school of nursing learning laboratory facilities for updating staff nurses' acute care skills. The staff developers from the health departments were clinical specialists in community health and taught the adaptation of the acute care skills for the home to their staff. In return for this collaboration between educational facility and agency, the agency provides clinical experiences for the students.

Another example is a hospital-based home health care program staffed by nurses who acquired acute care skills through participation in an inservice program in the hospital. This same agency is collaborating with a graduate program in nursing by providing experiences for clinical specialist students in both acute care and home health care nursing. In return for the experiences, there is consultation from the graduate faculty and collaborative research activities between nursing service and education.

For the most part, teaching–learning strategies for the professional development of nurses are in the hands of nurse educators in the academic settings and care providing agencies. Continuing education programs are usually administered by nurse educator experts. These same experts serve as consultants for health care agencies who need training for paraprofessional staff. In these instances, formal classes, intensive workshops, practice laboratories, and on-the-job training are indicated. The principles that guide teaching and learning activities still apply.

## Evaluation

Evaluation techniques of teaching–learning activities for staff and paraprofessionals in home health care settings are related to acquisition of nursing skills. Evaluation is directly related to quality assurance in the delivery of client care. Evaluation of the individual staff member's knowledge and skills can be tested through written examination, competency-based evaluation, and observations of actual practice. Behaviors are measured against the predetermined goals and objectives of the educational program. Quality assurance measures are based on the goals and outcomes set for delivery of care and include client satisfaction. Supervision of the staff's nursing skills is conducted through individual conferences, record review, observation of practice, client interviews, client progress toward improved health status, and client satisfaction indices.

## Learning Needs and Educational Strategies for Home Health Care Clients

When providing nursing care for clients requiring home health care, the nurse first identifies the nursing diagnoses related to the referral and the admission medical diagnoses and/or health problem(s). Frequently, these diagnoses relate to the same health problems facing the client and family and/or primary health care providers. During the assessment phase of the nursing process, specifically on the first home visit, the nurse must determine which diagnoses best apply to the client's condition, the family members or support systems rendering care, and the home environment. As the diagnoses are identified and listed, other potential diagnoses are ruled out.

Once the list of nursing diagnoses is completed, the nurse and clients set them in order of priority. The nursing diagnosis identified as having high priority by the client, family, nurse, and other care providers is listed as first in order of care. Many times, the diagnosis listed first corresponds to meeting physiologic needs of the ill person and the related nursing care skills that will aid in the recovery process.

Initially, the client and family may expect the nurse to provide total care. Eventually, after their anxiety levels have decreased and they indicate a need to move toward independence, their learning needs and priority for assuming the care of the ill family member will increase. Nursing diagnoses closely related to these needs are coping, ineffective; family processes, alterations in; health maintenance, alterations in; home maintenance management, impaired; and knowledge deficit.

Unless the skills are highly technical, requiring professional care for client safety, the nurse should introduce the concept that the client and family will ultimately assume care. If the nurse continues to provide care, the client and family will become dependent on her or him, and this fosters a dependent relationship on the health care provider. Owing to the reality of the eventual loss of financial support for nursing care and the demands of other families in the nurse's caseload, the relationship must eventually terminate. In order to prevent a crisis situation, it is imperative that the nurse identify teaching–learning needs at very early stages of care and work with the client and the family in developing plans that will foster the family's or client's ability to assume responsibility for the care.

Home health clients are referred for services because they require nursing techniques to meet basic needs, maintain activities of daily living, cure and/or recover from a medical diagnosis or health problem, or receive palliative measures for a terminal disease. The client will need to learn self-care measures that will promote the level of wellness, including the need for psychosocial support in the time of crisis. The family and/or significant others of the ill client also need crisis intervention and will need to learn all or some of the techniques of care for the client while in the illness phase.

## Application of the Nursing Process in Learning Needs for the Home Health Care Client

### Assessment

Developing a list of teaching–learning needs at an early stage of care for the home health care client is essential for quality care and cost-effectiveness. Early intervention can prevent secondary diagnoses, complications, disability, and, in some cases, unwarranted death. Early intervention mandates communication systems between nurses and referring agencies to identify clients prior to their discharge home. Although not usually possible, it is ideal for the nurse to meet the client, referral agents, and the family prior to the actual implementation of care in the home. To accomplish this end, the nurse from a community-based agency builds a relationship with acute care agencies and health personnel who provide care for the population that the home health care nurse serves. Nurses in hospital-based home care units have the advantage of close proximity to the acute care setting and personnel and are more likely to accomplish this ideal situation.

If possible, the home health care nurse obtains a list of clients anticipating discharge from the acute care setting and visits them in that setting, visits the family in the home to conduct a home assessment, and contacts the physician or other health care provider for referral. Educational needs are identified at very early stages in the acute care setting, and care is planned and implemented in collaboration with acute care nurses.

Collaboration provides the opportunity for the home health care nurse to:

1.  Observe the care that is to be provided
2.  Practice the skills in the acute care setting
3.  Meet with the physician and other health care providers for direct consultation and development of therapeutic plans
4.  Anticipate problems related to care in the home
5.  Plan for home care

It also affords the opportunity for both home health care and acute care nurses to work with the family and client in teaching them skills to move them toward independence.

### Profile of Client and Family

The diagnosis of a knowledge deficit for home health clientele requires an assessment of the individual client, the family, and the community support system needs. Assessment data include the variables discussed under the section on etiology and defining characteristics of the diagnosis. The data are organized into categories and described succinctly through a profile of the client and family and/or significant others and their teaching–learning needs.

The profile includes the following:

1.  Nursing diagnosis of the client
2.  Medical diagnosis and prognosis
3.  Major medically prescribed therapeutic regimens
4.  Previous nursing care plan
5.  Client's age and developmental level

6.  General physical condition, including sensory perceptual deficits
7.  Significant past health history
8.  Mental status and outlook
9.  Education and occupation
10. Family and/or significant others
11. Providers of care
12. Home setting
13. Socioeconomic factors
14. Cultural and language variables
15. Financial support system for health problems
16. Available resources
17. Assistance from relatives, friends, neighbors, and the community

Collection of the data assists the nurse in defining the nursing diagnosis(es) from the diagnostic cluster, setting realistic goals based on the client's characteristics and health condition, listing the major care providers, and identifying potential agencies or helpers to provide supplementary care and/or respite care for the family.

## Planning and Implementation

After the diagnosis of a knowledge deficit is established and the profile of the client and family is outlined, a mutually agreed upon goal for meeting the knowledge deficit is set. The goal is the expected outcome of the teaching–learning activities on the part of the client, family, and nurse. It is broadly stated in terms that measure the success of the plan for reaching the goal at some reasonable point in time. Because of the financial constraints of home health care reimbursement, the goal is usually no longer than 1 month in duration. After the major goal or client-centered outcome for learning is mutually agreed upon by nurse and family, the short-term goals or objectives to reach the goal are outlined. The time frames for short-term goals (objectives) are usually expressed in terms of days or weeks, leading toward the long-term goal of 1 month.

It is at this point in the nursing diagnosis of knowledge deficit that the nursing care plan becomes a teaching plan. Short-term goals (objectives) are stated in behavioral terms. They serve as criteria to measure the progress toward solution of the problem at hand and also guide the means through which the goal will be accomplished. In addition to behaviorally stated verbs that direct the learning activities of the client and care giver, they list what will be done, to what extent success will be measured, when and how often the prescribed activity will be carried out, who will participate in the activities, and when the objective is expected to be accomplished.

The use of behaviorally stated verbs for educational purposes was developed by Mager in 1975. Since that time, many teachers have adapted the method for developing curricula and instructional plans. Nurse and client educators use behaviorally stated objectives in their teaching activities. Examples of some of the verbs that apply to home health care are presented in Table 5-1.

The verbs are organized into the domains of learning identified by Bloom (1969). The cognitive domain includes those behaviors that demonstrate acquisition of facts, concepts, and theories necessary to gain knowledge. The psychomotor domain contains behaviors that demonstrate application of knowledge to neuromuscular skills and techniques. The affective domain includes those behaviors that demonstrate change in attitudes, values, or appreciation. The three domains of learning have application to the home health care situation by virtue of the client's and family's learning needs for knowledge of the health problem and its treatment, methods for coping with a crisis situation, and changes in lifestyles and health behaviors that require change in attitudes and values.

### The Teaching Plan

#### Content

The diagnosis of knowledge deficit requires a written teaching plan. It is recognized that nurses providing care have limited time in the practice setting. However, teaching plans can be brief and provide a guide for the nurse, client, family, and other care providers that provides for continuity of care, a record of the client's progress toward the goal or outcome, a method for assessing the client's condition if complications arise, and a method to evaluate nursing care.

The case study at the end of this section presents an example of a teaching plan, description of the client situation, profile of the client systems, an

**Table 5-1.** *Sample List of Verbs Applying to the Teaching–Learning Needs of Home Health Clientele According to the Domains of Learning**★*

| Cognitive | Psychomotor | Affective |
|-----------|-------------|-----------|
| discuss | administer | accept |
| develop | apply | advocate |
| identify | bathe | cope |
| initiate | feed | express |
| list | change | grieve |
| record | demonstrate | prevent |
| report | massage | promote |
| teach | position | relax |
| write | transfer | rest |

★ (From Bloom B: Taxonomy of Educational Objectives: Handbook 1: Cognitive Domain. New York, David Mackay Co, Inc, 1969)

overall goal or outcome of care, and objectives. Examples of objectives are care provider (the family member) or client centered and include the extent to which they are expected to be accomplished and when. Objectives are written to assist the nurse, care provider, and client in carrying out care and recording the activities. Each objective can serve as a guide for outlining content and teaching methods.

The outline of content in the teaching plan is specific to the learning needs of the client. It assists the nurse in identifying the knowledge and skills necessary for the client and/or provider to gain in providing care. The nature of the knowledge and skills indicates the type of teaching method that would best suit the learning material. For example, bedside care techniques usually require a demonstration and explanation on the part of the nurse. Because such techniques require psychomotor skills of the learner, the nurse includes return demonstrations by the client or care provider. Periodic review of the techniques helps to provide quality assurance in the event that the learner has misunderstood or forgotten certain aspects of the technique.

### Method

When the client must gain new knowledge about the diagnosis, prognosis, and rationale for treatment, the cognitive domain of learning is involved. Learning is achieved through discussion, audiovisual programs such as videotapes, written materials, and interviews to learn the extent of knowledge that is present and that is retained. Affective learning is accomplished through group interactions with other clients in similar circumstances, counseling sessions, and, in some cases, psychotherapy. Psychomotor skills require a review of factual materials and practice with the new skills. Special teaching methods are indicated when the client has sensory-perceptual deficits or alterations in thought processes. Examples of teaching methods include large-print written instructions, audiotapes for the visually impaired, videotapes for the hearing impaired, and behavioral modification techniques.

It is helpful to have a list of health agencies that provide teaching and educational materials. Having commonly used pamphlets, brochures, films, video- and audiotapes, audiovisual materials in languages other than English, and other learning aids on file is an additional advantage. The development of standard teaching plans that can be adjusted to the individual client for common home health care nursing diagnoses helps to facilitate the learning process and economizes the nurse's time. Examples of sources of standard teaching plans in addition to the nurse's own repertoire include nursing texts and materials from the American Red Cross, the American Cancer Society, The American Heart Association, and many other organizations.

## Evaluation

Measuring the outcome of the teaching plan is easily accomplished if the goal and objectives have been stated behaviorally and contain a time frame; the extent of knowledge, skill, or behavior to be attained; and an outline of the content. Table 5-4 (see page 124) presents examples of objectives derived from Tables 5-2 and 5-3 based on a hypothetical learning situation. Only a brief written plan is necessary, with emphasis on the objectives as guidelines for teaching amd measuring the level of understanding. Since they are mutually developed with the client, the client should have a copy to track progress on the attainment of the objectives. The written plan acts as a guideline for all health care providers involved in the home care situation. Goals and objectives serve as criteria to measure the success and quality of the care delivered.

### CASE STUDY

*DESCRIPTION OF CLIENT SITUATION*

Mr. C., age 65 years, has a medical diagnosis of a bleeding peptic ulcer treated surgically by gastric resection with a gastrostomy tube in place for feeding. He was discharged from the hospital with medical orders for gastrostomy tube feedings every 2 hours during the day, care of the incision, prophylactic antibiotics for 5 days, I.V., and medication for relief of pain as necessary. Modified bedrest: Mr. C. may be up in a chair for 2 hours in the morning, afternoon, and evening. Medical prognosis is favorable if nutritional balance can be achieved and no infections or complications arise.

Mrs. C, age 62 years, is in good health. She recently retired because of her husband's illness and is anxious to care for him at home. They have two adult children, many miles distant. Mr. and Mrs. C. live in a rented apartment; Mrs. C. drives the family car; and they are close to stores for providing basic necessities. Their retirement benefits and health insurance, in addition to Medicare, have been adequate for meeting their present health and medical care needs. The hospital from which he was discharged has a home care unit with nurses who have assumed his care at home after referral from the physician and acute care nurses. The hospital and home care nurses spent 2 days prior to his discharge teaching Mrs. C care of the gastrostomy and tube feeding methods. Major nursing diagnoses during hospitalization included

> Self-care deficits: feeding, bathing, toileting, activities related to debilitating reaction to bleeding peptic ulcer and surgery

Potential for infection related to open surgical incision

Alteration in nutritional status; less than body requirements related to peptic ulcer and complications

Alterations in comfort related to pain derived from surgical procedure and confinement to bed

Grieving related to loss of independence and disease process

Knowledge deficit related to medical diagnosis, nursing care management, and changes in lifestyle.

It is the latter diagnosis that pertains to both Mr. and Mrs. C. The following profile lists the specific learning needs that serve as the data base for the teaching plan as an example of the information that the nurse would collect for the nursing diagnosis of "knowledge deficit related to: . . . ."

## PROFILE

Mr. and Mrs. C. live in a 1-bedroom apartment on the second floor. Mr. C. was discharged today with a medical diagnosis of gastric ulcer, with gastric resection and gastrostomy tube in place. Nutritional support has been ordered through tube feedings q 2 hours; IV antibiotics b.i.d; and codeine p.r.n. for pain. Mr. C. is on bedrest, but may be up in a chair for 2 hours three times each day. The home health care nurse will visit the home twice each day during the first week. A home health aide can be in the home for 20 hours per week. Mrs. C. has return-demonstrated tube feedings twice in the hospital before Mr. C's discharge.

The client and his wife know the diagnosis to some extent. Mrs. C. had no instruction on bedbath, occupied bedmaking, toileting needs, skin care, care of the gastrostomy, transfer techniques, pain control, and nutritional needs. Mr. and Mrs. C. have indicated their desire to assume as much of his care as possible in the home setting. Some of their close neighbors have offered assistance.

The following teaching–learning needs have been diagnosed by the nurses in the acute care and home health care setting, a nutritionist, the client, his wife, and the physician. Mr. and Mrs. C. have knowledge deficits for facts concerning the medical diagnosis, prognosis, and treatment. Mrs. C. has a knowledge deficit for

1. Prescribed medical care for condition
2. Gastrostomy tube care
3. Bedside care, including feeding, bedbath, toileting, transfer, skin care
4. Need for respite from care giving activities.

Mr. and Mrs. C. and the home health care nurse agree on long-term goals: Two months from discharge date, Mr. C.'s health status will improve to the extent that he will gain 6 lbs, be well enough to have the gastrostomy closed, and be able to carry out activities of daily living independently. He will not experience complications or unwarranted death.

**Table 5-2.** *Examples of Behaviorally Stated Objectives Relating to Long-Term Goals**

| Person | Verb | Extent and Time |
| --- | --- | --- |
| **Activities of Daily Living** | | |
| *Hygiene:* | | |
| The client, with assistance from the care provider | will bathe | each day in the morning |
| The care provider | will massage | the client's back |
| *Nutrition:* | | |
| The care provider | will feed | the client q 2 hours through the gastrostomy tube |
| *Activities:* | | |
| The care provider | will transfer | the client to a chair for 2 hours twice each day |
| **Therapeutic Regimen** | | |
| *Medications:* | | |
| The visiting nurse | will administer | prescribed IV antibiotics b.i.d. |
| *Treatments:* | | |
| The care provider | will change | the gastrostomy dressing q.i.d. |
| | using | aseptic technique |
| **Psychosocial Needs** | | |
| *Care Provider:* | | |
| The care provider | will relax | at least once a week away from the home |
| *Client:* | | |
| The client | will participate | in planned social activities at least once a week |

* At the end of 2 months, the client's health status will improve to the extent that he will (1) gain 6 lbs, (2) have gastrostomy closed, and (3) carry out activities of daily living independently.

**Table 5-3.** *Examples of Teaching Plans, Including Content Outline and Teaching Method, Derived from Objectives Listed in Table 5-2*

| Objective | Content | Method |
|---|---|---|
| The client, with assistance from the care provider, will bathe each day in the A.M. | Bedbath | Demonstration by nurse Return Demonstration by client's wife |
| The care provider will massage the client's back and skin t.i.d. | Massage technique Skin care | Demonstration and return demonstration by wife |
| The care provider will feed the client q 2 hours during the day by the gastrostomy tube. | Care of gastrostomy tube Feeding method | Written instructions Discussion |
| The client will demonstrate adequate nutritional status through weight gain. | Nutritional needs | Demonstration and return by wife |
| The care provider will transfer the client to a chair for 2 hours twice each day. | Body alignment Body mechanics Transfer techniques | Demonstration Written instructions Discussion |
| The care provider will change the gastrostomy dressing q.i.d. using aseptic technique. | Aseptic technique Dressing change Observation of wound | Discussion Written instruction Demonstration with return demonstration by wife |
| The care provider will relax at least one time during the week away from home. | Relaxation benefits Community resources | Discussion Pamphlets Contact with neighbors |
| The client will participate in planned social activities at least once a week. | Socialization benefits Community resources | Discussion Pamphlets |

Table 5-2 presents a few examples of objectives that would apply to this situation and are relevant to the long-term goals agreed upon. Table 5-3 lists objectives from Table 5-2 and demonstrates how they may serve to outline the content in the teaching plan and the appropriate teaching methods relating to the content and the situation.

*Selected Diagnosis From Sensory Perceptual Patterns:
Comfort, Alterations in. Related Diagnoses:
Knowledge Deficit; Sensory Perceptual Alterations;
and Sexual Disfunction*

The experience of pain is a complex, multidimensional phenomenom, highly subjective and unique to each individual. According to McCaffery (1979), pain is "whatever the experiencing person says it is, and exists when he says it does" (p 81). In 1979, the International Association for the Study of Pain (IASP) developed a taxonomy of pain terms and definitions for use as a minimal standard vocabulary. Pain was defined by the IASP as "an unpleasant sensory and emotional experience associated with actual or potential tissue damage, and described in terms of such damage" (p 249).

The current leading theory of pain perception is the gate control theory, proposed by Melzack and Wall in 1965. It challenges the adequacy of the specificity and pattern theories of pain (Fig. 5-1) and postulates that the pain experience is determined by the interactions among three spinal cord systems. Peripheral stimulation activates nerve impulses to the substantia gelatinosa (SG) in the dorsal horn of the spinal cord, where these cells modulate the afferent impulses (known as the "gate control mechanism"). Next, afferent patterns in the fibers of the dorsal column act as a central control

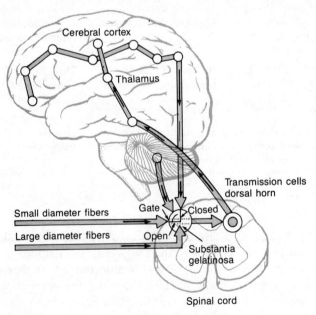

Figure 5-1. The gate-control theory of pain

trigger that activates selective brain processes, influencing the modulating gate control properties of the SG. Finally, transmission ("T") cells in the dorsal horn activate the neural mechanisms responsible for the perception and the individual's response to pain.

Neurons in the SG have the capacity to facilitate or inhibit transmissions. Impulses generated by low-intensity, mechanical (carried by large fibers) stimulation can close the "gate" in the SG to pain impulses (carried by small fibers). Chronic pain occurs when input from small-diameter fibers persists and keeps the gate open to pain transmissions. Memories, emotions, and attention can result in transmission of impulses by fast-conducting, large-diameter fibers to the thalamus, brain stem, and SG. These impulses can close the gate to ascending pain impulses if the individual is distracted or can enhance pain conduction if the individual is anxious (Yasko, 1983).

Melzack and Casey (1968) proposed a new conceptual model of pain, describing three dimensions of the pain experience using the principles of the gate control theory. Pain experienced by the individual is a complex sequence of behaviors determined by sensory, motivational, and cognitive processes acting on the motor mechanism. Therefore, pain is defined as a function of the interactions of all three determinants but cannot be ascribed to any one of them.

Based on their extensive research, Melzack and Wall (1982) contend that it is premature to formulate a definition of pain, because pain may actually represent "a category of experiences, signifying a multitude of different unique experiences having different causes, and characterized by different qualities varying along a number of sensory and affective dimensions" (p 71).

Ahles and associates (1983) have developed a multidimensional pain model based on Melzack and Casey's research and the client's interpretation of pain. Ahles' model identifies five separate components of the total pain experience:

1. Physiologic—organic etiology, physiologic response (i.e., vital signs, sleep deprivation)
2. Sensory—factors such as intensity, location, quality, quantity
3. Affective—factors such as depression and anxiety
4. Cognitive—meaning of the pain experience, influence on thought processes, communication and interaction patterns
5. Behavioral—functional ability, activity level, analgesia consumption
*6. Environmental—factors such as setting, climate, noise, and lighting

* A sixth component, environmental, has been added by the authors to further conceptualize the pain experience in the home setting. The model serves as a reference in assisting the client, family, significant other, and/or health care provider to assess all dimensions of the pain experience.

Recent research on endorphins and enkephalins indicates that these protein substances are activated subconsciously and serve as a natural mechanism to suppress pain. It is postulated that these endogenous opiates are released when pain is anticipated or experienced and that they block transmission of pain impulses. There may also be a relationship between pain intensity and endorphin activity. Endorphins and enkephalins have been

**Table 5-4.** *Examples of Recording and Measuring Success of a Teaching Plan Using Objectives as Criteria (Examples From Objectives in Table 5-3)*

| Objective (Criterion) | Date Met | Comment |
|---|---|---|
| The client, with assistance from the care provider, will bathe each day in the A.M. | Partially; 2 weeks after admission to service | Care taker must prepare husband for health care provider visit in A.M. Client is bathed each night before sleep. |
| The care provider will massage the client's back and skin t.i.d. | Partially; 2½ weeks after admission to service | Care provider massages back in A.M. after breakfast; in the afternoon after client returns to bed; and massages back and skin in the evening during the bath. |
| The care taker will feed the client q 2 hours during the day by the gastrostomy tube. | Yes; 4 days after admission to service | After demonstration, discussion, and 3 return demonstrations, provider safely feeds client. |
| The care provider will transfer the client to a chair for 2 hours three times a day. | Yes; 3 days after admission to service | After demonstration and return demonstrations, provider safely transfers the client to a chair. |
| The care provider changes the dressing using aseptic technique | Yes; 1 week after admission to service | After demonstration and return demonstration, provider changes dressing q.i.d. using aseptic technique. |
| The care provider will relax at least one time during the week away from home. | No; since admission | There is no other provider of care; search continues. |
| The client will participate in planned social activities at least one time each week. | Yes; priest visits every Sunday afternoon | Other activities are being explored. |

linked to noninvasive pain relief mechanisms such as application of heat and/or cold, distraction, biofeedback, hypnosis, and invasive pain control measures such as acupuncture, and transcutaneous electrical nerve stimulation (TENS). For example, warmth and warm weather stimulate serotonin production, and cold and cold weather stimulate norepinephrine. Unfortunately, recent research has shown that the administration of narcotics inhibits the release of these endogenous narcotic-like substances and prolongs the experience of pain (Kenner et al, 1985).

Pain relief methods are generally classified as noninvasive or invasive/systemic. Noninvasive pain relief measures are external techniques such as distraction, imagery, relaxation–visualization, and hypnosis. Invasive/systemic pain relief measures include the administration of medications, anesthetics, use of acupuncture, and neurosurgical procedures (Table 5-5).

Pain is a universal, yet unique, experience for each individual. About one third of all Americans will experience persistent or recurring pain that will necessitate medical intervention at some time in their life. More than 50 million Americans are partially or totally disabled by pain, losing more than 700 million workdays annually and costing about $60 billion in health care, compensation or litigation, and sick time. Chronic back disorders and arthritis account for the most frequent and expensive pain problems in the United States (Bonica and Chapman, 1980).

Pain relief measures become a prerequisite for living, especially for the individual experiencing chronic, unrelenting pain. The individual feels helpless, anxious, fearful, and out of control. To continue living may only represent further pain, greater physical and moral deterioration, and destruction. The individual experiencing pain must gain a sense of mastery or control over the pain experience. Assisting the individual, family, and significant other to understand, assess, and perform noninvasive and invasive pain reduction measures is essential to coping with a potentially overwhelming situation in the home.

## Etiology and Defining Characteristics

Alteration in comfort: related to pain as defined by Carpenito (1983) is "a state in which the individual experiences an uncomfortable sensation in response to a noxious stimuli" (p 112). Etiologic and contributing medical factors may include acute or chronic illnesses (cancer, cardiac, and vascular disorders), trauma, inflammation, musculoskeletal disorders, diagnostic tests, and surgery.

Acute pain is associated with a specific precipitating event, with a duration of from 1 second to less than 6 months. It is time-limited and is usually triggered by trauma, diagnostic testing, or surgical procedures. Acute pain usually subsides when the cause or stimulus is removed and/or when healing occurs.

**Table 5-5.** *Classification of Pain Reduction/Relief Methods (Based on Gate-Control Theory of Pain)*

| Pain Reduction/Relief Method | Local | Systemic | Thalamic | Cortical |
|---|:---:|:---:|:---:|:---:|
| **Noninvasive** | | | | |
| Biofeedback | | | x | x |
| Breathing exercises | x | | x | x |
| Cold | x | x | | |
| Distraction | x | | | x |
| Electrical stimulation | | x | x | |
| Education | | | | x |
| Heat | x | x | | |
| Humor | x | | x | x |
| Hypnosis | | | x | x |
| Imagery | x | | x | x |
| Massage | x | | x | |
| Massage with menthol ointments | x | | x | |
| Meditation | x | | x | x |
| Music therapy | x | | x | x |
| Pressure | | x | | |
| Relaxation | x | | x | x |
| Tactile stimulation | x | x | | |
| TENS | | x | x | |
| Vibration | x | x | | |
| **Invasive/Systemic** | | | | |
| Medications | | | | |
|   Anesthetics | x | x | x | |
|   Antidepressants | | | x | x |
|   Anti-inflammatory agents | x | | | |
|   Antispasmodics | x | x | | |
|   Narcotics | | x | ? | x |
|   Non-narcotics | x | | | |
|   Steroids | x | | ? | ? |
|   Tranquilizers | | | ? | |
| Neurosurgical procedures | x | x | x | x |

**Suggestions for use:**

1. If the client can point to the site of pain, the pain is localized, cutaneous, and/or superficial. *Local and systemic* interventions are recommended initially.

2. If the client cannot localize the pain and/or the pain has several sites, *systemic, cortical, and/or thalamic* interventions are recommended.

3. Combining noninvasive and invasive interventions may act synergistically to reduce and/or minimize the pain.

Chronic pain may be intermittent or constant and persists longer than 6 months. Chronic pain leads to changes in personality, lifestyle, functional ability, and coping. Pain may persist without an identifiable cause or may continue even when the apparent cause is removed.

## Focus of Nursing Care

The focus of nursing care for the assessment and management of pain is noninvasive and invasive pain intervention strategies. Traditional and non-traditional approaches for reduction of acute and chronic pain are included.

## Outcome Criteria

The following outcome criteria are specific for the client experiencing acute or chronic pain. The person and/or family member and/or health care provider will

Acknowledge the uniqueness of the pain experience
Acknowledge or verbalize alterations in comfort/pain
Verbalize/identify location(s) and rate quantity of discomfort/pain
Identify associated factors that intensify the pain experience
Identify associated factors that decrease or minimize the pain experience
Discuss principles and concepts of noninvasive and invasive pain reduction techniques
Perform noninvasive pain reduction strategies
Utilize invasive pain reduction strategies
Verbalize/identify reduced pain

## Application of the Nursing Process

### Assessment of the Client

The client who has acute or chronic pain needs continual ongoing assessment by the care provider. Assessment of the client experiencing pain provides the foundations on which interventions are built (Donovan, 1986). Based on the previously discussed pain model by Ahles and colleagues and adapted by Keating and Kelman, six essential parameters will form the basis for pain assessment: (1) physiologic, (2) sensory, (3) affective, (4) cognitive, (5) behavioral, and (6) environmental.

The home health care nurse assesses the client and/or family's

1.  Interest and potential ability to assess pain
2.  Ability to assess pain based on the six identified parameters of the total pain experience

3.  Knowledge of principles of noninvasive and invasive pain reduction techniques
4.  Ability to perform noninvasive pain reduction strategies
5.  Ability to use invasive pain reduction strategies
6.  Ability to recognize potential complications and react knowledgeably

## Pain Assessment Parameters

### Physiologic

The client/care provider (when appropriate) will assess

1.  Physiologic response to pain
2.  Vital sign patterns as baseline and monitoring data
3.  For side-effects related to pain treatment modalities

Pain can be caused, for example, by inflammation, nerve compression owing to tumor enlargement, fluids and/or hemorrhages, diminished blood supply, obstruction, chemical nerve irritation, muscle spasm, infection, trauma, distention, bone infiltration, or tumor metastases. Cutaneous pain is usually well localized, whereas deep somatic and/or visceral pain is more diffuse and referred to other tissues.

Vital signs are useful as baseline data to assess effects of intervention strategies. Clients and families need to know that chronic pain does not elicit a sympathetic nervous response but that in acute pain, changes in vital signs are common. Families should become familiar with the client's respiratory rate patterns and be aware that with pain relief, sleep, and relaxation, normal respirations may range from 8 to 12 breaths per minute. If clients are receiving narcotics, bowel function is assessed routinely to prevent constipation.

A change in activity level, including sexual activity and alterations in sleep/rest patterns, is assessed. If clients have been uncomfortable for an extended period of time, the spouse or significant other may assume that sexual activity would increase their discomfort. However, if this has not been discussed, the client may feel rejected or perceive that the partner no longer loves him or her. This emotional pain of perceived rejection can be as distressing as the actual pain. The nurse must be sensitive to the emotional needs of the client and significant other in assessing this important area. Nutrition and elimination patterns are also reviewed with the client to assess the impact of the present pain on his or her lifestyle.

Age is a factor in pain communication. Young children may not have the vocabulary and understanding of functions and sensations of various parts of their bodies to communicate their "hurt." The elderly may have reduced or impaired communication skills related to illness and augmented by the aging process.

*Sensory*

The client or care provider (when appropriate) will

1. Identify location of site(s) of pain
2. Verbalize quantity of pain experienced

Location and quantity of pain are all factors related to the sensory pain component. If the individual is able, ask him or her to point with one finger to the site or site(s) of pain. The person can also indicate on a diagram of a human body where the pain is and attempt to describe the pain (Fig. 5-2).

Quantity of pain includes the quality and duration of the pain experience. Visual analog scales are commonly used by the client to rate or quantify the pain experience. The client is asked to rate the pain experienced by placing a mark on the scale that represents the intensity of his or her pain (Fig. 5-3). These techniques are recorded by the client or family at specific intervals in a daily pain journal to be used as a basis for evaluation of pain intervention strategies (Display 5-1).

Children are asked to rate the quantity of pain using colors. They are asked to choose a color that they associate with the "biggest hurt" they have ever had. Then they select corresponding colors based on "bigger hurts" to "little hurts" to "not hurting at all." Children can then color a

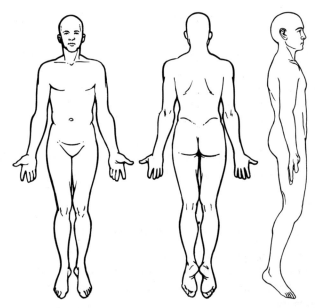

Figure 5-2. Human figure diagrams that can be used to identify pain locations. The client (adult or child) is asked to point to the areas on the diagram where they are experiencing pain or place an X on or choose a color to shade the areas of pain.

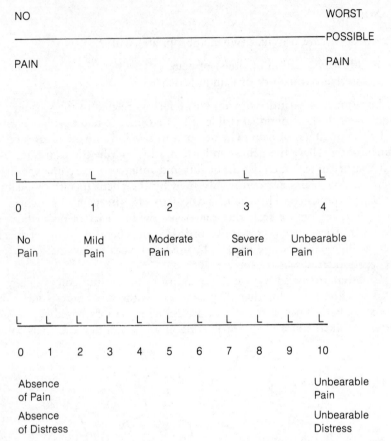

Figure 5-3. Visual analog scales used to quantify the pain experience. Clients are asked to rank the pain they are presently experiencing by making a mark at the point they feel best describes or represents the intensity of the pain.

figure using the colors to describe their "no hurts," "little hurts," and "big hurts" and identify the location and quantity of their pain.

### Affective

The client or care provider (where appropriate) will

1. Verbalize presence of fear, anxiety, and/or depression
2. Identify factors that may intensify the pain experience
3. Verbalize attitudes toward pain experience and pain treatment modalities

Fear, anger, anxiety, and depression are common examples of factors that intensify the pain experience. The nurse and/or health care provider

*Display 5-1*
**Pain/Comfort Journal**

| Date: Time | Comfort/Pain Estimate★ | Activity | Pain-Reducing Used | Measures | Meds Adm | Comfort/Pain Estimate★ |
|---|---|---|---|---|---|---|
| 8 A.M. til Noon | | | | | | |
| Noon til 4 P.M. | | | | | | |
| 4 P.M. til 8 P.M. | | | | | | |
| 8 P.M. til midnight | | | | | | |

*Observations/Comments:*

*Directions:*

Enter date, estimate comfort/pain level for time period indicated, and briefly describe activity level. If comfort/pain measures are used, specify measure and length of time used. If medication is administered, indicate drug, dosage, route, and time given. Estimate comfort/pain level 30–60 minutes after pain-reducing measures have been provided, and record.

★ Estimate pain on a scale of 0–4:

No pain 0   1   2   3   4 Pain   Unbearable

must assess attitudes and any misconceptions that the client and/or family have regarding the pain experience and pain management, and re-emphasize that pain is an unique experience to each individual. Mood state and present pain coping strategies used by the client and family are also assessed. Derogatis et al (1976) demonstrated that care-givers routinely overestimate a client's anxiety levels, while grossly underestimating the level of depression the client experiences.

## Cognitive

The client or care provider (when appropriate) will

1. Assess the understanding of the organic etiology of pain (if known) and expected physiologic responses
2. Identify the meaning of the pain experience on current lifestyle
3. Identify the impact of pain on thought processes, communication, and interaction patterns

It is important to determine whether the physician and/or members of the health care team have fully explained to the client or care providers the physiologic basis of the pain (if known). For many people, knowledge is control. Explanations of pain and pain management techniques may provide the client with some intellectual control and may be helpful in eliciting the client's assistance in managing his or her pain.

The meaning that pain has for an individual is associated with cultural and religious factors, past experiences, social expectations, and future expectations. Zborowski's (1952) research found wide variations in overt pain behaviors that evolved from ethnic expectations that held constant through second and third generation immigrant groups. This research provides a framework for understanding cultural variations in the pain response, but caution must be exercised to prevent stereotyping.

The meaning of the pain experience is explored with the client, for example, when pain is associated with the loss of control, independence, and fear of becoming a burden to family and loved ones. Other real fears might include financial worries and concerns about providing for others if they should not be able to return to work or if they should die. Some individuals believe that pain is punishment for a wrongdoing and may not actively seek relief from the pain until penance has been performed.

Chronic pain interrupts the client's and the family's ability to communicate, spend time together, and come to terms with present and future losses, and pending separation. Family and care givers may feel angry, guilty, vulnerable, helpless, and impotent in their efforts to reduce the relentless pain that may persist sometimes until death (Coyle et al, 1986).

## Behavioral

The client or care provider (when appropriate) will

1. Assess impact of pain on activity level and functional ability
2. Assess attitudes to noninvasive and invasive pain reduction strategies
3. Assess behavioral responses to current pain treatment modalities, including analgesia consumption

Baseline information is essential to determine the impact pain has on activity level and functional ability. For example, can the client ambulate, has there been a change in appetite, and how does the client sleep? It is also important to determine the client and care provider's attitudes toward various pain intervention strategies. For example, if the client is skeptical about hypnosis or biofeedback and not receptive to these techniques, it is not the best decision to select these methods for intervention with the client. Assess the pain treatment modalities that the client is currently using, including analgesia, and determine whether alternative treatment modalities should be suggested.

## Environmental

The client or care provider (when appropriate) will

1. Assess how family and/or significant others, friends, and members of the health care team interact with the client
2. Assess for factors in the client's environment that may reduce or intensify the pain experience

It is important to determine whether significant others are available to assist the client, yet also allow time for privacy and rest. Determine whether the environment is conducive to rest and if equipment is readily accessible. Control of environmental factors, such as noise, temperature, and light is an important consideration. For example, if clients are on bedrest, do they prefer the bed away from family? Or would they actually prefer to have the bed placed in the living room so that even if they do not have the energy to move out of bed, they could still observe what is happening throughout the day? Consider whether they need assistive devices, that is, eating devices, wheelchair, hospital bed, walker, cane, commode, overhead trapeze, and/or hoyer lift.

The presence of music, radio, or television may serve as a distraction or an annoyance, depending upon the individual. Accessibility to a telephone may be an alternate method of communication if the client is too uncomfortable for visitors but is able to talk to friends for brief periods of time.

## Planning and Implementation

The nurse will use the information obtained from assessing the client in the home environment to determine which aspects of pain reduction techniques and strategies need reinforcement and to review what additional information needs to be discussed with the patient and family. Short-term goals will then form the basis for the nursing care plan (prescription).

The nurse will implement the care plan, monitor the client's status, and revise the care plan accordingly (Display 5-2). A specific care plan focusing on the needs of a client receiving intrathecal (epidural) morphine is presented. Figure 5-4 illustrates the epidural catheter and pump placement.

### Monitoring of Client Status

Potential complications of pain management can often be avoided or minimized if the client or significant other and health care provider systematically monitor the following assessment parameters routinely as part of the prescription for the client with pain. Any abnormal signs and symptoms should be reported immediately to the appropriate health care individual and/or agency. These may include

1. Visual changes
2. Alterations in gastrointestinal function (persistent vomiting, constipation)
3. Alterations in level of consciousness, that is, difficulty in arousing client, presence of hallucinations
4. Urinary retention or decrease in output
5. Unusually slow or significant change in heart rate, or significant variations in blood pressure (if being monitored)

(*Text continues on p.138*)

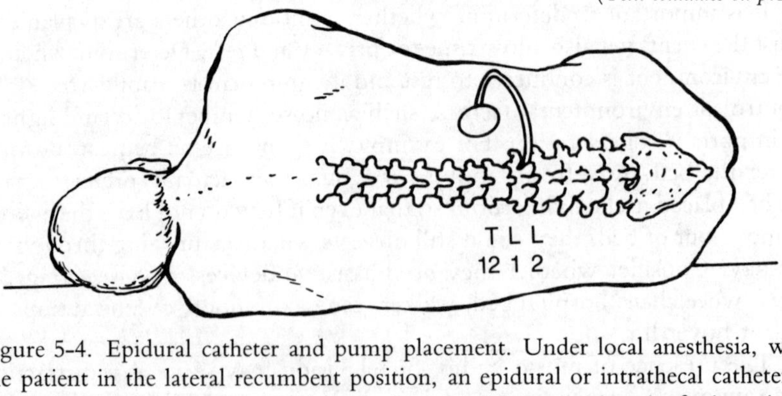

Figure 5-4. Epidural catheter and pump placement. Under local anesthesia, with the patient in the lateral recumbent position, an epidural or intrathecal catheter is inserted under fluoroscopy usually at the T12, L1, L2 area (easiest site for insertion). The catheter is then tunneled under the skin to the abdomen. The pump (which has been filled with a preservative-free morphine) is implanted into a subcutaneous pocket in the abdominal wall (Paice, 1986).

*Display 5-2*
## Sample Care Plan: Comfort/Pain Reduction Measures

Chronic pain management: Noninvasive techniques and epidural (intrathecal) morphine

### Long-Term Goals (Outcomes)

At the end of 4 weeks, the client (includes individual/family member/ significant other) will:

* Practice principles and concepts of noninvasive pain reduction techniques (distraction)
* Implement principles and concepts of invasive pain reduction technique (intrathecal morphine)
* Identify complications of pain reduction methods and appropriate interventions
* Use pain reduction techniques
* Demonstrate ability to correctly use the drug administration device and supplemental equipment for intrathecal morphine infusions
* Verbalize/identify reduced pain

Demonstrate or verbalize reduced anxiety and fear related to loss of control, change in lifestyle, self-concept, fear of the unknown

### Short-Term Goals (Objectives) for Priority Problems

Asterisks (*) indicate priority problems selected for this sample care plan but will vary according to each client or family and their learning needs. Additional problems can certainly be identified, but, for the purpose of this care plan, the most commonly encountered problems in the home environment will be addressed to serve as a reference for the home health care nurse.

**Week I.**
The client will:

1. Verbalize to the nurse the major principles and concepts of intrathecal morphine infusions and distraction techniques
2. Verbalize to the nurse instructions regarding pump function and administration of supplemental narcotics
3. Record comfort level daily in journal

*(continued)*

*Display 5-2 (Continued)*
**Sample Care Plan: Comfort/Pain Reduction Measures**

**Week II.**
In the home setting, the client will:

1. Verbalize signs and symptoms associated with complications of intrathecal morphine infusions
2. Verbalize appropriate interventions to manage complications and when to notify health personnel
3. Practice one distraction technique twice daily

**Week III.**

1. The epidural catheter will remain intact with no evidence of infection or catheter-related complications.
2. The client will continue to experience reduced discomfort or pain and maintain and/or increase his or her activity level.
3. The client will continue to practice distraction techniques at least three times daily.
4. The client will evaluate the effectiveness of intervention(s).

*Nursing Care Plan (Prescription)*

**Week I.**
In the home, the nurse will:

1. Review with the client and family the principles and concepts of intrathecal morphine infusion and distraction techniques, including:
    *a.* A diagram and discussion of intrathecal morphine infusion, including review of catheter and pump placement (Fig. 5-4)
    *b.* Review of titration of drug and dosage adjustments
    *c.* Review of pump function and drug supplements, including dose titration
    *d.* Review equipment and supplies needed with specific instructions as to what is needed and where it can be purchased
    *e.* A specific review of one distraction technique (Display 5.3)
2. Review pain assessment, how to record and use the daily comfort/pain journal.

**Week II.**
In the home, the nurse will:

1. Review with the client potential complications of intrathecal morphine infusion and signs and symptoms, including:
    *a.* Infection
    *b.* Catheter malfunction
    *c.* Pump malfunction
    *d.* Fever

*(continued)*

*Display 5-2 (Continued)*

  *e.* Urinary retention
  *f.* Pruritus
  *g.* Drug tolerance
2. Provide the client with a list of suggested interventions to follow if they suspect complications
3. Observe the client perform one distraction technique and offer feedback
4. At the end of the session with the nurse, the client will verbalize:
  *a.* Signs and symptoms of intrathecal morphine infusion–related complications
  *b.* Suggested interventions to follow, including when and who to contact

**Week III.**
The nurse will:

1. Review with the client recording(s) from the comfort/pain journal and make suggested revisions in comfort measures if indicated
2. Review frequency and amount of supplement medication with the client and adjustments (dosage) to implement if indicated
3. Review distraction techniques and evaluation of effectiveness of pain relief measure and client's perceived comfort/discomfort level. If indicated, alternate distraction techniques are introduced and reviewed.
4. Encourage the client to address any new or continued concerns related to intrathecal pain management and/or use of pain distraction techniques.
5. Provide client with information regarding additional community resources and services that can be provided if appropriate, e.g., Meals on Wheels, Hospice, Emergency Communication Systems

*Evaluation*

Evaluation is based on outcomes established and continuing needs, including:
1. Client's ability to manage procedures
2. Comfort level of client
3. Health status of client
4. Specific concerns identified by either client or health care provider
5. Availability of insurance/health coverage

6. Alteration in activity, sleep, nutrition, and elimination related to pain
7. New site of pain or persistent pain with no relief from pain intervention strategies
8. Malfunction of equipment used with pain relief method

Complications may include equipment malfunction and side-effects of pain reduction techniques and/or medications. Complications and interventions with implications for clients in the home setting will be discussed briefly.

## Maintenance of Equipment and Supplies

Numerous pain management devices are now available to the client for use in the home care setting. It is essential that the client and/or significant other have a thorough understanding of the operation of the equipment and have either a back-up system available and/or direct 24-hour access to a health care agency and/or vendor that will service and repair the equipment if there is a malfunction. General suggestions include

1. Know *who* and *how* to contact an appropriate individual or agency if problems arise
2. Select the appropriate drug administration device, and know the purpose and function of the specific device being used. Examples include
   a. Venous catheters
      i. External (Hickman, Groshong catheters)
      ii. Implanted (Infusaid, Port-a-Cath)
   b. Venous/atrial pumps
      i. External (Cormed, Autosyringe)
      ii. Implanted (Infusaid)
3. If an ambulatory or portable (external) infusion pump is used to store and deliver the medications, the individual needs to
   a. Read the pump meter, and adjust the pump flow rate
   b. Change the drug delivery bag and tubing
   c. Prime the tubing
   d. Change and/or recharge the battery
   e. Administer "rescue" doses of parenteral narcotics (if indicated)
4. If a transcutaneous electrical stimulation (TNS or TENS) is used, the individual needs to
   a. Apply conductive jellies
   b. Place electrodes in the proper position and tape correctly
   c. Know "how" and "when" to adjust voltage, pulse width, and frequency controls
   d. Change and/or recharge the battery
5. Always have extra batteries available

6. Know what additional supplies will be needed (tubing, medication bags, needles, syringes, etc.), and *always* have an extra 2–3 day supply on hand
7. Know complications and side-effects, and review specific interventions for management
8. Verify with the pharmacy and/or the vendor that drug(s) are available and in the appropriate route, dosage, concentration, and volume. (Epidural morphine must be preservative free.)

## Side-Effects and Precautions With Pain Reduction Techniques

Distraction techniques will usually temporarily increase pain tolerance and decrease pain intensity, but, after the distraction technique is over, the client may have increased awareness of pain and fatigue. Distraction will work best for brief periods of time and with milder forms of pain. Distraction is not an effective method with chronic pain but can be beneficial if used intermittently. Some distraction techniques useful for the home health care client and his or her family are given in Display 5-3.

Massage is never used for calf pain or if a thrombus is suspected or present. Range of motion and positioning can be effective if muscle tension or spasm are reduced, but *initial* movement may temporarily increase the pain. This can be partially controlled by avoiding sudden jerky movements and using smooth, continuous motion when positioning or exercising. The care provider and client need to continually assess whether pain is being aggravated by fatigue or the presence of tissue injury.

Heat is contraindicated in the first 24 to 28 hours after trauma or if edema, hemorrhage, and/or pruritus are present. Application of heat is not usually indicated for cancer lesions and metastatic sites. Extreme caution is used when applying heat to individuals with decreased circulation and/or impaired sensation. Maximal effects of local heat application occur within 20 to 30 minutes, and application for more than 1 hour will cause vasoconstriction and may produce thermal injury. *Dry* heat may be tolerated better than *moist* heat, because water is a better conductor and slows evaporation. If the client is diaphoretic, tolerance to heat will decrease.

Cold is contraindicated more than 48 hours after trauma and in individuals with decreased or impaired sensation. Prolonged application produces vasodilation; local application at short intermittent intervals is generally recommended. It may be most beneficial if application of cold is between 30 and 60 minutes, followed by 60 minutes of rest. Application for more than 60 minutes will produce vasodilation, increase circulation, and potentiate pain.

*Note:* Avoid *any* application of heat or cold over a pump site or prolonged bath or sauna (greater than 45 minutes), because they can affect pump function and drug distribution.

*Display 5-3*
**Distraction Techniques**

*Introduction and Preparation*

Initially, it is important to remember that noninvasive techniques such as distraction are for short-term benefit and, in addition, may have a synergistic effect when used with other pain reduction measures. McCaffery (1979) emphasizes that prior to using a technique, it is most important to understand how the client perceives his or her problem and assess the client's attitude or reaction to the use of distraction techniques. Once that has been determined, the individual can begin the technique *if* the client is willing to participate.

*Note:* This technique should be taught to another family member or friend in addition to the individual; it may be used several times daily. Involving significant others evokes a feeling of active participation to help reduce the client's pain and improve comfort. It also provides the client and family with an increased sense of control over the current situation.

*Preparation*

1.  Try to assist the client to relax before beginning distraction techniques.
    a.  Ask the client to rate present tension/discomfort using one of the visual analog scales, and describe what it feels like
    b.  Ask the client what he or she thinks is causing tension/discomfort
    c.  Ask the client where he or she would like to be spending time right now and what activity he or she would like to be doing
2.  Reduce environmental distraction; have the client assume as comfortable a position as possible; ask the client to concentrate and focus attention on either an object, thought, idea, stimulus (voice, music). Some individuals will close their eyes, whereas others may stare at an object.
3.  There are many "scripts" to use with relaxation; however, this author suggests that the focus on the script be individualized to the client. For example, begin with:
    a.  "Take a deep breath with me. Hold it. Let the air out slowly and think about relaxing. Try it again." Repeat sequence several times.
    b.  Have a specific focus from the person's life that was identified as a pleasurable experience, and either "paint the scene" or

*(continued)*

---

*Display 5-3 (Continued)*

"relive the event" with the client, providing input when needed. For example

  i. A mother may wish to recall her daughter's wedding or her own.
  ii. A person may recapture an exciting sports event in which he or she enjoyed participating.
  iii. Another individual may wish to sing along with a musical tape and clap or tap out a rhythm.
  iv. A person may recall a visit with a close friend, sharing activities they experienced together.

4. In ending the distraction/relaxation technique,
  a. The facilitator reminds the person how (hopefully) comfortable, happy, or calm, he or she feels recounting the past experience and suggests using the technique again when he or she is tense or uncomfortable.
  b. Usually the person is asked to count down, take several deep breaths, and reorient to the present.

---

## Side-Effects and Precautions with Pain Medication

Table 5-6 lists common non-narcotic and narcotic analgesics used in the home care setting and briefly reviews common routes, equianalgesic doses, duration of effects, and comments regarding client and home care implications. Additional suggestions for the client or health care provider to cope with the side-effects are briefly discussed in the following paragraphs.

*Nausea and vomiting* may occur for the first few days after initiating narcotic therapy. An antiemetic should be prescribed, but, if symptoms persist, consideration is given to changing the narcotic.

*Constipation* can be minimized by diet, fluid intake, and exercise, if possible. High fiber and roughage such as whole-grain breads and cereals, fresh fruits, and vegetables are encouraged. Eight to 10 8-ounce glasses of fluid should be consumed daily, and, if permitted, a regular daily activity should be encouraged. The client is advised to discuss the use of laxatives with the physician before using over-the-counter preparations.

*Respiratory depression* and *drowsiness* are expected side-effects of narcotics and may be more pronounced initially. If they persist for more than several days, the physician may reduce the dose. Remind the person that the goal is to reduce or alleviate the pain but, at the same time, encourage him or her to try to resume a productive lifestyle. If drowsiness still continues after dose reduction, the physician may consider prescribing another medication.

*Note:* If there is an abrupt or continual change in level of consciousness, a continued decrease in the rate and depth of respirations, the presence of Cheyne–Stokes asthma, and the client is confused or difficult to arouse, the client may need to be seen immediately in the emergency room. Depending upon the client and the drug regime, Narcan may be administered 0.4 mg– 0.8 mg, either intravenous (IV) push or intramuscular (IM). The dose may be repeated for 2 to 3 doses every 2 to 3 minutes in order to reverse the effects of respiratory depression if it has been determined that it was caused by narcotic therapy.

Depending upon the narcotic ordered and the route, some physicians will suggest that clients have Narcan at home for emergency use only. If Narcan is administered, it will reduce *all* analgesia effect and the client will

(*Text continues on p.145*)

**Table 5-6.** *Pain Medications*

| Drug | Route | Dose (mg) | Duration (hours) | Comments |
|------|-------|-----------|------------------|----------|
| **Non-Narcotic Analgesics for Mild to Moderate Pain Relief★** | | | | |
| **Aspirin** (Bayer, Empirin, A.S.A.) (available as suppl) | PO | 650 | 4–6 | Anti-inflammatory, G.I., and hematologic side-effects; use with caution in cancer clients. Hemorrhage is uncommon if dose is *less* than 1 g/day. Take with food or ample fluid. |
| **Acetaminophen** (Tylenol, Tempra, Datril) (available as a suppl) | PO | 650 | 4–6 | Weaker anti-inflammatory drug than aspirin. Not recommended for long-term use in clients with anemia, cardiac, renal, hepatic, or pulmonary disease. (Suggested maximal daily dose should not exceed 2.6 g.) |
| **Proxyphene hydrochloride** (Darvon) | PO | 65 | 4–6 | Additive effect when used with CNS depressants or alcohol. Euphoric effect; potential for abuse; caution not to drive or operate machinery. (Suggested maximal daily dose should not exceed 390 mg.) |

**Table 5-6.** *Pain Medications (Continued)*

| Drug | Route | Dose (mg) | Duration (hours) | Comments |
|---|---|---|---|---|
| **Ibuprofen** (Motrin) | PO | 300–600 | 2–4 | G.I. side-effects; use caution if aspirin-related sensitivity. May be used with renal impairment, partial excretion by biliary system. Bone marrow depression and CNS side-effects. (Dosage should not exceed 2.4 g/day.) Administer with food or milk. Also use caution in cardiac and hepatic dysfunction. |
| **Indomethacin** (Indocin) | PO<br>PO | 25–50<br>75 | 4–6<br>8–12 | G.I. and hematologic side-effects. Use with *extreme* caution in elderly and in impaired renal, hepatic function. (Dosage should not exceed 200 mg/day.) Administer with food or milk. |
| **Naproxen** (Naprosyn) | PO | 250–750 | 12–15 | Side-effects, precautions are the same as for indomethacin. Also potentiates G.I. toxicity if aspirin and steroids are being given. (Dosage should not exceed 1100 mg/day.) |

**Narcotic Analgesics for Mild to Moderate Pain\***

| Drug | Route | Dose (mg) | Duration (hours) | Comments |
|---|---|---|---|---|
| **Codeine** | PO | 32 | 4–6 | Additive effect when used with aspirin. Orthostatic hypotension, drowsiness, constipation. Caution its use in head injury, hepatic, renal, hypothyroidism, Addison's disease, and CNS-related disorders. |
| **Meperidine** (Demerol) | PO | 50 | 4–5 | Increased analgesia effect with thorazine. Same side-effects as codeine, and, in addition, contraindicated with MAO inhibitors, supraventricular tachycardia, and prostatic hypertrophy. |

**Table 5-6.** *Pain Medications (Continued)*

| Drug | Route | Dose (mg) | Duration (hours) | Comments |
|---|---|---|---|---|
| Pentazocine (Talwin) | PO | 30 | 4–6 | Has both analgesic and opiate properties. PO dosage should not exceed 60 mg/day. Use caution in clients with CNS, renal, hepatic, and cardiac diseases. If switching from a narcotic to Talwin, observe for withdrawal, because Talwin has narcotic antagonist properties. |
| **Narcotic Analgesics for Severe Pain†** | | | | |
| Morphine, Morphine SO₄, Morphine HCL, MS Contin, Roxanol (available as supp.) | IV IM PO | 5 10 60 | 2–4 4–5 4–5 | † Also available in slow-release tablets (MS Contin) and concentrated solutions (i.e., Roxanol 100 mg/ml). Respiratory and circulatory depression are major hazards. Observe also for nausea and vomiting, constipation, CNS changes, tolerance, dependence, hypotension, urine retention. † *Caution*: Clients may sleep for hours initially; this may *not* represent an excessive dose, but may indicate relief for the client. If respiratory function and vital signs are stable, it is recommended to wait 3 days before dose reduction is implemented. |
| Codeine | IM PO | 130 200 | 4–6 4–6 | (See Comments under Part I.) |
| Oxycodone Hydrochloride | IM PO | 15 30 | 3–5 3–5 | Synthetic narcotic with similar side-effects as morphine. Observe for any aspirin- or acetaminophen-related side-effects. (See Comments under Part I.) |

(Percodan includes addition of aspirin, phenacetin, and caffeine)
(Percocet 5 or Tylox includes addition of acetaminophen)

**Table 5-6.** *Pain Medications (Continued)*

| Drug | Route | Dose (mg) | Duration (hours) | Comments |
|---|---|---|---|---|
| **Levorphanol** (Levodromoran) | IV IM PO | 1 2 4 | 3–4 4–5 4–6 | Protect drug from light; pill has bitter taste. Drug accumulates, requires some titration with initial doses. Similar side-effects as morphine. |
| **Hydromorphone** (Dilaudid) (also available as supp.) | IV IM PO | 1 1.5 7.5 | | More soluble than morphine. Higher injectable concentrations available (10 mg/ml). Similar side-effects as morphine. |
| **Meperdine** (Demerol) | IV IM PO | 2–3 2–4 3–4 | | Incompatible with *any* IV drug; pain at injection site; may cause phlebitis after IV administration. Similar side-effects as morphine. |
| **Oxymorphone** (Numorphan) (available as supp. and IV) | IM PR | 1 10 | 4–6 4–6 | Well absorbed rectally. Similar side-effects as morphine. |
| **Methadone** (Dolophine) | IV IM PO | 5 10 20 | 3–4 4–6 4–6 | Dosage highly individualized; drug accumulates, and marked sedation can occur; monitor client closely. Other side-effects similar to morphine. |

\* Potency of drugs compared with aspirin 650 mg. *except* the following drugs:
  Ibuprofen (Motrin)
  Indomethacin (Indocin)
  Naproxen (Naprosyn)
† Potency of drugs compared with morphine 10 mg. I.m.

awake with excrutiating pain. The client will need support and an explanation that the situation is temporary; when stable, he or she can receive some medication to relieve the pain.

## Evaluation

The outcome criteria presented at the beginning of this section are used to evaluate the client's progress, make recommendations, and revise the nursing care plan. Criteria are also reviewed in relation to the client and family satisfaction and standards of home health care.

## References

Ahles TA, Blanchard EB, Ruckdeschel JL: The multidimensional nature of cancer related pain. Pain 17:22–28, 1983

Bloom B: Taxonomy of Educational Objectives: Handbook 1: Cognitive Domain. New York, David MacKay Co, Inc, 1969

Bonica J, Chapman CR: Chronic Pain: Current Concepts. Kalamazoo, Michigan, The Upjohn Company, 1985

Carpenito LI: Nursing Diagnosis Application to Clinical Practice. Philadelphia, J.B. Lippincott, 1983

Coyle N et al: Continuous subcutaneous infusions of opiates in cancer patients with pain. Oncology Nursing Forum 13(4):53–57, 1986

Derogatis LR, Abeloff M, McBeth CD: Cancer patients and their physician in the perception of psychological symptoms. Psychosomatics 17:191–201, 1976

Donovan M: Nursing assessment of cancer pain. Seminars in Oncology Nursing 1(2):109–115, 1986

IASP Subcommittee on Taxonomy: Pain terms: A list with definitions and notes on usage. Pain 6:249–252, 1979

Kenner CV, Guzetta CE, Dossey BM: Critical Care Nursing: Body-Mind-Spirit. Boston, Little, Brown and Co, 1985

Knowles MS: The Modern Practice of Adult Education: Andragogy Versus Pedagogy, 2nd ed. Chicago, Follett Publishing Co, 1980

Mager RF: Preparing Behavioral Objectives for Instruction, 2nd ed. Belmont, California, Frearon, 1975

McCaffery M: Nursing Management of the Patient with Pain. Philadelphia, JB Lippincott, 1979

Melzack R, Casey KL: Sensory, motivational, and central control determinants of pain: A new conceptual model. In Kenshalo D (ed): The Skin Senses, p. 423–429. Springfield IL, Charles C Thomas, 1968

Melzack R, Wall PD: Pain—new mechanisms: A new theory. Science 150:971–979, 1965

Melzack R, Wall PD: The Challenge of Pain. New York, Basic Books, 1982

Paice J: Intrathecal morphine infusion for intractable cancer pain: A new use for implanted pumps. Oncology Nursing Forum 13(3):41–47, 1986

Yasko J: Guidelines for Cancer Care. Reston, VA, Reston, 1983

Zborowski M: Cultural components in response to pain. J Soc Issues 8:16–30, 1952

# 6

# Diagnostic Cluster: Circulatory and Ventilatory Patterns

Advances in technology, including improved diagnostic testing and treatment, coupled with early discharge from acute care settings, have created a need for care of the client with both acute and chronic respiratory and cardiovascular disorders. This chapter will focus on the application of the nursing process in the home care setting related to the diagnostic cluster of circulatory and ventilatory patterns. The first section of the chapter will address home health care nursing concepts and interventions for airway and ventilation therapy, including apnea monitoring. The second section will discuss home health care measures for cardiac rehabilitation, pacemaker monitoring, and stroke rehabilitation.

## Nursing Diagnoses

Activity intolerance
Cardiac output, alterations in
Comfort, alterations in
Communication, alteration: verbal
Home maintenance management, impaired
Mobility, impaired
Knowledge deficit
Respiratory functions, alterations in
Self-care deficit
Sexual dysfunction
Tissue perfusion, alterations in

## Selected Diagnosis from Ventilatory Patterns: Respiratory Function, Alterations in

In 1984, the American Association of Respiratory Therapy conducted a survey in 20 states to identify the number of hospitalized ventilator-assisted clients whose medical conditions were stable enough to be managed at home. More than 2200 clients were identified. Hospital care costs per client per year were estimated at $220,000, compared with home care costs approximated at $21,000 per client per year (1984). It is obvious that maintaining ventilator-assisted clients in the home environment reduces health costs substantially and offers the client and family the option for returning home on a part-time or extended basis. Assisting the individual/family/ significant other to understand principles related to treatment, including utilization and maintenance of equipment, provides them with the knowledge and skill to confidently care for the person who requires ventilatory assistance in the familiarity and comfort of the home environment.

Disorders that require some form of assisted ventilation may include chronic obstructive pulmonary disease (COPD), neuromuscular diseases, trauma or spinal cord injury, and chest wall deformity (Johnson, 1986). There are three major ventilation devices used to assist or provide ventilation:

1. *Diaphragmatic manipulators* elicit movement of the diaphragm through electrical stimulation of the phrenic nerve or mechanical pressure on the diaphragm. The diaphragmatic pacer, rocking bed, and pneumobelt are the most commonly used diaphragmatic devices. One advantage of a diaphragmatic device is that an artificial airway is not required; however, only clients that have effective diaphragmatic muscle movement will benefit.

2. *Negative pressure ventilators (NPV)* apply negative pressure around the thorax during inspiration creating a pressure gradient within the thoracic cavity and causing air to flow into the lungs. Examples include the body tank (iron lung), chest cuirass or shell, and plastic wrap. An artificial airway is not needed, but tidal volume cannot be controlled, and blood may pool in the abdominal area.

3. *Positive pressure ventilators (PPV)* apply positive pressure during inspiration causing air to flow into the lungs. There are two PPVs available: the pressure-cycled or pressure-limited ventilator, and the volume-cycled or volume-limited ventilator. A pressure-cycled or pressure-limited ventilator ends inspiration when a pre-set pressure is achieved. A volume-cycled or volume-limited ventilator ends inspiration when a pre-set volume has been delivered. The volume-

cycled or volume-limited ventilator is the most frequently used ventilation device in the home because of the consistency of tidal volume delivered. PPVs usually require the use of an artificial airway.

The ventilator has several modes of operation:

1. *Assist mode* is used when the client initiates each breath but may not be able to achieve an adequate tidal volume; the machine cycles in response to the client's inspiratory effort, which triggers the ventilator to deliver a pre-set volume.
2. *Control mode* is used for clients whose respiratory drive is absent or excessive. The machine delivers a breath at a pre-set rate, regardless of the client's inspiratory effort, or lack of it. (This mode is seldom used.)
3. *Assist/control mode* is used most frequently for clients whose respiratory rates are erratic. The machine assists the client in response to independent inspiratory efforts but takes over and initiates the breathing if the client becomes apneic. However, the client can resume independent regulation of the respiratory rate at any time.
4. *Intermittent mandatory ventilation (IMV)* is used to deliver a predetermined number of breaths (mandatory breaths) and allows the client to breathe independently between machine breaths. IMV allows time for reconditioning of respiratory muscles and is used to "wean" clients from the ventilator to eventually resume breathing on their own (Fuchs, 1979).

Positive end-expiratory pressure (PEEP) is used in some clients to prevent atelectasis and keep alveoli open while surfactant is being produced. Lack of surfactant collapses alveoli and thus decreases the functional reserve capacity (FRC) and area available for gas exchange, and arterial oxygen pressure will fall. PEEP is used to treat acute respiratory distress syndrome (ARDS), pulmonary edema, or any condition in which intrapulmonary fluid is a problem (Fuchs, 1979).

There are four primary ventilator settings to monitor:

1. *Fraction of inspired air* ($F/O_2$) is a fixed number set by a dial on the ventilator (assessed daily by an oxygen analyzer or monitor which is purchased for the home setting and requires instruction). $F/O_2$ is expressed as a percentage (i.e., 40%) and is prescribed by the physician based on the lowest possible amount needed to promote adequate oxygenation.
2. *Respiratory rate* is a rate set by a dial on the ventilator to provide adequate ventilation. Count the client's respiratory rate with the set ventilatory rate, and assess and compare findings based on ventilator's mode of operation (see previous section).

3. *Inspiratory pressure* reflects lung function, and a continual increase may indicate fluid overload and pulmonary edema. Temporary increases can be eliminated if the client is suctioned or equipment is assessed and corrected for kinks, water, or obstruction.

4. *Tidal volume* reflects the amount of gas expired during ventilation (also referred to as exhaled air) and is an indicator of lung compliance. Spirometers can be used to measure ventilator-set tidal volumes to determine whether the pre-set rate is being delivered to the client or whether there is any complication, such as leakage from the machine or airway cuff.

If supplemental oxygen is needed, there are three major types of oxygen delivery systems available:

1. *Oxygen concentrators* remove dust particles and nitrogen from room air and concentrate and store the remaining oxygen to be used when needed. This is the least expensive home oxygen system if a client uses low-flow oxygen for more than 15 hours a day. Concentrators usually have a flow rate range of 0 liters to 7 liters per minute at 75% to 96% oxygen. They operate on 115-V AC, 60-Hz current and will increase the electric bill by approximately $10 to $20 a month, depending upon usage (Wyka, 1984). There is little maintenance other than keeping the bubble humidifier filled with sterile water and cleaning the filter weekly. Flow rates, percentage of oxygen, and pressures should be checked monthly. A back-up oxygen cylinder (D or E) with a regulator for emergency use should be available during a power failure or if the client is away from home. Oxygen cylinders are made from aluminum and are available with portable carts or pouches. Noise from the concentrator can be reduced by placing it on a mat or pad. Since concentrators generate heat, there must be adequate ventilation. Alarms are battery operated and need to be checked routinely. Concentrators will continue to decrease in size and weight; battery-operated models will soon be available.

2. *Liquid oxygen* is safer, yet more expensive than oxygen cylinders (tanks). Liquid oxygen is used when a low flow of oxygen is required for only several hours during the day. The oxygen is stored in a liquid state in metal thermos-like containers. When the oxygen is used, it changes from a liquid to a gas state as it leaves the container. One advantage of the system is that a smaller portable unit can be refilled from the larger tank. The portable unit can be carried over the shoulder or on a cart. A portable unit can supply 5 to 6 hours of oxygen at 2 liters/min and weighs only 10 lb when full. The liquid system should be well vented, because "spillage" is common when a portable unit is filled from the main tank (Hogstel, 1985).

3. *Oxygen cylinders (tanks)* are the cheapest system when the patient requires oxygen less than 15 hours a day. A cylinder stores oxygen gas under pressure, which is indicated by a pressure gauge attached to the tank. A flow meter can be set to deliver the amount of oxygen prescribed by the doctor. The client monitors the amount of oxygen left in the tank so that a new supply can be ordered in advance. A back-up or extra tank should always be available, as well as a smaller, portable cylinder for travel or ambulation. Since oxygen cylinders are high-pressure tanks, it is advisable to avoid tipping or knocking the tank over. The supplier should provide a stand to secure the tank.

Apnea monitors are used in the home setting to monitor respirations in place of a disconnect alarm in clients on ventilators and in apneic infants to prevent hypoxic events. Infants at risk include pre-term infants, infants diagnosed with apnea, siblings of sudden infant death syndrome (SIDS), and those who have experienced "near miss" SIDS episodes (Norris-Berkemeyer and Hutchins, 1986).

Respirations are monitored by motion detectors, thoracic impedance, or a thermistor at the nares or mouth (Johnson, 1986). Since the monitor alarms only when central apnea occurs and will not alarm if there is obstructive apnea, heart rate is monitored in addition to respiratory rate.

Tracheostomy tubes are available in a variety of styles. The tube should be large enough to accommodate ventilatory needs but small enough to avoid tracheal wall damage. The tube should conform to the anatomic shape of the individual's trachea, end at least 2 cm above the carina, yet be long enough to remain in the trachea. A cuff may be required to prevent aspiration or provide PPV.

Use of a cuff may lead to tracheal wall damage, including stenosis, but the introduction of double cuffs (large-volume and low-pressure) has reduced the incidence of complications. Tracheal wall pressure is also reduced by the minimal leak technique (MLT) and minimal occluding volume (MOV). MLT adjusts the volume of the cuff to allow for a minimal air leak around the cuff at the end of inspiration. MOV uses the smallest volume of air to inflate the cuff and prevent air leak around the cuff (Johnson, 1986).

Additional tracheostomy features include presence of an obturator, inner cannula, detachable cuffs, adjustable neckplates, and speech devices. Sizes generally range from an inside diameter (ID) of 3 mm to 14 mm to an outside diameter (OD) of 14 to 43 French. Prices vary from approximately $15 to $100, depending upon size and the addition of a cuff and pressure regulating valve. Selection of a tracheostomy tube will depend upon the client's age, neck anatomy, present health status, prognosis, activity level, means of ventilator assistance, volume and consistency of secretions, and whether or not speech is requested (artificial airways that permit speech).

Additional airway and ventilation accessories that are needed include tracheostomy care supplies, suction supplies, resuscitation bags (AMBU bag), humidification, alarms, percussors, vibrators, air cleaning units, and deionized water systems.

## Etiology and Defining Characteristics

Alteration in respiratory function as defined by Carpenito (1983) is "the state in which the individual experiences a real or potential threat to the passage of air through the respiratory tract, and to the exchange of gases ($O_2$–$CO_2$) between the lungs and the vascular system" (p 346). Etiologic and contributing factors may include surgery, COPD, emphysema, cerebral vascular accident (stroke), other neuromuscular disorders, neoplasms, neonatal- and infant-associated respiratory disorders, decreased lung function with aging, and associated environmental factors, including tobacco, chemical agents, and toxic fumes.

## Focus of Nursing Care

    Airway and ventilation therapy
    Home apnea monitoring

## Outcome Criteria

The person or family/care provider will:

1. Demonstrate increased air exchange and maximal pulmonary function
2. Demonstrate understanding of principles and concepts related to respiratory function
3. Demonstrate understanding of principles and concepts related to:
    Airway and ventilation therapy
    Apnea monitoring equipment
4. Use equipment competently and confidently
5. Identify complications of therapy and appropriate interventions in the home care setting
6. Maximize self-care activities and optimal level of functioning
7. Demonstrate reduced anxiety related to lack of knowledge and fear of the unknown

## Application of the Nursing Process

### Assessment

The client who requires ventilatory assistance in the home has usually been unable to be weaned from ventilatory support in spite of repeated attempts or suffers from a disease or injury that is chronic and progressive in nature. Families can provide excellent care to these persons if they are given the opportunity to learn the principles and procedures involved. The home health care nurse collaborates with the client, family, and referring agency through a contract to assess, monitor, and evaluate the plan of care. The nurse assesses:

1. Suitability of the home environment where procedures are performed and care is administered
2. Safety of home environment (electrical capacity, hazards of oxygen therapy)
3. Preparation, handling, storage, and disposal of sterile, clean, and contaminated equipment
4. Cleaning and disinfecting of reusable equipment
5. Ability of the family to demonstrate:
   Respiratory assessment
   Knowledge of ventilator functions
   Troubleshooting ventilator problems
   Suctioning
   Tracheostomy care
   Bagging technique
6. Ability of the family to recognize potential complications and react knowledgeably and effectively
7. Community resources and communication systems for notifying utility services, telephone company, ambulance, fire, police, hospital, physician, and home health care agency
8. Impact of illness on the client and family's lifestyle, interactions with others, and coping strategies used
9. Availability of "back-up" or other care providers to assist family if necessary
10. Availability of community respite services and support groups
11. Ability of client/family to communicate (i.e., by assistive devices)
12. Availability of equipment, services, and supplies provided by community and local vendors
13. Family knowledge and ability to perform cardiopulmonary resuscitation (CPR).
14. Ability of family to administer medications and feed client

15.  Potential client needs related to nutrition, hydration, elimination, immobility, skin integrity, and growth and development.

## Planning and Implementation

The nurse uses the information obtained from assessing the client in the home environment to determine what aspects of respiratory care procedures need reinforcement and review and what additional information needs to be discussed with the patient and family. Short-term goals form the basis of the prescription for the care plan, which is presented in Display 6-1. The nurse, client, and family implement the care plan and revise the plan accordingly.

### Monitoring of Client Status

Safety guidelines for monitoring and maintenance of respiratory equipment are included in Display 6-2.

Potential complications of ventilatory therapy can be avoided if the client's nursing prescription includes assessment for the conditions listed below. Any abnormal signs and symptoms should be reported immediately to the appropriate health care person or agency.

1.  Airway obstruction/alteration in respiratory pattern (change in respiratory rate, retractions, nasal flaring, wheezing, cough, anxiety, clammy skin, cyanotic lips, fingernails)
2.  Fever above 101°F
3.  Alterations in color, odor, and consistency of secretions (presence of foul odor, yellow or green mucus, presence of blood in sputum)
4.  Alterations in appetite, behavior, fluid, and elimination patterns
5.  Alterations in intake and output
6.  Equipment malfunction

### Complications and Suggested Interventions

Respiratory complications include airway obstruction, tracheal damage, infection, tension pneumothorax, fluid and elimination problems, gastrointestinal bleeding, and equipment malfunction. Complications and interventions for complications for clients in the home setting are briefly discussed in the following paragraphs.

**Airway Obstruction.**   If airway obstruction occurs, the family/care providers must know how to perform respiratory assessment, including

1.  Vital signs
2.  Recognition of normal and abnormal variations in client's breathing patterns, including shortness of breath and apnea (Jackson, 1986)

(*Text continues on p. 160*)

*Display 6-1*
**Sample Care Plan: The Client Requiring Ventilatory Assistance in the Home Setting**

*Long-Term Goals (Outcomes)*

At the end of 3 weeks, the client (individual and/or family/significant other) will:

1. Demonstrate increased airway exchange and maximal pulmonary function.
2. Demonstrate understanding of principles and concepts related to respiratory function.
3. Demonstrate the ability to perform ventilator-assisted care correctly and confidently, including
   Respiratory assessment
   Ventilator checks
   Suctioning
   Tracheostomy care
   Bagging technique
4. Identify complications of therapy and appropriate interventions in the home care setting.
5. Utilize safety measures related to oxygen therapy.
6. Maximize self-care activities and optimal level of functioning.
7. Demonstrate reduced anxiety related to lack of knowledge, change in lifestyle, and fear of the unknown.
8. Utilize available community resources for persons and families with altered respiratory function.

*Short-Term Goals (Objectives)*

**Week 1**

1. The client/care provider will verbalize the major principles and concepts of respiratory function as they relate to ventilator-assisted care.
2. The client/care provider will demonstrate the ability to
   Assess respiratory status
   Perform ventilator checks
   Suction the client
   Perform tracheostomy care
   Perform manual resuscitation bagging technique
3. The client/care provider will identify persons in the neighborhood available to assist in an emergency.

*(continued)*

*Display 6-1 (Continued)*
**Sample Care Plan: The Client Requiring Ventilatory Assistance in the Home Setting**

*Short-Term Goals (Objectives)*

**Week 2**

1. The client/care provider will verbalize factors that increase ventilator-assisted complications.
2. The client/care provider will verbalize safety issues related to ventilator care.
3. The client will verbalize a plan of action in the event of a power failure.

**Week 3**

1. The client/care provider will verbalize interventions to treat ventilator-assisted complications.
2. The client will maintain optimal respiratory function, and lungs will be free of infection.
3. The client will verbalize knowledge of available community resources for persons and families with alterations in respiratory function.

*Nursing Care Plan (Prescription)*

**Week 1**

1. In the home, the nurses will review with the client and family the principles and concepts related to ventilator care, including
   Written information describing the client's specific respiratory disorder
   A list of equipment and supplies that will be needed (including what, where, approximate price, how to order, how *much* to order for at least a 2-week supply, and a list of available vendors)
   A list of community services available and specific assistance they offer (American Lung Association, American Heart Association, American Cancer Society)
   Step-by-step procedures of specific respiratory and ventilator care
2. In the home, the nurse will demonstrate to the client/care provider step-by-step procedure of respiratory assessment, ventilator checks, suctioning, tracheostomy care, and bagging technique.

*(continued)*

*Display 6-1 (Continued)*

*Nursing Care Plan (Prescription)*

3. In the home, the nurse will provide the client/care provider with the opportunity to ask and answer their questions.
4. In the home, the client/care provider will perform correctly all the ventilator-assisted care procedures reviewed.
5. The client/care provider will inform the nurse of persons who are willing to participate or assist as back-ups and discuss how they can receive instructions

**Week 2**

1. In the home, the nurse will review with the client/care provider ventilator-assisted complications, including
   List of complications, including signs and symptoms
   Safety guidelines related to ventilator care (especially oxygen and electrical hazards)
   Suggested guidelines for action in the event of a power failure
2. At the end of the session, the client will verbalize:
   Signs and symptoms related to ventilator care complications
   Safety guidelines for potential ventilator care hazards
3. At the end of the session, the client/care provider will perform ventilator therapy, and the nurse will provide verbal feedback and suggestions.

**Week 3**

1. In the home, the nurse will review with the client/care provider
   A list of specific interventions for ventilator-related complications
   A checklist for reordering supplies
2. Auscultation of the lungs will demonstrate improvement in respiratory function and no presence of respiratory infection.
3. The client's tracheostomy stoma will be free of skin irritation or infection.
4. At the end of the session, the client/care provider will
   Verbalize specific interventions for ventilator-related complications.
   Indicate at least one community resource that they will contact in the next week.

*Display 6-2*
**Safety Guidelines for Respiratory Equipment**

*Oxygen Safety Guidelines*

Notify the local fire department that oxygen is in use in the home. Keep an all-purpose fire extinguisher available.

If an oxygen tank is used, store upright to prevent an explosion.

Keep the oxygen supply at least 5 feet away from a heat source and electrical applicances.

Never use a fireplace for heat while using oxygen.

Do not smoke when oxygen is being used (this applies to all persons, not just the client!)

Do not use oxygen around a stove (including wood-burning stoves), space heater (kerosene heater), radiators, heat ducts, steam pipes, or any other heat sources.

Do not use electric blankets and electric heating pads.

Do not use matches, cigarette lighters, candles, sparking or mechanical toys, and electrical equipment that generates heat (blow dryer, curling iron).

Avoid the use of flammable products such as moisturizers, hair sprays, hair oils, and ointments that contain oil and alcohol. Oxygen can remain in bed linen and clothing for as long as 3 to 6 hours after use (Oxygen Therapy, 1986).

Do not place oxygen tubing under clothing, furniture, carpets, or bed linen.

Avoid synthetic clothing.

Avoid creating static electricity. Wear 100% cotton clothing, and use all-cotton sheets and blankets.

Turn off oxygen flow regulators when not in use to avoid oxygen leaks.

Do not recharge batteries in the same room in which oxygen is stored or used.

Never place or store oxygen in the trunk of a car.

Use only the oxygen flow rate prescribed by the doctor.

Keep oxygen units out of the reach of children.

*Apnea Monitor Safety Guidelines*

Three-prong outlets or electrical adaptors are mandatory. Home monitor must contain fuses to protect the monitor from power surges.

*(continued)*

*Display 6-2 (Continued)*

*Apnea Monitor Safety Guidelines*

Position monitor where alarm or indicator lights are easily visible.

The client's residence must have 24-hour communication access. A back-up plan is developed if needed (access to emergency communication services).

A portable light source with necessary equipment and supplies is placed close to the monitor for easy access.

Do not bathe the client while attached to the monitor.

Assess if the client needs supervision or restraints to avoid chewing or tampering with monitor wires (Apnea Monitor Alert, 1985).

Avoid placing monitor on surface that muffles the alarm sound (e.g., mattress, carpeting, against draperies or wall)

Avoid showering, vacuuming, using noisy electrical equipment if only one person is home, because he or she may not hear alarm. An intercom should be purchased to permit the apnea alarm sound to be audible throughout the client's residence (Norris-Berkemeyer, 1986).

Remove leads from the patient unless they are attached to the monitor.

Unplug power cord from the wall if it is unplugged from the monitor.

*Community Safety Guidelines*

The follow agencies should be informed of the patient's health status and potential emergency needs:

Telephone company
Electrical, power, gas company
Fire department
Emergency medical services/ambulance services
Police department
Vendor/rental company
Primary physician/health service
Hospital/emergency room

3. Amount, color, and consistency of secretions (including presence of blood in secretions)
4. Presence of cough or change in nature in cough
5. Distress signs such as anxiety, diaphoresis, pallor, cyanosis, nasal flaring, retractions, and wheezing

If these signs and symptoms are present, the care provider should first suction the client. It may be recommended to preoxygenate the patient using an AMBU bag and instilling normal saline prior to suctioning. If the airway continues to be obstructed with mucus and the mucus cannot be removed by suctioning, the tracheostomy should be changed immediately. Mucous plugs are a common cause of airway obstruction in the home. If the client is on a ventilator and is still experiencing problems, check any tubes for water accumulation or accidental disconnection.

If the client has a cuffed tracheostomy, assess for an airway leak by placing a hand close to the client's nose and mouth to detect air or auscultate over the trachea with a stethoscope. The cuff can be deflated and reinflated, and the client can be reassessed. The cuff could have a leak or could be moved over the end of the opening of the tracheostomy to occlude the opening. This situation necessitates changing the tracheostomy tube immediately. Assess the position of the tracheostomy tube, observing for any pulsation or bleeding around the tracheostomy. If the client is still experiencing respiratory difficulty, disconnect the client from the ventilator and AMBU him or her with oxygen connected to the AMBU bag. If his or her respiratory status improves or is relieved, notify the person responsible for servicing and repairing the machine. Continue with the AMBU bag and oxygen until the back-up system is in place or until the machine is repaired. If the client is still in respiratory distress, continue to manually ventilate him or her with a resuscitation bag, transport him or her to the nearest emergency care facility, and notify the physician.

Thick secretions are often related to inadequate humidification or dehydration. Dehydration decreases normal pulmonary fluids, creating thick secretions. Ventilated air should always be humidified and heated to body temperature. Observe for signs of dehydration such as decreased secretions when suctioning, dry lips, dry tongue, decreased skin turgor, and thirst. Humidification is more often a problem with children, because water more frequently accumulates in the small-bore tubing. Bleeding is another complication and may be indicative of excessive suctioning, incorrect suctioning technique, or lack of humidification.

Additional complications that cause airway obstruction can occur during the changing and insertion of tracheostomy tubes. The tube may accidentally be misplaced anteriorly and into the space between the skin and the tracheal wall instead of in the trachea. Decannulation and inability to replace a tracheostomy tube can occur. Although it is difficult, the care provider must first remember to *stay calm*. If the client is coughing and becomes further agitated, bronchospasm may occur. It is recommended that *two* persons be available to change a tracheostomy. If it is difficult to reinsert a tracheostomy tube that is being changed or one that has been pulled or "coughed out," instill a few drops of saline, wait a brief period of time, and attempt to insert the tube. If you are not successful, insert a tracheostomy tube that is one or two sizes smaller until the client relaxes enough to reinsert the prescribed size.

Bronchodilators and steroids are medications often used to decrease airflow obstruction and prevent or reverse bronchospasm. The base for all bronchodilator therapy is aminophylline, which is available in a variety of preparations. Clients should be aware that nausea and vomiting are common signs of aminophylline toxicity and that long-term steroid therapy can impair thought processes. The nurse is advised to consult a pharmacology text and carefully review possible side-effects with clients and families.

**Tracheal Damage.**    Increased pressure on the tracheal wall from the tracheostomy tube and cuff may result in tissue ischemia, which can lead to irritation, ulceration, and necrosis. Tracheoesophageal fistula, tracheostenosis, and tracheitis may occur. Proper size, length, and cuff selection were discussed earlier in this chapter. The use of MLT, MOV, and periodic cuff deflation (if indicated) reduces the possibility of tracheal complications. Any continued tracheal pressure or discomfort is discussed with the physician for further evaluation.

**Infection.**    Most persons who have a tracheostomy will, at some time, become colonized with certain organisms. It does not necessarily imply serious infection but may indicate that the person is harboring and growing certain common organisms, for example, *Pseudomonas* (Czarniecki, 1985). Warning signs of a serious respiratory infection include fever, chills, change in general behavior, and change in color, odor, and consistency of secretions (presence of yellow or green mucus with a foul odor and increase in consistency and amount). The person may also complain of increased coughing or change in the nature of cough, shortness of breath, fatigue, sore throat, change in appetite, and fluid balance.

Intervention includes immediate notification of appropriate health care personnel. If infection is present, the client may be treated at home with antibiotic therapy. Clients are reminded to finish the antibiotic prescription, even if they feel better, to prevent developing resistant organisms. Fluid intake is increased to prevent dehydration as well as the thick secretions that become a breeding ground for bacteria.

All respiratory equipment, including tubing, humidifiers, suction machines, tracheostomy tubes, and other accessories must be cleaned and disinfected frequently. Policies and procedures will vary, but most agencies recommend cleaning them every 24 to 48 hours. Periodic cultures of the equipment are recommended if the client has frequent respiratory infections (Display 6-3).

*Display 6-3*
## Guidelines for Cleaning Respiratory Equipment

1.  Choose one area of the house to disassemble, wash "dirty" or contaminated equipment with a mild liquid detergent and hot water, and rinse thoroughly. It is recommended that the "cleaning area" and "disinfecting area" for equipment be in two separate areas or receptacles. Toothbrushes are helpful for cleaning tubing lumens and small parts. Bottle brushes are helpful for cleaning wide tubing.
2.  The washed equipment is disinfected by soaking it in an acetic acid solution for 20 to 30 minutes. All equipment should be fully submerged for contact with the solution. A 3.0% acetic acid (vinegar) solution can be made by adding: 1 part vinegar to 3 parts water {2 cups vinegar + 6 cups of water = ½ gal of 3% solution} (Johnson, 1986).
3.  Rinsing with tap or distilled water is recommended after disinfecting the solution. However, some agencies do not recommend rinsing the acetic acid solution; thus, it is wise to check agency policy.
4.  Air drying of equipment is essential to control bacterial growth and prevent infection.
5.  The equipment should be stored and reassembled in a clean, dry work area.

*Suggestions for Specific Equipment*

Review manufacturer's cleaning and maintenance instructions to become familiar with the instructions and guidelines.

1.  *Humidifier.* Water reservoir should be emptied, cleaned, and refilled daily to prevent bacterial growth.
2.  *Suction machine and tubing.* Empty, wash, and rinse container and tubing daily. Depending upon the amount of secretions, the container and tubing are sterilized and disinfected several times a week.
3.  *Intermittent positive pressure breathing apparatus (IPPB).* Nebulizers and mouthpieces should be cleaned in soap and hot water and rinsed after every treatment. Unused medications should not remain in the nebulizer between treatments.
4.  *Tracheostomy tubes.* Procedure for cleaning and sterilizing equipment:
    *Plastic tracheostomy tubes.* Clean with soap, hot water, pipe cleaners, and toothbrush, and rinse well. Soak for 8 hr in

*(continued)*

*Display 6-3 (Continued)*

hydrogen peroxide. Rinse first with 70% isopropyl alcohol, followed by sterile water or saline. Dry with a clean paper towel. Apply new twill tape, and store in a clean container. *Metal tracheostomy tubes.* Clean with soap, hot water, pipe cleaners, and toothbrush, and rinse with water. If tube is tarnished, apply silver polish with a toothbrush, rinse with water, and wash again with soap and water to remove any traces of polish. Add the tubes to boiling water for 15 minutes, then drain and cool. Apply new twill tape and store in a clean container (Hazinski, 1986).

*Reuse of disposable suction catheters*

The reuse of disposable suction catheters is a controversial area. Soaking and milking catheters with a disinfectant is the recommended cleaning procedure, but, in reality, the narrow lumen is impossible to brush clean, and the risk of infection related to mucous adherence and bacterial contamination is great. In addition, reuse may not be cost-effective if cleaning is time-consuming or results in an increased incidence of infection (Johnson, 1986).

Research problems include the lack of available data and clinical studies and inconsistency in definition and technique of clean vs sterile. One study by Harris and Hyman (1984) found a group of persons who use a "mixed technique," using both clean and sterile technique in the suctioning procedure. Harris and Hyman found that clean technique did not result in a higher infection rate than for the group who practiced sterile technique when suctioning clients with tracheostomies.

**Pneumothorax.** Clients who are mechanically ventilated are at risk for pneumothorax, especially persons ventilated with high levels of PEEP. Subcutaneous emphysema may develop over the chest and neck and appear prior to "blowing a lung." Other signs and symptoms indicative of a tension pneumothorax include tachypnea, tachycardia, hyperresonance to percussion, absent breath sounds, and sharp chest pain. The trachea may shift from the midline toward the unaffected side, and the affected side of the chest may be fixed in a maximal inspiratory position. The ventilator peak inspiratory alarm (PIP) may sound, since there is a significant increase in the amount of pressure to ventilate the client. If a pneumothorax is suspected, it is an emergency, and the care provider is instructed to immediately call an ambulance to transport the client to a hospital, disconnect the client from the ventilator, and ventilate manually with an AMBU bag until the ambulance arrives. Relief of intrapleural pressure can best be achieved by the insertion of a chest tube (Fuchs, 1979).

***Fluids, Nutrition, and Aspiration Complications.***   Dehydration can cause secretions to thicken and make it difficult for the client to raise the secretions or remove them by suctioning. Signs of dehydration include decreased secretions on suctioning, decreased skin turgor, dry mouth, dry or cracked lips, dry tongue, decreased urinary output, concentrated urine, and increased thirst. The appropriate health care provider is notified so that treatment can be discussed and initiated. The usual recommended treatment is to increase fluid intake, preferably by the gastrointestinal tract or, if necessary, intravenously.

Enteral nutrition with either flexible small-bore nasogastric or gastrostomy tubes is the preferred route if the gastrointestinal tract is functioning. A nasogastric tube may be used initially. It should be determined from the appropriate health care provider whether the endotracheal or tracheostomy cuff is to be inflated or deflated during the procedure. When infusing the formula, the head of the bed is elevated prior to feeding and the fluid should be at room temperature and instilled slowly (200 ml–250 ml of feeding takes 20 to 30 minutes). Too rapid a rate will lead to abdominal distention, nausea, vomiting, and diarrhea. Water is administered with every feeding to hydrate the client, keep the tube patent, and prevent bacterial growth. If possible, to prevent aspiration or regurgitation, the client is kept in an upright position for 30 to 60 minutes after a feeding. If aspiration occurs repeatedly, a gastrostomy tube may be indicated.

If the client aspirates, suction immediately to prevent aspiration pneumonia. Secretions can be tested for the presence of formula by using a glucose test strip, because glucose is *not* normally found in respiratory secretions. Adding a few drops of food coloring to the formula and then assessing suctioned pulmonary secretions will also indicate whether aspiration has occurred.

Overhydration can occur, especially in clients with chronic lung disease who are susceptible to right-sided heart failure (cor pulmonale). The care provider who is skilled in auscultation may hear fine crackles in the dependent areas of the lung if the fluid has shifted into the alveoli. The client on a volume-cycled ventilator is observed for increased inspiratory pressure. If there are signs and symptoms of overhydration, the appropriate health care provider is notified. Treatment usually consists of specific orders to monitor intake and output, assess for dependent edema (sacrum, ankles), and continue to assess renal and cardiac function (Carroll, 1986).

About 25% of all ventilator clients develop gastrointestinal bleeding. The care provider routinely observes stools and gastrointestinal secretions for presence of bleeding. Occasional hemetesting of stools is recommended. If any findings are positive, the physician or health care agency is notified immediately.

*Equipment Malfunction.* There are various models of ventilators, airways, oxygen equipment, and accessories available. The client and care provider in the home care setting must possess a comprehensive understanding of the function, operation, maintenance, and trouble-shooting of the equipment. A back-up system must be available, and direct 24-hour access to a health care agency or vendor is mandatory for delivery, service, and repair of equipment. General suggestions for trouble-shooting ventilators, tracheostomy tubes, and apnea monitors are presented in Display 6-4.

The care provider should be aware that if an alarm sounds on a piece of equipment, the client should *always* be assessed first. How does the client appear? Is he or she experiencing any respiratory distress? The problem may be with the equipment and not with the client. If the cause of an alarm cannot be determined on a piece of respiratory equipment (ventilator), the client should be removed from the ventilator, manually ventilated with a resuscitation bag, attached to a flow meter and oxygen source, and transported to a hospital.

Additional considerations for the client and care provider are the tremendous alterations in lifestyles that occur and the mandatory 24-hour surveillance and monitoring by qualified persons. Anxiety, fear, and loss of control are feelings commonly experienced by the client and care provider. Support groups assist families to express their feelings and to share in their concerns. Only babysitters, family, or friends who are certified in cardio-pulmonary resuscitation (CPR) are qualified to care for persons with respiratory problems.

Travel is encouraged for both the client and the care provider but requires extensive planning. Portable, battery-operated ventilators are available. Other necessary equipment for travel include portable suction equipment, catheters, solution, oxygen, spare airway (trach, scissors, ties), paper towels, manual resuscitation bag, medications, and receptacle for used equipment and supplies. If commercial transportation is used, it is wise to contact appropriate company representatives to make specific plans. Although not feasible for all clients, travel is encouraged for those able in order to increase the opportunity to change the environment, interact with others, and improve one's quality of life.

## Evaluation

The effectiveness of the nursing care plan for the client with respiratory function alterations is measured in terms of meeting pre-set long-term goals

*Display 6-4*
**Troubleshooting Ventilators, Tracheostomy Tubes,**
**and Apnea Monitors**

I.   Ventilators. If a ventilator is to be used in the home setting, the individual must monitor and understand
   A.   Fraction of inspired oxygen ($FiO_2$)
   B.   Respiratory rate
   C.   Inspiratory pressure
   D.   Exhaled volume
   E.   Inspiratory and expiratory times
   F.   Positive end–expiratory pressure (PEEP)
   G.   Mode of ventilation:
      1.   Assist
      2.   Control
      3.   Assist-control
      4.   Sigh
      5.   Intermittent mandatory ventilation (IMV)
   H.   Alarm Checklist (Fuchs, 1986)
      1.   *High-pressure alarm* may indicate:
         a.   Increased airway resistance (client needs suctioning)
         b.   Kink, obstruction (client lying , biting on tube)
         c.   Water in tubing
         d.   Pneumothorax
         e.   Client coughing or holding breath while ventilator delivers breath
         f.   Displacement of artificial airway
         g.   Herniation of cuff over artificial airway
         h.   Increased airway resistance (bronchospasm)
         i.   Decreased pulmonary compliance
      2.   *Low-pressure alarm* may indicate:
         a.   Leak in system (tubing disconnected, leak in tubing)
         b.   Leak in/around airway cuff
         c.   Leak at humidifier
      3.   *Low-exhale volume alarm* (indicated by high or low pressure readout or spirometer alarm) may indicate:
         a.   Breath not being delivered due to leak in system
         b.   Spirometer not attached/disconnected
         c.   Client's respirations on IMV are no longer spontaneous
   I.   Emergency measures

*(continued)*

*Display 6-4 (Continued)*

    J.   Care provider anxiety/support system
    K.  Communication

II.  Tracheostomy Tubes. If a tracheostomy is to be used in the home care setting, the individual/care provider must assess and monitor
    A.  The need for suctioning
    B.  Suctioning technique
    C.  Tracheostomy care
    D.  Peristomal care
    E.  Changing the tracheostomy
    F.  Accidental cannulation
    G.  Bleeding
    H.  Emergency procedures
    I.   Humidification
    J.   Communication with client
    K.  Care provider anxiety/support system
    L.  Travel

III.  Apnea Monitors. If the client is using an apnea monitor in the home care setting, the individual/care provider must monitor and assess
    A.  Attaching the individual to a monitor (lead or belt placement)
    B.  Measurement technique (heart rate, motion detector)
    C.  Features including
        1.  Sensitivity adjustment
        2.  Breath indicator
        3.  Apnea delay setting
        4.  Bradycardia alarm setting
        5.  Line voltage/battery-type
        6.  Operating time on portable battery
        7.  Alarm silencer
    D.  Malfunction (Norris–Berkemeyer and Hutchins, 1986)
        1.  Loose or detached leads
        2.  Improper lead or belt placement
        3.  Dry electrodes
        4.  False alarms
        5.  Sensitivity adjustment
    E.  Emergency measures
    F.  Family/client anxiety
    G.  Family support/resources
    H.  Travel

and objectives. The ability to maintain the client at home with ventilatory assistance is the desired outcome of home respiratory therapy. Less frequent hospitalizations and a comfortable death at home, if the client is in the final stages of progressive respiratory or cardiac disease, are other measures of success for home health care nursing intervention.

The outcome criteria listed in the beginning of the chapter and the objectives for the nursing care plan listed in Display 6-1 are examples of criteria that may be used by the home health care nurse for measuring the success of the nursing care plan. These criteria must be adjusted to the individual client situation, the primary provider of care, the family's health needs, and the community's role in meeting the needs of the at-risk population. They will serve as initial standards of care for home health care problems related to alterations in respiratory function.

## Selected and Related Diagnoses From Circulatory Patterns: Cardiac Output, Alterations in; Tissue Perfusion, Alterations in

The current emphasis on prevention and rehabilitation for cardiovascular health problems has expanded the role of the nurse in caring for persons with these types of illnesses. The home health care nurse is often responsible for coordinating and facilitating cardiac and stroke rehabilitation programs. The following section focuses on concepts of cardiac and stroke rehabilitation in the home. Suggested outcome criteria with specific interventions for the client, family, and health care provider in the home setting are included.

Cardiovascular diseases are the leading cause of death in the United States. More than 42 million Americans are currently diagnosed with one or more of the following cardiac disorders: hypertension, coronary heart disease, rheumatic heart disease, and cerebrovascular accident. In addition, cardiovascular diseases are a major cause of disability and chronic illness costing Americans more than $40 billion annually.

Advanced technology, including improved diagnostic imaging studies, surgical techniques, medical therapies, and pharmaceutical agents offer realistic hope and improved quality of life for people with cardiovascular disease. The home care nurse is faced with the challenge of assisting the client and family in developing a realistic plan of care focused on prevention and treatment of further disease. Intervention strategies include limitation of disabilities, psychosocial support, and education of the client for lifestyle modification through risk reduction behaviors and rehabilitation.

Regardless of the causative factors, that is, myocardial ischemia, vascular abnormalities, conduction defects, and so on, the sequence of events in cardiovascular diseases is very similar. When blood flow to the myocardium is reduced, contractility decreases, and stroke volume and cardiac output fall. Left ventricular end diastolic volume increases, and the ejection fraction decreases. Compensatory mechanism responses include sympathetic stimulation and constriction of peripheral circulation to increase heart rate and contractility and improve stroke volume and cardiac output. Reduced renal blood flow activates secondary compensatory mechanisms (renin-angiotensin-aldosterone [RAA] feedback system), which increases renal reabsorption of sodium and water and increases blood flow to the heart (*Cardiovascular Disorders*, 1984).

If myocardial ischemia is severe, the normal compensatory mechanisms will be unable to support adequate cardiac output, arterial pressure, or renal perfusion. Left ventricle hypertrophy, which is a response to prolonged myocardial tension, may temporarily improve contractility. In addition, cardiac drugs (digitalis) and diuretics are used to improve renal perfusion and reduce fluid retention. If these compensatory and support mechanisms fail, cardiogenic shock will lead to multisystem failure and death unless the pumping mechanism of the heart can be restored.

Myocardial ischemia, if prolonged, causes irreversible tissue necrosis and is referred to as an infarct, or myocardial infarction. Depending upon which coronary artery is occluded, the infarct may occur in the anterior, lateral, septal, or diaphragmatic or inferior wall of the myocardium. An infarct damaging the full thickness of the cardiac wall is described as transmural, whereas a partial thickness infarct is described as nontransmural or subendocardial. During an ischemic attack, the client may experience pressure under the breastbone that may radiate to the arm (most often the inner aspect of the left arm), neck, jaw, or other areas of the upper torso.

*Many* clients (approximately 25%) *never* experience specific pain; they may relate their discomfort to indigestion, bladder, or dental problems, or they may experience dyspnea with no discomfort. Associated signs and symptoms can also include cool, clammy skin; cyanosis; decreasing blood pressure; weak thready pulse; and decreased urinary output. Major risk factors include hypertension, hypercholesterolemia, and cigarette smoking. Contributing risk factors include age, obesity, sedentary lifestyle, left ventricular hypertrophy (caused by hypertension), family history, Type "A" personality, stress, gender (males), race (blacks), glucose intolerance (diabetes), gout, and use of oral contraceptives (Kenner et al, 1985).

Conduction defects can severely compromise cardiac output, leading to syncope, convulsions, and death. Indications for permanent pacemaker insertion include those clients with complete, intermittent, or incomplete atrioventricular block with Stokes-Adams syncope or congestive failure, sinus bradycardia, sinus arrest or symptomatic sinoatrial block, permanent postoperative surgical heart block, or uncontrollable tachydysrhythmias (Sager, 1984).

Pacemaker selection will depend upon the client's dysrhythmia, cause of the dysrhythmia, and functional and conduction status of the myocardium. Components of a permanent pacing system include a pulse generator (energy source) and one or more pacing cathether electrodes (which can be bipolar or unipolar). The pacing electrodes may be positioned surgically using an endocardial implant through a transvenous approach (preferred method) or implantation of an epicardial implant. The energy source may be either lithium batteries or a nuclear battery. The half-life of the nuclear battery (plutonium 238) is more than 86 years, but the system is designed to last 10 to 20 years. Lithium batteries with copper sulfide and iodine cathodes appear to outlast other units; however, pacemakers have been reported to last from 18 months to 8 years. Nuclear pacemakers are not as common as the lithium batteries because of controls established by the Food and Drug Administration (FDA) and the Nuclear Regulatory Commission (NRC).

A pacemaker consists of a pacing circuit, sensing and program circuitry, a mode of response to sensed impulse, and tachyarrhythmia functions. A five-letter code has been designed by the Intersociety Commission for Heart Disease to facilitate communication between the manufacturers of pacemakers and health professionals who select pacemakers (Millar, 1985). The code is written on the pacemaker to clearly identify the system being used (Display 6-5). Most clients requiring cardiac pacing are given ventricular inhibited pacing (VVI) systems.

A cerebral vascular accident (CVA) is a neurologic dysfunction that interrupts cerebral circulation owing to a spasm, occlusion, or hemorrhage of a blood vessel. Symptoms manifested depend upon the location and extent of cerebral ischemia. Symptoms persist more than 24 hours in contrast to transient ischemia attacks (TIAs), which generally last *less* than 24 hours. Symptoms may include subtle changes such as memory lapse, numbness, tingling of extremities, and gait and balance disturbances. Classic

---

*Display 6-5*
**Code for Pacemakers**

*First Letter—Chamber paced*

A = atrium
V = ventricle
D = double (dual) chamber
S = single chamber

*(continued)*

*Display 6-5 (Continued)*

*Second Letter—Chamber sensed*

A = atrium
V = ventricle
D = double (dual) chamber
S = single chamber

*Third Letter—Mode of response to sensed impulse*

I = inhibited
T = triggered
D = double
O = none
R = reverse

*Fourth Letter—Programmability*

P = programmable rate or output
M = multiprogrammability
O = none

*Fifth Letter—Tachyarrhythmia functions*

B = burst
N = normal rate compensation
S = scanning
E = external
O = none

**Examples of pacing systems commonly used**
AOO = atrial asynchronous (fixed rate)
AAT = atrial triggered (atrial demand)
AAI = atrial inhibited (atrial demand)
VAT = A–V synchronous
VOO = ventricular asynchronous (fixed rate)
VVT = ventricular triggered (ventricular demand)
VVI = ventricular inhibited (ventricular demand; most common system)
VDD = atrial synchronous (ventricular inhibited)
DOO = A–V sequential (fixed rate)
DVI = A–V sequential (ventricular inhibited)
DDD = fully automatic dual chamber (A–V universal)

symptoms include convulsion, fever, vomiting, headache, coma, aphasia, and hemiplegia, dysphagia, and incontinence (Steffl, 1984). Predisposing factors include age, family history, hypertension, diabetes, atherosclerosis, sex (postmenopausal women) and ethnicity (blacks).

Both of these cardiovascular disorders require immediate hospitalization for stabilization, followed by a comprehensive rehabilitation program that begins in the hospital and continues in the home care setting using a multidisciplinary team approach. The nurse in the home care setting facilitates the client's and family's rehabilitation with emphasis on exercise, medications, diet, and lifestyle modifications that include stress reduction strategies, behavior modification, relaxation techniques, and specific coping strategies.

## Etiology and Defining Characteristics

Decreased cardiac output, alterations in: decreased as defined by Carpenito (1983) is "the state in which the individual experiences a reduction in the amount of blood pumped by the heart, resulting in compromised cardiac function" (p 104). Alteration in tissue perfusion as defined by Carpenito is "the state in which the individual experiences or is at risk of experiencing a decrease in nutrition and respiration at the cellular level due to a decrease in capillary blood supply" (p 477).

Common etiologic and contributing factors may include cardiovascular disturbances such as a CVA, myocardial infarction (MI), congestive heart failure (CHF), hypertension, shock, diabetes, COPD, TIAs, arteriosclerotic vascular disease (ASVD, ASHD), atherosclerosis, and anemia.

## Focus of Nursing Care

Cardiac rehabilitation
Pacemaker monitoring
Stroke rehabilitation

## Outcome Criteria

The person (or family/care provider) will

1. Demonstrate increased/improved cardiac output
2. Demonstrate increased/improved peripheral circulation
3. Demonstrate understanding of principles and concepts related to cardiac rehabilitation and stroke rehabilitation, including
   Lifestyle modifications
   Diet
   Medications
   Exercise

4. Demonstrate behaviors that reflect lifestyle changes consistent with the prescribed rehabilitation program(s)
5. Identify complications of therapy and specific interventions for the client at home
6. Maximize self-care activities and optimal level of functioning
7. Utilize measures/behaviors to conserve oxygen and energy during sexual activity
8. Demonstrate reduced anxiety and fear by using effective coping patterns

## Application of the Nursing Process

### Assessment

The client recovering at home from MI, pacemaker insertion, or CVA and his or her family/care provider initially need support and reassurance that they can competently manage their situation at home. The home health care nurse assesses, monitors, and evaluates the plan of care that was established in the hospital and determines whether it is realistic for the client and family. (It is important to note, however, that many rehabilitation programs in larger urban areas are hospital-based and home visits may not be reimbursable or covered by insurance or Medicare.) In this section we address the major components of rehabilitation programs and the health care provider's role in assisting the client at home to achieve an optimal level of functioning and maximize self-care activities. Common parameters for cardiac and stroke rehabilitation will be presented, with a specific care plan for cardiac rehabilitation discussed in Display 6-6 and a specific care plan for stroke rehabilitation discussed in Display 6-7.

The nurse in the home care setting assesses the

1. Client's knowledge of goals of the rehabilitation program
2. Client's present cardiovascular risk factors and contributing factors
3. Ability of the individual/care provider to perform activities of daily living
4. Client's need for assistive devices
5. Client/care provider's knowledge of medications administered, including route, action, frequency, and dosage to be administered, expected side-effects, and toxic effects
6. Client/care provider's ability to purchase, plan, and prepare meals according to recommended diet
7. Client's ability to participate in exercise program prescribed by physician and health care team based on established guidelines
8. Client/care provider's ability to use stress reduction and relaxation techniques
9. Awareness of community support programs

10. Awareness of vendors, surgical suppliers, and equipment
11. Impact of illness on the client and family's lifestyle and interactions with others
12. Family's knowledge and ability to take a pulse and blood pressure
13. Family's knowledge and ability to perform CPR
14. Family's ability to recognize potential complications and react knowledgeably and effectively

## Planning and Implementation for Cardiac Rehabilitation

A brief review of the components of a cardiac rehabilitation program is presented to facilitate home health care planning. The goal of cardiac rehabilitation is to assist the client and family to achieve and maintain an optimal state of health. The three components of the program include exercise, education, and psychological support. The clients must want to achieve the goal through active participation and behavior modification. Candidates for the program include persons diagnosed with recent myocardial infarction, stable angina pectoris, coronary artery bypass surgery, and clinical manifestations of ischemic heart disease.

### Phases of Cardiac Rehabilitation Program

The program is divided into three or four phases, and clients may enter a program by physician referral only.

*Phase I* begins while the client is hospitalized and continues until discharge. Activity progresses from 4 to 16 stages or steps of activity. Clients are usually at 3 to 5 METs at discharge.* Clients and families/significant others are educated about heart disease, risk factor modification, prescribed medications, diet, and home activities.

---

* METs or metabolic equivalents of a task measure the work load of various activities on the pulmonary and cardiovascular system. They are used to measure aerobic exercise, ability and performance of healthy persons involved in endurance training, and in the rehabilitation of pulmonary and cardiovascular clients (Guzetta and Dossey, 1984).

The MET formula is

$$1 \text{ MET} = 3.5 \text{ ml } O_2/\text{kg body weight/minute}$$

Lying at rest quietly = 1 MET of energy expenditure; climbing a flight of stairs = 3.5–4.0 METs; sexual intercourse in a comfortable position with one's usual partner = 3.5–4.0 METs.

An exercise or stress test measures a person's ability to perform work. A treadmill or ergometric bike is used, and the workload is changed every few minutes according to established scientific protocol. Each protocol stage is equivalent to a stated number of METs. The MET numbers then represent the average energy expenditure measured by testing the oxygen content of the air expired by the subject and the body weight of the subject.

*Phase II* begins at the time of hospital discharge and lasts approximately 3 months. The client exercises 2 to 5 times per week under professional supervision and monitoring and should be able to perform 10 METs or more at the time of discharge, with a heart rate goal of 70% to 85% of the rate safely achieved on the initial stress test. Clients and families continue to receive information about heart disease, ways to maintain positive behavior lifestyle changes, and continued emphasis on risk factor reduction and modification.

*Phase III* begins after completion of the training program (Phase II) and should continue for life. This phase is more independent, and the client maintains a level of training by exercising 2 or 3 times per week and adhering to previous changes in lifestyle for continued health promotion behaviors. This phase is designed to maintain physical and cardiovascular fitness and emotional well-being.

The nurse collaborates with other members of the comprehensive rehabilitation team to help the client plan a realistic program. The level of activity following a patient's discharge is individually tailored. The nurse can facilitate the client's rehabilitation by determining what specific aspects of the plan need reinforcement and review and any additional information that should be discussed with the patient and family. Short-term goals will then form the basis for the care plan which is included in Display 6-6.

A general guideline/careplan for the individual at home recovering from a CVA is included in Display 6-7.

## Monitoring of Client Status

Potential complications of cardiac and stroke rehabilitation can be minimized if the client or family/care provider monitor the following parameters. Any abnormal signs and symptoms should be reported immediately to the appropriate health care individual or agency.

1. If angina is experienced for the *first* time, notify the physician for instructions. If the client has nitroglycerin tablets or spray, he or she can take as many as three pills or can use a spray application, each taken 3 minutes apart; if there is no relief, the physician should be notified. If angina occurs during rest, sleep, or a period of inactivity, use nitroglycerin as directed and notify the appropriate health care provider or agency within 12 hours. If pattern, location, severity, or duration of angina changes, use nitroglycerin as directed and notify the appropriate health provider or agency. If any associated symptoms occur for the first time, such as shortness of breath, dizziness, faintness, or unusual weakness, notify the appropriate health care provider or agency.
2. Side-effects of medication are included in Table 6-1.

(*Text continues on p. 184*)

*Display 6-6*
**Cardiac Rehabilitation Care Plan for Client at Home**

*Long-Term Goals (Outcomes)*

At the completion of the cardiac rehabilitation program, the client/care provider will

1. Maximize self-care activities and optimal level of functioning.
2. Demonstrate increased/improved cardiac output.
3. Demonstrate increased/improved peripheral circulation.
4. Demonstrate behaviors that reflect lifestyle changes consistent with the goals of the rehabilitation program.
5. Utilize measures/behaviors to conserve oxygen and energy during activity.
6. Demonstrate reduced anxiety and fear by using effective coping patterns.

*Short-Term Goals (Objectives for Priority Problems)*

**Phase I**
(During hospitalization)

1. Client demonstrates awareness of principles and concepts related to disease, risk factors, behavior modification, and role of exercise.
2. Client demonstrates awareness of diet and prescribed medications.
3. Client verbalizes fears and anxieties regarding recovery and fear of recurring cardiac disease.

**Phase II**
(Begins with discharge from the hospital and lasts up to 3 months)

1. Client demonstrates positive lifestyle changes and modifies risk factors.
2. Client can exercise at a target heart rate goal of 70%–85% of the rate achieved on the initial stress test and remain asymptomatic or perform at 10 METs or greater 2 to 5 times per week.
3. Client uses coping strategies to effectively deal with anxiety, depression, and grief.

*(continued)*

*Display 6-6 (Continued)*
*Short-Term Goals (Objectives for Priority Problems)*
**Phase III**
(After completion of Phase II, and continues indefinitely as an integral part of client's lifestyle)
1. Client continues to maintain total body–mind fitness.
2. Client uses available community resources to maintain fitness.

*Nursing Care Plan (Prescription)*

Only Phase II will be addressed, because Phase I occurs in the hospital setting prior to discharge.

**Initial Visit**

1. In the home, the nurse will review with the client and family the principles and goals of Phase II cardiac rehabilitation, including
   Assessment of client and family's current level of understanding regarding management and treatment of the disease/illness
   What the client considers to be essential to know to cope with the present situation
   Warning signs that need prompt medical attention
   Availability of ambulance and transportation if an emergency arises
   Client's identification of current risk and contributing factors in current lifestyle
2. In the home, the nurse will
   Ask the client to demonstrate taking a pulse and will validate it
   Ask the client to plan a menu based on the prescribed diet
   Ask the client to review medication schedule and actions of drugs.
   Encourage the client to verbalize fears, anxieties, and concerns that he or she is experiencing and explore present coping strategies
   Contract with the client to select *one* risk factor he or she is willing to change
   Provide the client with a list of available community resources to assist with his or her lifestyle changes (e.g., American Cancer Society, American Lung Association, or American Heart Association for smoking cessation programs)

*(continued)*

*Display 6-6 (Continued)*
**Cardiac Rehabilitation Care Plan for Client at Home**

*Subsequent Visits*

1. The nurse
   Communicates with the rehabilitation team and client to assess progress, provide nursing input, review care, and revise goals if necessary.
2. In the home,
   Ask client to prepare a grocery list based on his or her specific diet
   Ask the client to review side-effects/precautions of medications and encourage the client to ask questions that he or she may have
   Ask client to count his or her pulse and validate it with the nurse
   Ask the client to review how he or she has modified or changed *one* risk factor since the last visit
   Contract with the client to continue work on his or her lifestyle modifications, and have the client select one more risk factor to modify or eliminate
   Ask the client if he or she has any questions or concerns about resuming sexual activity. The following guidelines may be helpful:
   · It may be helpful to dispel myths, fears, and concerns about sexual activity and cardiac function. Research has shown that a person with cardiac disease who has intercourse with the usual partner in a comfortable environment has a heart rate of only 120 per minute during a normal 15-second orgasm (Nemec, 1976). This is comparable to climbing one or two flights of stairs or taking a brisk walk (3.5–4 METs). Thus, if a person can tolerate stair-climbing or a brisk walk, sex should not be a problem.
   · It is advised that the client and partner be well rested, wait an hour or two after a heavy meal, choose comfortable positions, and rest afterward.
   · Oral sex places no additional strain on the heart, but anal sex may cause vagal stimulation, which could be dangerous to persons with arrhythmias. Consultation with the physician prior to resuming anal intercourse is advised.

*(continued)*

*Display 6-6 (Continued)*

- It is not uncommon for angina to occur during or after intercourse. The client should follow instructions for nitroglycerin, but remember that the partner may experience the side-effects if they kiss after use. Effects may also be experienced by the partner if a sublingual tablet, spray, or uncovered transdermal paste placed on the chest is used. A plastic wrap may be used to cover the paste. If chest pain or other symptoms persist, the client should notify the physician or appropriate health care provider.
- Tobacco, marijuana, and alcohol should be avoided prior to intercourse.
- Beta blockers, antihypertensives, vasodilators, tranquilizers, and antidepressants may decrease sexual drive or performance. Both the client and his or her partner may need reassurance.

3. Provide reinforcement and encouragement to the client and family to continue health-promoting behaviors and to use all available resources to assist in maximizing their potential.

*Display 6-7*
**CVA (Stroke) Rehabilitation Care Plan
for the Client at Home**

*Long-Term Goals (Outcomes)*

At the end of 3 weeks, the client (client includes individual and/or family/significant other) will

1. Maximize self-care activities and optimal level of functioning.
2. Demonstrate improved ability to express self.
3. Demonstrate reduced anxiety related to lack of knowledge, change in lifestyle, and fear of the unknown.
4. Utilize available community resources for individuals and families recovering from a CVA.
5. Utilize safety measures related to ambulation and self-care.
6. Demonstrate movement toward reconstruction of an altered body image.

*(continued)*

*Display 6-7 (Continued)*
**CVA (Stroke) Rehabilitation Care Plan
for the Client at Home**

*Short-Term Goals (Objectives)*

**Week 1**

1. The client/care provider will verbalize understanding of the major goals of the rehabilitation program.
2. The client/care provider will identify people in the neighborhood who are available to assist in an emergency.
3. The client care provider will demonstrate the ability to perform range of motion (active or passive, based on location and extent of CVA), management of bowel and bladder function, and maintenance of safety.

**Week 2**

1. The client will (considering type of CVA experienced) demonstrate increased ability to communicate.
2. The client/care provider will demonstrate range-of-motion joint exercises, at least 2 to 3 times per day (active or passive, based on condition and health status).
3. The client/care provider will demonstrate understanding of assistive devices used for the client's rehabilitation.

**Week 3**

1. The client/care provider will actively participate in the stroke rehabilitation program.
2. The client will verbalize knowledge of available community resources, including assistive devices and equipment for individuals and families recovering from a CVA.

*Nursing Care Plan*

**Initial Visit**

1. In the home, the nurse will review with the client and family the principles and goals of stroke rehabilitation, including
   Assessment of client and family's current level of understanding regarding management and treatment of their disease/illness
   Written information describing client's specific medical condition

*(continued)*

*Display 6-7 (Continued)*
*Nursing Care Plan*

> A list of assistive devices and equipment that will be needed (including what, where, approximate price, how to order, and a list of available vendors)
> Availability of ambulance or transportation if an emergency arises

2. In the home, the nurse will instruct the client/family member in regard to
   Feeding
   Bathing
   Grooming
   Toileting
   Transfer procedures
   Ambulating
   Range-of-motion exercises (active and passive)

3. In the home, the nurse will provide the client with a list of
   Available community resources to assist with his or her life-style changes and support groups that are available
   Any medications or treatments that the client is receiving, and will encourage questions

4. If communication is impaired, the nurse will review communication interventions that
   Provide alternatives to communication, including verbal, written, gestural approaches, or electronic devices
   Demonstrate and acknowledge the client's frustration
   Promote comprehension

**Subsequent Visits**

1. The nurse will refer, coordinate, and facilitate collaboration with other members of the health care team, including
   Physical therapist
   Occupational Therapist
   Speech pathologist
   Physician

2. The nurse will assess progress, provide input, review care, and revise goals if necessary with client/family. (This should also include a frank discussion with the care provider, assessing his or her coping strategies, and determining whether assistance in the form of respite care, home health aids, and so on, will support the caregiver's role.)

3. Educate and continue to monitor the safety of the client's environment, emphasizing, especially for the client who is regain-

*(continued)*

*Display 6-7 (Continued)*
## CVA (Stroke) Rehabilitation Care Plan for the Client at Home

ing ambulation, skills to
    Provide and evaluate the client's and family's ability to safely and correctly use prescribed assistive devices such as side-rails, handrails, and ramps, raised toilet seats, shower chairs, walkers, and canes
    Re-emphasize safety measures such as removal of scatter rugs and wearing of flat shoes
    Evaluate client's ability to feed him- or herself and avoid foods that may precipitate choking, such as soft breads, semi-cooked vegetables, large pieces of meat, and mashed potatoes
4. Provide reinforcement and encouragement to both the client and family, and continue to use all available resources to assist the client and family to maximize their potential.

**Table 6-1.** *Common Cardiac Medications*

| Drug Classification: Beta Blockers | | Action | Common Side-Effects |
|---|---|---|---|
| **Generic Name** | **Trade Name** | | |
| Nadolol | Corgard | Decrease the workload of | Dizziness, fatigue, |
| Proranolol HCL | Inderal | the heart, lower blood | dyspnea, depression, |
| Metoprolol Tartrate | Lopressor | pressure, antiarrhythmia | bradycardia, vivid dreams |
| Atenolol | Tenormin | | (Abrupt discontinuation can cause rebound angina.) |
| **Drug Classification: Calcium Blockers** | | | |
| **Generic Name** | **Trade Name** | | |
| Diltiazem | Cardiazem | Vasodilator, increases | Dizziness, fatigue, |
| Nifedipine | Procardia | coronary blood flow, | constipation, diarrhea, |
| Verapamil | Calan, Isuptin | helpful in treating angina caused by vasospasm antiarrhythmias | hypotension |
| **Drug Classification: Diuretics** | | | |
| **Generic Name** | **Trade Name** | | |
| Furosemide | Lasix | Reduce total body volume | Weakness, fatigue, |
| Hydrochlorothiazide | Hydrodiuril | of water and salt by | hypotension, nausea, dry |
| Chlorothiazide Sodium | Diuril | increasing urinary | mouth, skin rash |
| Triamterene | Diazide | excretion | (Potassium loss may cause leg cramps; instruct client to supplement diet with citrus fruit, raisins, and bananas.) |

**Table 6-1.** *Common Cardiac Medications (Continued)*

**Drug Classification: Cardiotonic Glycosides**

| Generic Name | Trade Name | | |
|---|---|---|---|
| Digoxin | Lanoxin | Increases cardiac output (strengthen pumping action of heart) | Nausea, decreased or loss of appetite, blurry vision or other visual changes, headaches (Instruct client to take pulse prior to taking medication; if pulse less than 60 or greater than 100, notify physician.) |

**Drug Classification: Antiarrhythmias**

| Generic Name | Trade Name | | |
|---|---|---|---|
| Procainamide HCl | Procan, Pronestyl | Prevent, treat, and control arrhythmias by interfering with conduction of impulses | Dizziness, fatigue, diarrhea, nausea, vomiting |
| Quinidine | Cin-quin | | |
| Disopyramide phosphate | Norpace | | |

**Drug Classification: Antihypertensives**

| Generic Name | Trade Name | | |
|---|---|---|---|
| Methyldopa/ Methyldopate HCl | Aldomet | Lowers blood pressure by vasodilation and relaxation of smooth muscle, and diuretic effect | Dizziness, orthostatic hypotension, rash, tachycardia (Instruct client to change position from lying to sitting, or sitting to standing, slowly.) |
| Hydralazine HCl | Apresoline | | |
| Captopril | Capoten | | |
| Prazosin hydrochloride | Minipress | | |
| Clonidine Hydrochloride | Catapres | | |

**Drug Classification: Anticoagulants**

| Generic Name | Trade Name | | |
|---|---|---|---|
| Aspirin | ASA, Ecotrin, | Use in acute MI is questionable; primary indication for prevention of venous thromboses, pulmonary emboli, and reocclusion of arteries opened by surgery | Observe for sites indicative of bleeding: gums, stools, urine, nosebleeds (Remind clients to keep appointment for blood studies to monitor drug levels.) |
| Dipyridamole | Persantine | | |
| Warfarin sodium/ | Coumadin Sodium | | |
| Warfarin potassium | Panwarfin | | |

**General Suggestions for Clients Taking Cardiac Medication**

1. Take medication as ordered.
2. If nausea or vomiting is experienced for more than 24 hours, notify physician. Serious side-effects can occur if drugs are omitted or abruptly withdrawn.
3. If one dose of a drug is accidentally skipped or missed, *do not* double the next dose. Take only single dose as prescribed.
4. If any new or different side-effects are experienced, contact the physician or appropriate health care person. It is helpful if the client notes any change in routine, schedule, diet, etc.
5. Check with the nurse/physician before taking any medication not prescribed by the physician, including over-the-counter (OTC) preparations. *Ask about food/drug interactions.*
6. Keep a list of medications that are being taken. A sample sheet might include the following information: *Date Drug Dosage/Frequency/Day Specific Times Instructions/Comments.*
7. When going to the doctor or if admitted to the hospital, bring this record with you.

3. If symptoms of exercise intolerance persist, notify the physician immediately. Report chest discomfort, lightheadedness, shortness of breath, dizziness, nausea, palpitations, irregular heartbeat, or increasing fatigue.
4. Pacemaker malfunction and related complications are explained in Table 6-2.

**Table 6-2.** *Troubleshooting Pacemakers in the Home*

| Potential Problems | Signs and Symptoms | Suggested Intervention |
| --- | --- | --- |
| Alteration in skin integrity related to surgical incision and pacemaker insertion | Pain, tenderness, redness, swelling, drainage, fever, bleeding | Notify physician; apply prescribed medications; monitor incision |
| Alteration in comfort related to incisional pain and reduced movement of upper extremity | Pain, restricted range of motion "frozen shoulder" | Perform range-of-motion position, relaxation, guided imagery |
| Knowledge deficit related to | | |
| Environmental and equipment precautions | Interference may be manifested by awareness of slowed pacemaker rate and transient dizziness | *Avoid electromagnetic interference:* microwave oven, arc welding, electric motors, gasoline engines, some burglar alarms, power transmitters, antennas for TV and radio. If symptoms are experienced, move away from area and notify physician. |
| Activity precautions temporary restrictions | Dizziness, weakness, shortness of breath, former symptoms will recur | No automobile driving, lifting, sports such as golf, bowling, swimming for 1 month (may dislodge pacing lead) |
| Permanent restrictions | Vibration can cause thrombosis of vein where lead is positioned; venous congestion of extremity may occur | Avoid all contact sports, equipment that produces an arm vibration, lawn mower, snow blower, serving overhand (tennis). Avoid use of electric shaver directly *over* generator. |

***Table 6-2.*** *Troubleshooting Pacemakers in the Home (Continued)*

| Potential Problems | Signs and Symptoms | Suggested Intervention |
|---|---|---|
| Anxiety related to fear of syncope episode, malfunction, and lack of knowledge about pacemaker function | If malfunction occurs former symptoms will recur | Encourage client to verbalize anxiety and fears. Instruct client about signs and symptoms of pacemaker malfunction. Instruct client to take pulse periodically. Give client card with pacemaker settings. (Phone monitoring is available for homebound clients.) Physician will need to monitor pacemaker's "end of life indicator". |

## Evaluation

The outcome criteria presented at the beginning of this section are used to evaluate the client's progress, make recommendations, and revise the care plan. Criteria are reviewed in relation to client/family satisfaction and standards of home health care. It is important for the client and the care provider to understand that cardiovascular disease is a chronic, progressive illness; there will be periods of remission, but there is also disease progression. The nurse needs to offer realistic hope and attainable goals to assist the client in maximizing his or her optimal health potential.

## References

American Association of Respiratory Therapy Times 8:28–31, 1984

Apnea Monitor Alert. Am J Nurs 85(10):1051, 1985

Cardiovascular Disorders. Springhouse, PA, Springhouse Corporation, 1984

Carpenito L: Nursing Diagnosis Application to Clinical Practice. Philadelphia, JB Lippincott, 1983

Carroll P: Caring for ventilator patients. Nursing 86, 2(16):34–39, 1986

Czarniecki L: Caring for a young child with a tracheostomy. Caring 4(5):30–32, 1985

Fuchs P: Understanding continuous mechanical ventilation. Nursing 79, 12(9):26–33, 1979

Guzetta C, Dossey B: Cardiovascular Nursing: Bodymind Tapestry. St Louis, Mosby, 1984

Harris R, Hyman R: Clean vs sterile tracheostomy care and level of pulmonary infection. Nursing Research 2(33):80–84, 1984

Hazinski M: Pediatric home tracheostomy care: A parents guide. Pediatric Nursing 1(12):41–48, 69, 1986

Hogstel M: Home Nursing Care for the Elderly. Bowie, Prentice-Hall, 1985

Jackson D: Nursing care plan: Home management of children with BPD. Pediatric Nursing 12(5):342–348, 1986

Johnson D: Ventilator-Assisted Patient Care. Rockville, Aspen, 1986

Kenner CV, Guzetta C, Dossey B: Critical Care Nursing. Body-Mind-Spirit. Boston, Little, Brown and Co, 1985

Millar S: AACN Procedure Manual for Critical Care. Philadelphia, WB Saunders, 1985

Nemec E: Heart rate and blood pressure responses during sexual activity in normal males. American Heart Journal 92:274, 1976

Norris-Berkemeyer S, Hutchins K: Home apnea monitoring. Pediatric Nursing 4(12):259–262, 304, 1986

Oxygen Therapy. Springhouse, PA, Springhouse Corporation, 1986

Sager D: The person requiring cardiac pacing. In Guzetta CE, Dossey BM: (eds): Cardiovascular Nursing: Bodymind Tapestry. St Louis, Mosby, 1984

Steffl B (ed): Handbook of Gerontological Nursing. New York, Van Nostrand Reinhold Co, 1984

Wyka K: Oxygen concentrators. Rx Home Care 6(12):60–74, 1984

# 7

# Diagnostic Cluster: Fluid, Nutrition, and Elimination Patterns

The introduction and availability of advanced health care in the home care setting combined with early discharge from the hospital have resulted in the use of sophisticated technology to treat hydration and to provide drug therapy and nutritional support to the client in the home care setting. The client, family and/or support system, and home health nurse must understand the principles related to treatment and to utilization and maintenance of equipment in the home care setting.

## Nursing Diagnoses

Nursing diagnoses identified with the diagnostic cluster and related to the selected focus of nursing care are listed here so that they may be incorporated into a plan of care for the client at home.

Bowel elimination, alterations in
Fluid volume deficit
Fluid volume excess
Infection, potential for
Knowledge deficit
Nutrition, alteration in, less than body requirements
Nutrition, alteration in, more than body requirements
Sexual dysfunction
Skin integrity, impairment of
Urinary elimination, alteration in

# Parenteral Therapy

Increasing numbers of patients who require parenteral and enteral infusions are discharged from the hospital. This section focuses on the principles and concepts of parenteral therapy, with emphasis on continuous and intermittent intravenous therapy, including discussion of infusion control devices, and vascular access devices. Suggested outcome criteria with specific interventions and troubleshooting action for the person, family, and health care provider in the home setting are included for each of the three selected areas.

## Selected Diagnoses From Fluid and Nutritional Patterns Related to Parenteral Therapy

Fluid volume deficit
Infection, potential for
Nutrition, alteration in, less than body requirements
Knowledge deficit

When an individual is unable to ingest food or fluid orally, the most common method of replacement is intravenous infusion therapy. Intravenous therapy may be administered on a continuous or on an intermittent basis. Continuous intravenous therapy is usually indicated for the individual who requires prolonged fluid and nutritional support. Intermittent therapy is usually indicated for short-term treatment and may include the administration of medications. Intermittent devices or heparin wells, however, reduce the risk of circulatory overload and electrolyte imbalance. In addition, intermittent devices may increase client comfort and mobility.

The selection of a specific parenteral fluid is dependent upon the individual's normal requirements and present health and hydration status. Major parenteral fluids are listed in Table 7-1, with key points briefly discussed.

## Parenteral Therapy Solutions

*Hypertonic solutions* are dextrose-based solutions commonly used to replace electrolytes and to bring about a fluid shift from within the cells to the plasma. Slow administration of these solutions reduces the chance of circulatory overload. Dextrose 5% in 0.9% saline, dextrose 5% in lactated Ringer's solution, and dextrose 10% in lactated Ringer's solution are commonly used hypertonic solutions.

*Hypotonic solutions* are usually saline-based solutions employed to shift fluid from plasma into the interstitial fluid. Half-normal saline (0.45% NaCl) is a commonly used solution.

*Isotonic solutions* may be dextrose-, saline-, or electrolyte-based and expand extracellular fluid volume. Lactated Ringer's solution, dextrose 5% in water, and normal saline (0.9% NaCl) are the solutions most commonly used in the home setting.

## Infusion Control Devices

The use of electronic infusion control devices to assist in monitoring intravenous fluid administration is becoming more common in the home. Electronic infusion control devices (ICDs) are proving to be more consistent than manual clamps and may be safer because of their built-in alarm systems. In addition, they may help to ensure that the patient is receiving the prescribed amount of solution and/or medication at the correct rate. However, no device replaces the continued need for observation and monitoring of the IV site, equipment, and patient responses to treatment. There are only *two* types of ICDs: the **gravity controller** and the **infusion pump**. Both are available in volumetric or nonvolumetric models (Koszuta, 1984).

*Gravity controllers* are basically electronic flow clamps that use the force of gravity to infuse fluid into a vessel by applying and releasing pressure on the tubing until a preset rate or volume is met. Electronic sensors count the drops as they fall. Gravity controllers are used *more* often than infusion pumps, because gravity usually provides the fluid pressure necessary to overcome the resistance of the patient's pressure. *Caution:* Infiltration will *not* be detected by use of a controller alone unless the flow rate or volume decreases. (That is, the IV catheter or needle may have punctured the vessel wall and may be infusing solution interstitially. As long as the flow rate or volume remains the same, the alarm will not sound and the solution will continue to flow. However, the alarm will sound when the solution container is empty, when air is present in the system, or when there is a change in the flow rate.)

*Infusion pumps* infuse fluid by generating their own positive pressure to overcome the resistance of the patient's pressure (Huey, 1983). They are not affected by container height. Infusion pumps can be used when a low or a high fluid rate is required (Koszuta, 1984). Most infusion pumps are volumetric models, although they are also available in nonvolumetric models.

Infusion pumps may be classified according to their delivery mechanism and may include syringe, peristaltic, and cassette pumps. *Caution:* Infusion pumps may not detect infiltrations unless enough back pressure is present to trigger the alarm. In the presence of other complications, such as a line occlusion, to compensate for the resistance, the infusion pump will increase

*Table 7-1.* Intravenous Fluids

| Solutions | Nonelectrolyte Constituents | Cations/Liter | | | Anion/Liter | | Calories/Liter | pH | Tonicity | Comments |
|---|---|---|---|---|---|---|---|---|---|---|
| | | Na | K | Ca | Cl | Lactate | | | | |
| **Dextrose in water** | | | | | | | | | | |
| Dextrose 5% | Dextrose | | | | | | 170 | 4.8 | Isotonic | Does not replace electrolytes or correct fluid deficit; irritates veins; hemolyzes red cells |
| Dextrose 10% | Dextrose | | | | | | 340 | 4.7 | Hypertonic | |
| Dextrose 20% | Dextrose | | | | | | 680 | 4.8 | Hypertonic | |
| **Dextrose in Saline** | | | | | | | | | | |
| Dextrose 5%/saline 0.2% | Dextrose | 34 | | | 34 | | 170 | 4.6 | Isotonic | Provides calories, Na, water, and |
| Dextrose 5%/saline 0.45% | Dextrose | 77 | | | 77 | | 170 | 4.6 | Hypertonic | |

| Solution | Additive | Na | K | Ca | Cl | Lactate | Calories | pH | Tonicity | Uses |
|---|---|---|---|---|---|---|---|---|---|---|
| Dextrose 5%/saline 0.9% | Dextrose | 154 | | | 154 | | 170 | 4.4 | Hypertonic | |
| Dextrose 10%/saline 0.9% | Dextrose | 154 | | | 154 | | 340 | 4.8 | Hypertonic | Cl; treats hypovolemia and promotes diuresis if dehydrated |
| **Saline** | | | | | | | | | | |
| 0.45% Sodium chloride | | 77 | | | 77 | | | 5.9 | Hypertonic | Supplies daily salt and water; used as routine electrolyte replacement |
| 0.9% Sodium chloride | | 154 | | | 154 | | | 6.0 | Isotonic | |
| **Multiple Electrolytes** | | | | | | | | | | |
| Ringer's | | 147 | 4 | 4.5 | 155.5 | | | 6.0 | Isotonic | Replaces Na, Cl, K, Ca similar to ECF concentration used in vomiting/G.I.; provides calories |
| Lactated Ringer's | | 130 | 4 | 3 | 109 | 28 | 9 | 6.5 | Isotonic | |
| 5% Dextrose/LR | Dextrose | 130 | 4 | 3 | 109 | 28 | 179 | 5.1 | Hypertonic | |
| 10% Dextrose/LR | Dextrose | 130 | 4 | 3 | 109 | 28 | 349 | 4.9 | Hypertonic | |

pressure in an attempt to deliver the solution. If this is unsuccessful, an alarm will sound.

Gravity controllers and infusion pumps, as mentioned previously, are available in volumetric and nonvolumetric models. Volumetric ICDs deliver a specific volume of fluid at a specific rate. This device is used most often for long-term or continuous infusions (i.e., hyperalimentation). Volumetric devices are also more accurate than nonvolumetric models. Nonvolumetric ICDs deliver fluids at a specific drop rate. They are used most often for short-term therapy but are considered less accurate than a volumetric device, because the drop size is affected by density, viscosity, temperature, and surface tension of the fluid.

## Venous Access Devices

Recent developments in venous access devices have resulted in increased mobility and greater freedom for the client who once required prolonged hospitalization for hydration, medication, and nutrition. There are basically two types of venous access devices (VADs): the *external venous access device* and the *implantable access device*, which is also referred to as subcutaneous venous access device or implantable port.

Generally, the external venous access devices include the silicone silastic atrial catheters (e.g., Hickman/Broviac, Corcath, Raaf, and Groshong) and the small-gauge central venous catheters (e.g., Intrasil and Centrasil). The atrial catheters, however, are most commonly used in the home setting and will be discussed briefly.

The silicone silastic atrial catheters have several common characteristics. The catheters are single or double lumen with a Dacron polyester fiber cuff to anchor the catheter subcutaneously and reduce the risk of ascending infection. Insertion of the catheter is done under local or general anesthesia. A small incision is made in the neck region (insertion site) to access either the cephalic, internal, or external jugular vein, although any vessel large enough to accommodate the catheter can be used. Forceps are used to form a subcutaneous tunnel from the incision to about the level of the fourth or fifth intercostal space on the chest (approximately between the sternum and the nipple). The tips of the forceps, when brought out through the skin, create a catheter exit site. The catheter is grasped and gently pulled through the tunnel, with the Dacron cuff being positioned subcutaneously. An estimation of the catheter length needed to reach the right atrium is made; the catheter is then trimmed and inserted into the vessel. Correct placement is verified by x-ray (catheter is radiopaque) or fluoroscopy. The incision (insertion site) used to initially isolate the vessel is closed, and, at the exit site, a single stitch may be used to secure the catheter until the Dacron cuff is anchored by tissue growth (Figure 7-1).

Until recently, most central line catheters were open-ended and required

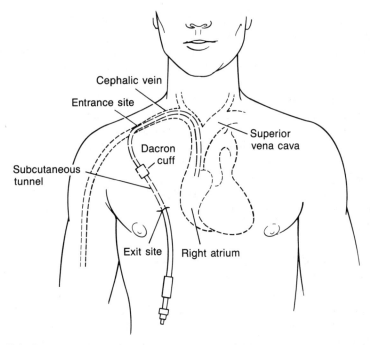

Figure 7-1. Position of external venous access device (Hickman catheter) on the chest wall.

heparin locks and routine flushes. However, the Groshong central venous catheter incorporates a unique closed-end tip design. A two-way slit valve is in the sidewall of the catheter adjacent to the tip. The slit valve opens outward during fluid infusion and inward for sample withdrawal. The two-way valve on the catheter closes when not in use, preventing blood from entering the catheter and eliminating the need for routine heparin irrigations. Unlike open-ended catheters, the valve design prevents air embolism caused by the venturi effect of blood flowing around the tip of the catheter. The potential for air embolism or blood loss during a temporary catheter disconnection is reduced greatly (Cath Tech, 1985).

Implanted infusion ports or subcutaneous venous access devices consist of a self-sealing septum encased in a port made of metal or plastic attached to a catheter (Winters, 1984). The port is a one-piece unit (e.g., Infuse-a-Port, MediPort) or a two-piece unit (e.g., Port-a-Cath). The ports are single or dual, and the catheters vary in lumen diameter (Wilkes et al, 1985).

Catheters are placed in a vein or artery. Venous access is used for fluids, drug therapy, blood products, and blood samples, whereas arterial ports are used for specific regional drug therapy. Use of an implantable venous access device for home total parenteral nutrition (TPN) or hyperalimentation is usually *not* recommended because of the frequency of daily needle puncture, potential complications of skin breakdown and infection, and additional cost of equipment.

Insertion of the implantable venous access device is usually done under local anesthesia as an outpatient procedure. The catheter is tunneled to various sites, for example, by means of a vein to the right atrium or by way of the hepatic artery for arterial placement. Additional sites may include the peritoneal cavity or epidural space. A subcutaneous tunnel is created from the catheter insertion site to a subcutaneous pocket in the anterior chestwall that holds the port. Optimally, the port is created over a bony prominence usually near the distal third of the clavicle. In obese or large-breasted clients, the port may be inserted where there is less adipose tissue, that is, more midline, near the clavicle. In women, however, to avoid irritation from a bra strap, the port is not placed at the mid-clavicular line (Figure 7-2).

## Etiology and Defining Characteristics

Fluid volume deficit as defined by Carpenito (1983) is "the state in which the individual experiences or is at risk of experiencing vascular, cellular, or intracellular dehydration," (p 185). Etiologic and contributing factors may include diabetes, dehydration, shock, cancer, infection, fever, burns, surgery, vomiting, diarrhea, difficulty in swallowing or in feeding oneself.

## Focus of Nursing Care

Continuous and intermittent intravenous therapy, including use of
Infusion control devices
Vascular access devices

## Outcome Criteria

The person (or family or care provider) will

1. Identify the principles and concepts related to intravenous therapy
2. Identify the principles and concepts related to vascular access devices
3. Demonstrate the ability to use intravenous therapy equipment competently and confidently
4. Demonstrate the ability to use vascular access devices competently and confidently
5. Identify complications of intravenous therapy and appropriate interventions in the home care setting
6. Identify complications of vascular access devices and appropriate interventions in the home care setting
7. Maintain an intake of a minimum of 2000 ml to 2500 ml daily

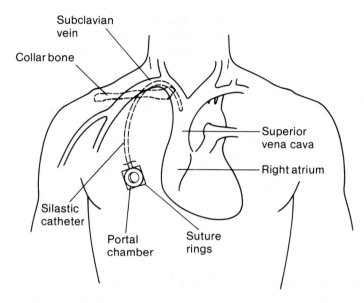

Figure 7-2. Venous access device: Implanted infusion port.

## Application of the Nursing Process

### Assessment

Total body water (TBW) in the adult constitutes 55% to 60% of total body weight. Body water, however, will vary with age, sex, weight, and lean body mass. To approximate fluid replacement in an individual who, for example, has lost 3 lb in 2 days, consider that 60% of 3 lb is about 2 lb, or 1000 ml of fluid, that needs to be replaced in addition to minimal daily fluid requirements.

A brief systems review assessing the individual for fluid balance deficit may reveal dry conjunctiva, decreased tearing, dry mucous membranes, increased viscosity of saliva, and dry, cracked tongue, with generalized decreased skin turgor, change in temperature (may be increased or decreased), and increased or decreased pulse rate, with a narrow or decreased pulse pressure. For systolic blood pressure to drop, however, a 15% to 25% volume deficit must occur. Postural blood pressure changes are indicative of volume depletion and may appear before other cardiovascular changes. A postural decrease is defined as a drop of 15 mm Hg in either systolic or diastolic pressure, or a pulse increase of 20 beats per minute when the patient sits or stands.

Fluid balance excess may be reflected by periorbital edema, a bounding pulse, jugular vein distention, increased respiratory rate, dyspnea, dependent edema, and warm moist skin. Weight losses or gains of greater than 5% of total body weight suggest dehydration or overhydration.

Once it has been determined that the client will need to receive intravenous therapy, the nurse will need to assess

1. Client-related factors that may affect ability to administer intravenous therapy at home safely and competently (Display 7-1).
2. Suitability of home environment to perform procedure(s)
3. Literacy skills, availability of telephone, and transportation
4. Availability of "back-up person" for assistance when needed
5. Preparation, handling, storage, and disposal of sterile, clean, contaminated, and used equipment

(*Text continues on p. 198*)

---

*Display 7-1*
### Checklist: Planning for Home IV Therapy

*Client-Related*

Age:
Present diagnosis:
  Health status:
  Cardiac
  Renal (including baseline 24-hour urinary output)
Present condition:
Vital signs:
Movement, activity level:
Preferred venipuncture site:
Vessel patency
  (Hx phlebitis, extravasations)
Ability to perform self-care, level of understanding, literacy skills:
Financial resources/constraints:

*Environment*

    Family or care provider literacy skills (e.g., ability to read, tell
      time):
    Family ability to perform care and use equipment correctly and
      safely:
    Assistive resources:
      Ability to summon help (i.e., telephone, neighbor,
      communications system hookup with hospital or health
      care agency)

*continued*

*Display 7–1 (Continued)*

*Environment*

> Availability or professional home care staff
> Availability of space for use and storage and for disposal of equipment
> Availability of vendors, surgical supply houses
> Back-up system if electrical power fails

*Equipment*

> Solution: type, volume, rate, temperature, viscosity potential for extravasation
> Container: height, pressure, vented or nonvented
> Catheter/needle: length, gauge, accessories
> Intermittent device (heparin well):
> Filter:
> Tubing (diameter and length):
> Venous access devices (external or implanted):
> > Site
> > Needles for accessing devices, if indicated
> > Tubing
> > Additional equipment/accessories
> Infusion control devices:
> > Pump (volumetric or nonvolumetric)
> > Controller (volumetric or nonvolumetric)
> > Amount of fluid in drip chamber
> > Drip sensor position
> > Cassette (i.e., is priming necessary)
> > Loading/attaching set to venipuncture
> > Purge mode
> > Rate setting (ml/hr = volumetric)
> > (gtt/min = nonvolumetric)
> > Alarm features, which can indicate:
> > > Low battery or battery failure
> > > Empty solution container
> > > Air or line detection
> > > Clot formation
> > > Infiltration
> > > Malpositioned catheter/needle
> > > Clogged filter
> > > Malpositioned drop sensor
> > > Flow or rate variation

6. Ability of the client or care provider to recognize potential complications and react knowledgeably
7. Impact of intravenous therapy on client or family lifestyle and coping ability

## Planning

The client or care provider considers the following when planning to use IV therapy. (Display 7-1 serves as a guide for planning intravenous therapy.)

### General Equipment Considerations

1. Make arrangements with a pharmacy or surgical supply company or vendor to purchase solutions. Consider the cost, operating hours, delivery, and related equipment rental.
2. Containers and solutions are verified for correct solution, strength, volume, and expiration date.
3. Bottles and/or bags are examined for cracks, leaks, or punctures.
4. Solution should be clear. (If discolored or cloudy or if precipitate is present, discard, and select a new solution.)
5. Port on bag or cap over port on bottle is secure and intact (unless medication was previously added, in which instance the bottle or bag would be labeled).
6. Selection of tubing will depend upon the amount of fluid to be delivered, the client's health status, and the type of solution. A microdrip system (1 ml = 60 drops) may be used if a small amount of fluid is to be delivered. A macrodrip system (10 drops = 1 ml, or 15 drops = 1 ml) will deliver solutions in larger quantities and faster rates than will microdrip systems. *Note:* The drop factor is always indicated on the tubing box.
7. Venting
   a. A standard bottle with no built-in air vent requires vented tubing.
   b. A bottle with a built-in air vent requires *non*vented tubing.
   c. Plastic bags may require nonvented tubing because the bag will compress as the solution flows out.
8. Tubing
   a. Primary tubing is used with continuous solutions and usually contains ports to add medications or piggyback solutions or medications.
   b. Secondary tubing is shorter in length, is usually attached to a primary line by a needle, and is used to infuse medications or solutions intermittently.
   c. Extension tubing extends the existing tubing by 10 to 12 inches.

It is used for the attachment of a filter and/or for use with an infusion control device. In some instances, it provides greater movement and mobility for the patient.

9. IV stands or poles can be rented or purchased from surgical suppliers or vendors. However, the client or care provider may want to check insurance coverage first before purchasing these items. Depending upon the vendor, IV stands may be supplied with the equipment at no additional cost. Clients should also contact local volunteer organizations with loan closets (e.g., American Cancer Society) that lend equipment at no cost to the client. Local social service departments are also helpful in obtaining information about available resources. Some individuals are very innovative and create their own devices using coat racks, coat hangers, and other household items.

10. ICD selection should be based on the client's present medical condition; solution type, volume, and viscosity; whether or not positive pressure is indicated; size of needle or cannula being used; degree of accuracy needed and rate required, and availability of equipment (Display 7-2).

## Planning for Insertion of a Peripheral Line

When selecting the appropriate needle or catheter, the home health care nurse should consider

1. *Condition of veins.* Repeated venipunctures may cause inflammation, varicosity, scarring, or sclerosing. The vein selected should be soft, full, and unobstructed. Medications such as steroids and cancer chemotherapeutic agents may increase vessel fragility and hamper venous access.

2. *Health status of patient.* Age, activity level, and present nutritional status will affect venipuncture site selection. Avoid an edematous arm or lower extremities because of the risk of infection or phlebitis. Do *not* use an extremity that was previously used for a shunt or fistula if sensation is diminished (hemiplegia) or if a previous extravasation occurred. If a patient had a mastectomy, the arm on the operative site is not used for venipunctures or parenteral therapy.

3. *Length of therapy anticipated.* If long-term therapy is anticipated, choose a vein at the most distal site (preferably the hand) that allows for subsequent access sites in the forearm and antecubital fossa area if necessary. Consider the hand orientation of the patient, and try to select a site away from areas of flexion; otherwise, stabilize with an armboard. In patients younger than 60 years of age, the metacarpal veins are the best initial insertion site, because they are splinted by the bones of the hand. Long-term therapy, however, may ne-

(*Text continues on p. 201*)

*Display 7-2*
**Guidelines for Selecting Infusion Control Devices**

*Remember:* When making a decision, first determine whether a gravity controller or infusion pump is indicated. Then determine whether a volumetric or nonvolumetric model is indicated. (There may be circumstances in which either a pump or controller is appropriate, and one must consider which piece of equipment is the safest and most effective.

*Present Health Status of Client*

**Controllers**
These may be safer for specific populations, including children, the elderly, and cancer patients who have been receiving chemotherapy. Their vessels may be more fragile and more susceptible to infiltration. The infusion pump, however, has the ability to add pressure to an IV line to overcome resistance to flow. If the maximal pressure of the pump is not able to overcome the occlusion, the alarm will be triggered. However, an infiltration will *not* always cause enough pressure to set off the alarm, and the use of a pump could actually increase the severity of an infiltration. This is why the controller is often recommended rather than the infusion pump.

In addition, pumps are seldom recommended for peripheral lines. However, if the solution is viscous or if the patient's activity restricts gravity flow and a filter is in use with the IV, there may be indications for the use of a pump.

Patients with a cardiac or renal history may require an ICD with *volumetric* accuracy to restore or maintain fluid balance if they are receiving fluid over a long period of time (i.e., total parenteral nutrition).

**Solutions and Route**
Highly viscous solutions, such as hyperalimentation, may require the use of a pump, especially if the rate is greater than 100 ml/hour. Other factors that may decrease the flow rate and warrant the use of a pump rather than a controller include decreased temperature of solution to be infused, variable or increased vascular pressure (e.g., patients with congestive heart failure or pulmonary edema), and the use of a filter.

As mentioned previously, pumps are usually not used with peripheral lines. A pump is indicated, however, with the use of intra-arterial chemotherapy, such as hepatic artery infusions.

*continued*

*Display 7–2 (Continued)*

**Positive Pressure**

Infusion pumps are required to deliver intra-arterial chemotherapy, thus overcoming the resistance of arterial blood pressure. In addition, pumps may be recommended to administer viscous solutions such as hyperalimentation and when filters are in use to prevent clogging and backflow. Pumps have also been recommended in central line infusions (i.e., by a subclavian line). A *very* important word of caution, however; if pumps are used with central line catheters, such as Hickman or Broviac, a pump could exert enough pressure to "blow" the line. If an occlusion occurs within the catheter, the pump may continue to exert increased pressure to overcome the resistance, and, if there are any weakened areas within the walls of the catheter, added pressure may result in rupture, leakage, or severage of the catheter. An additional risk may exist if a filter is added to a central line, slowing the rate and possibly "clogging" the filter and increasing the pressure of the pump to overcome the resistance that may actually "blow" the line apart. If the IV becomes disconnected, the alarm on the pump will *not* sound if the pump is delivering fluid at a constant volume, whereas nonvolumetric models deliver fluid at a constant drop rate. Drop size, however, varies with the viscosity of the solution used, so that the flow rate will vary depending upon the solution being used. Generally, long-term infusions such as hyperalimentation, will use volumetric ICDs. Consideration should also be given to children, to the elderly, and to patients with any medical conditions that warrant close observation and maintenance of strict fluid and electrolyte balance (e.g., burns, cardiac or renal disorders).

Short-term drug administration may necessitate the use of a nonvolumetric model to deliver the medication at a constant drop rate in order to titrate the drug according to the patient's response.

cessitate the insertion of a central line and venous access device (Figure 7-3).

4. *Solution to be infused.* Large veins may be used for hypertonic, acidic, alkaline, highly viscous, or caustic (extravasating) solutions. The amount of solution to be infused is also considered. Rapid infusion necessitates larger veins or may require the use of a central vein.
5. *Needle selection.* When selecting a needle or catheter, the smaller the gauge number, the larger the size needle or catheter. Always use the smallest gauge IV device that delivers the infusion. Plastic catheters are more flexible and are less likely to puncture vessel walls

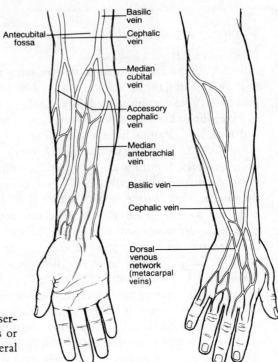

Figure 7-3. Sites for the insertion of intravenous needles or catheters for parenteral therapy.

than are steel needles. They are usually recommended for use in the home. Because plastic catheters are more likely to be used for a longer period of time, they increase the risk of phlebitis or infection. Plastic catheters introduce the risks of catheter embolism or allergic reaction. Steel needles *may* be recommended for intermittent or short-term therapy, because they cause less vessel trauma upon insertion and are less likely to produce an allergic reaction.

6.  *Venipuncture tips.* Explaining the procedure to the client and family helps reduce anxiety. Anxiety can produce a vasomotor response leading to venous constriction, which affects dilation of a vein. If it is difficult to locate a vein after applying a tourniquet, opening and closing the fist, or hanging the arm down and gently tapping the extremity, it may be helpful to have the client soak both arms in a sink filled with warm water. Other methods include the use of a hot pack, a heating pad, or a low heat dryer with the intent of selecting an appropriate site for venipuncture. If a heating pad or blow dryer is used, the nurse places her hand next to the patient's skin while the heat is applied to assess whether the temperature is too warm. Tapping or slapping of the hand or arm is done cau-

tiously, because this may be injurious to an individual with delicate vessels.

To reduce the incidence of phlebitis, the smallest gauge needle or cannula is used. It facilitates blood flow around the cannula within the vein and decreases irritation. Heparin locks also reduce the risk of phlebitis and are considered for use, especially with intermittent infusions. They decrease the amount of cannula manipulation and reduce the mechanical irritation of the vein.

Skin preparation materials are at room temperature to avoid vasoconstriction of the vein as the skin is cleansed. Some clients are allergic to iodine-containing compounds; thus, the skin should only be cleansed with alcohol.

## Implementation

### Venipuncture Technique

1. Explain the procedure to the client and family. Allow the opportunity for questions to decrease anxiety and to gain the client's trust and support. Briefly review the client's present health status and assess upper extremities for potential venipuncture sites. If soaking of the extremities is required, this should be initiated while gathering equipment.

2. Decide whether a local anesthetic will be used to reduce the pain of venipuncture. This remains a controversial issue, and a review of agency policy is recommended. Lidocaine is frequently the drug of choice. A 25- or 27-gauge needle is used to inject 0.1 ml to 0.2 ml of either 0.5% or 0.1% intradermally.

3. Select venipuncture site and apply tourniquet. The vein selected should appear and feel distended and swollen. *Note:* If the tourniquet is too loose, the vein will remain flat; if the tourniquet is too tight, the pulse is not palpable. In patients 60 years and younger, the metacarpal veins are the best initial insertion site, because they are splinted by the bones of the hand. However, if the infusion warrants a larger vein, the basilic or cephalic vein is a better choice. In patients older than 60 years of age, diminished sensation and decreased subcutaneous tissue in the hand necessitate selection of an IV site other than the hand, such as the basilic or cephalic vein. Avoid the median antebrachial vein, because this site is too near the radial nerve and radial artery.

4. Prepare the skin with providone-iodine or according to agency policy. Shaving the skin prior to venipuncture if the hair is excessive facilitates patency of the catheter dressing and reduces pain when removing the tape. If the client is immunosuppressed, has a low

platelet count, or is receiving anticoagulant therapy, discuss shaving with the physician, because it may be contraindicated or the use of an electric razor may be recommended. Shaving may actually cause abrasions and, in some cases, open the skin to infection.

5.  When performing the venipuncture, pierce the skin with the needle at a 20- to 45-degree angle, with the bevel upward and lateral to the vein. The skin is stretched below the intended puncture site to help stabilize the vein. Advance the needle through the skin, and, as the vein is entered, a slight resistance may be felt. When a blood flashback is observed behind the needle, the needle is tilted upward slightly before advancing to reduce the risk of puncturing the posterior vein. *Remember:* Once the venipuncture has been performed, blood flashback has been observed behind the needle, and the cannula has been stabilized, *release the tourniquet* and attach the administration set to the needle.

6.  Apply the antimicrobial ointment if indicated (this may vary according to agency policy), avoiding tension or pressure at the site that could dislodge the needle or catheter.

7.  Stabilize the needle or catheter and tubing to prevent irritation of the vein and reduce the risk of phlebitis.

8.  Apply a dressing to the IV site; this can be a dry sterile dressing or a polyurethane adhesive dressing. Polyurethane dressings may save time and reduce catheter manipulation. Polyurethane dressings such as Op-site and Tegaderm are sterile, transparent, and occlusive yet semipermeable. These dressings are waterproof and, because of their pliability, conform to the client's anatomic structure. Water vapor and air escape from the covered site, which reduces skin maceration, yet the dressing protects the skin from water or bacteria; thus, the dressing may be left in place for up to 72 hours or, in some instances, longer. The major advantage of the polyurethane dressing is that it is transparent and allows visualization of the site without removing the dressing and reduces the risk of infection and catheter manipulation.

    Additional suggestions for observation of clients:

    a.  Signs and symptoms of sensitivity to polyurethane dressings include generalized redness, skin reactions, itching, and discomfort, which should be reported to the appropriate health provider. Emphasize to the client or care provider to *first* rule out infection, then consider skin sensitivity.

    b.  Avoid placing tape to secure the IV line on the polyurethane dressing, because it will necessitate removing the dressing each time that the IV is retaped. When removing the polyurethane dressing, remind the client to use an alcohol wipe to moisten the edge of the dressing, which makes it easier to remove.

9. It is helpful to suggest the use of an armboard to stabilize the extremity if the client is active. A folded newspaper or magazine, ruler, or child's block wrapped with Kerlix or Kling works well. The hand is positioned over the end of the armboard. Remind the client or care provider not to flatten or extend the hand, because this may immobilize the hand in a nonfunctional position, and risk nerve damage.

## Insertion of Intermittent IV Devices

1. After gathering equipment, fill the injection cap and extension tubing (if used) with the heparinized solution to avoid introducing air into the system prior to performing the venipuncture.
2. Follow the suggested procedure previously reviewed in steps 3 through 6 of the venipuncture techniques for insertion of the catheter or needle. Then attach the primed injection cap and tubing to the catheter hub. (There is some equipment that is available with a catheter attached to the tubing and a heparin cap at the end of the tubing. Regardless of the type of equipment for an intermittent device, the emphasis is to prime the system with a heparinized solution to avoid introducing air.)
3. Before securing the needle or catheter, determine the patency of the vessel. Cleanse the injection port with an alcohol wipe and aspirate for a blood return and then slowly inject 1 ml to 2 ml of normal saline, observing for signs of infiltration. *Note:* If normal saline, rather than heparin, is used each time to assess patency initially, it will reduce the chance of further tissue irritation if infiltration is present.
4. If the IV is patent after the injection of normal saline, withdraw the syringe and reinsert a second syringe filled with 1 ml to 2 ml of heparinized solution and inject slowly to minimize irritation. The heparinized solution aids in preventing clot formation.
5. After injecting the heparinized solution, secure the catheter, apply the povidone ointment, and cover the site with a dry sterile dressing or transparent dressing.
6. The same procedure for labeling and recording information regarding the date, time, and size of catheter is followed.

   *Note:* Some agencies use different concentrations of heparinized solutions (e.g., 100 U/ml or 10 U/ml). To ensure accuracy, verify the prescribed solution with the physician. Because there are several brands of heparin solution prepared by different pharmaceutical firms, preservatives used in the heparin solution may vary. Patients have been known to develop a sensitivity that may be attributed to a particular brand of heparin solution.

The nurse must be aware of any complaints of burning, pain, discomfort, or skin or allergic reactions and should confer with the physician regarding any untoward findings. Some patients complain of increased site irritation and mild discomfort or pain during heparin administration. Greater discomfort may be experienced by patients receiving heparinized solutions 100 U/ml rather than 10 U/ml because of the increased concentration of drug in the saline solution.

Heparin is available in single or multidose vials or in pre-filled syringes. The multidose vial is the least expensive; however, it increases the risk for contamination. It is important to consider these factors when assisting the client and family for discharge from the hospital.

### Administration of Medication by an Intermittent Infusion Device

Prior to infusing any medication by an intermittent infusion device, the patency of the line is assessed and the IV site is evaluated. Cleanse the injection port with alcohol and insert a syringe filled with 1 ml to 2 ml of normal saline into the port. If the port is stabilized with one hand while inserting or withdrawing the needle, chances of dislodging the catheter are minimized. It is preferable to use a needle less than 1 inch in length (½ in.–⅝ in.), because anything longer may extend beyond the plasticized injection port or cap and perforate the catheter tubing. (This necessitates removing and restarting the IV.) Aspirate to assess for blood return.

*Caution:* Presence of blood return is *not* always a reliable method of determining patency. The catheter or needle may be the same size as the vein, and blood may not flow around the cannula or needle. A blood return may occur even in the presence of an infiltration if the needle or cannula has punctured the vessel wall allowing fluid to leak into the subcutaneous tissue, yet the cannula remains in the vein. Therefore, it is important to consider and evaluate all factors to determine vessel patency. If infiltration is suspected, it is safer to restart a new line rather than risk the danger of further infiltration and/or drug extravasation.

Once patency of the IV site has been established, inject 1 ml to 2 ml of normal saline and withdraw the syringe. (If resistance is met when attempting to inject the normal saline, do not apply excessive pressure; this may indicate clot formation at the tip of the catheter, and undue force may dislodge the catheter and precipitate an embolus. Withdraw the syringe, try to reposition the catheter, and try again. If there is still resistance, it is safer to discontinue the present IV and restart a new one.)

The medication is administered either by IV bolus or IV minibag or bottle. Again, consider needle length using only ½ in. to ⅝ in. to reduce piercing the catheter. Observe for any side-effects, monitor the rate of flow during administration, and assess the patency of the site. Following drug administration, withdraw the syringe or tubing and needle, cleanse the injection port, and insert a syringe with 1 ml to 2 ml of normal saline. This solution will flush the line. Withdraw the syringe, cleanse the port again with an alcohol wipe, and inject 1 ml to 2 ml of heparinized solution to maintain patency,

Because systemic therapy, that is, antibiotics, may include the administration of more than one drug, the risk of drug incompatibility is considered when using an intermittent IV infusion. To avoid this complication, always use separate tubing and needles with each drug infusion. Flush with 10 ml to 15 ml of normal saline between administration of different antibiotics to reduce the risk of precipitate formation within the catheter tubing. It is not necessary to administer heparin if the next antibiotic is administered immediately after the line has been flushed by normal saline. After the second antibiotic has infused, the line is flushed again with 1 ml to 2 ml of normal saline, and the heparin flush is administered.

## Monitoring of Intravenous Therapy

The nurse in the home care setting will need to collaborate with the individual and/or significant other to periodically assess and monitor and evaluate the plan of care (contract). Potential complications of intravenous therapy can be avoided if the client or care provider systematically monitor the following assessment parameters. Any abnormal signs or symptoms should be reported immediately to the appropriate health care individual or agency.

1. Pain, redness, swelling, coolness, or skin irritation at the IV site and/or surrounding area
2. Inability to infuse solution (try to reposition extremity, raise height of solution infusing first, then keep IV clamp open, notify appropriate personnel)
3. Leakage of solution/fluid from catheter site
4. Shortness of breath, hoarseness, cough, and/or bounding pulse and blood pressure

Access the individual's ability with a Hickman catheter to

1. Change and care for the exit site dressing
2. Maintain catheter patency by flushing the catheter line(s)
3. Change the injection caps
4. Secure the catheter lines
5. Demonstrate knowledge of signs and symptoms of infection and when to notify the agency or physician
6. Identify signs and symptoms of catheter malfunction (i.e., obstruction) and appropriate intervention
7. Temporarily secure or repair the catheter in the event of a catheter severing or breaking

*Flow Rate.*   Many factors related to the patient and to equipment affect flow rate. Patient factors include vessel diameter, venous pressure changes, client position, venous spasm following insertion, and venous obstruction. Equipment factors include IV container height, temperature and viscosity of solution, tubing position and length, and position of regulator clamp.

The IV container needs to be 2½ to 3 feet above the venipuncture site. Tubing should not hang or dangle below the IV site. If necessary, loop or tape tubing close to the client, (avoiding kinking or obstructing the flow) or use a shorter piece of tubing, but not so short as to restrict patient movement.

If the IV is not infusing at the prescribed rate, determine whether the container is empty, whether the drip chamber is less than half full, and whether the flow clamp has been regulated. It has been suggested that the regulator clamp be positioned on the tubing *higher* than the IV site. Check all connections to ascertain that the tubing is securely attached, especially at catheter and needle hub insertion sites. A wet site dressing indicates a loose connection or an infiltrated IV.

If the flow rate is still positional, reposition the needle or catheter by placing a sterile 2 × 2 over or under the catheter hub to change the angle. If the flow rate improves, stabilize the catheter or needle by retaping and/ or applying a splint to maintain the new position. Withdrawing the needle or catheter slightly (⅛ to ¼ in.) may change the position of the bevel of the needle or catheter and restore the flow rate. It is helpful to rotate the catheter as it is withdrawn; however, this should *not* be attempted with a steel winged–tip needle, because it might irritate or puncture the vessel wall causing an infiltration or phlebitis. *Never* advance the catheter or needle in the vein; this will increase the risk of infection.

If a clot is suspected, *never* irrigate the IV; this could dislodge a clot and greatly increase the risk of a life-threatening embolus. Clamp the IV, disconnect the tubing from the catheter or needle hub, attach an empty syringe, and try to aspirate the clot. If that procedure is not successful, discontinue the IV, select another vein, and restart the IV.

## Complications

Ongoing assessment of the client's condition while receiving IV therapy at home is essential in order to detect potential complications. Complications may include phlebitis and infiltration, which are most common, and also infection, circulatory overload, and catheter embolus.

*Phlebitis.*   One of the most common problems associated with IV therapy, phlebitis is defined as an irritation leading to inflammation of the intima of the vein, which may be bacterial, mechanical, or chemical. Signs and symptoms include warmth, which may be the only initial sign, followed by pain, tenderness, redness, and erythema. The venous cord may be palpable and indurated. The IV rate may decrease, and, when pressure is applied to the vein 1 in. to 2 in. distal to the cannula tip, the flow may stop.

*Note:* Normally pressure applied to the vein wall will stop an IV solution flow temporarily, but, if an infiltration is present, the IV will continue to flow, even if pressure is applied to the vein distal to the cannula tip.

**Infiltration.** Infiltration is an extravasation of IV fluid into the subcutaneous tissue resulting from a dislodged needle or catheter and/or puncture of the wall of the vein. Signs and symptoms include changes in skin temperature, especially decreased temperature or coolness surrounding the IV site, which may be an early sign of infiltration. Skin blanching and edema may occur.

If swelling is observed, it is important to rule out dependent edema and normal limb configuration; thus, both extremities are assessed. Feldstein (1986) suggests assessing swelling with the use of a penlight. Place the penlight on the swollen area and observe the size of the halo created. Place the penlight on the same area of the opposite extremity and observe the size of this halo. If the halo surrounding the IV site is larger than the halo observed in the opposite extremity, infiltration is strongly suggested, because increased fluid in the tissue causes a greater diffusion of light.

A partial infiltration owing to partial protrusion of the needle or cannula through the vein wall may occur and is manifested as diffuse swelling rather than a hard lump. Edema may occur at the insertion site because the tape is secured too tightly.

*Note:* Lowering the IV bag or bottle to verify blood return is *not* a reliable method of determining patency. If the cannula or needle inserted into the vein is the same size as the vessel, blood is not able to flow around the needle or cannula. Thus, even if the IV is patent, there will be no blood return when the IV solution is lowered. A blood return can occur, however, in the presence of an infiltration. The needle or cannula punctures the vessel wall, yet remains in the vein while fluid leaks into subcutaneous tissue.

If the client or family member or health care provider suspects an infiltration or phlebitis, he or she should notify the appropriate health care personnel and stop the infusion. The client and/or health care provider needs to know how to remove a catheter. To avoid further vessel damage, the client is instructed to avoid massaging or rubbing the affected extremity. Application of moist, warm compresses is usually recommended unless the infiltration was caused by a specific vesicant drug agent. Vesicants can be very painful and can cause serious complications. Specific recommendations should be discussed with the physician to treat an extravasation caused by a vesicant.

Additional complications of IV therapy include infection, circulatory overload, and embolism.

*Infection.*   Use of aseptic technique during insertion, tubing, solution changes, and site care prevents most infections. Handwashing is mandatory to minimize sources of contamination. Clients and care providers must be aware that hand lotions and bar soaps are potential sources of contamination. Skin preparations, including antiseptics, iodine-based solutions, and alcohol wipes should be used on a daily routine basis.

The effectiveness of the use of topical antibiotics at the insertion site is questionable, because alterations in skin flora can occur and result in infections (candidiasis). Tubing and needle changes are done on a routine basis but vary according to policy and research findings. The Centers for Disease Control recommends tubing changes every 24 hours for indwelling intravenous therapy.

Signs and symptoms of an infection include swelling, tenderness, erythema, and fever. The client or care provider should remove the catheter, apply a topical antibiotic ointment, and cover with a dry sterile dressing. Elevation of the extremity and application of a warm compress help to reduce pain and inflammation. A culture is recommended if the catheter used was plastic. If a systemic infection is suspected, the physician may prescribe a broad-spectrum antibiotic even before the culture and sensitivity is completed.

*Circulatory Overload.*   Circulatory overload should *not* be a common occurrence with the increased utilization of electronic infusion control devices. Clients with a cardiac or renal history/disorder are closely monitored. Generally, in an adult, continuous IV therapy is rarely infused at a rate faster than 4 ml/min. If there is impaired cardiac or renal function, the intravenous rate should not exceed 2 ml/min.

Signs and symptoms of pulmonary edema include a rapid bounding pulse, jugular venous distention, dyspnea, increased respirations, hoarseness, cough, rales, and increased blood pressure. If any of these symptoms occur, the agency or physician should be notified immediately. (Some agencies have developed standing emergency orders or protocols.) If the physician or health care agency cannot be reached within a reasonable period of time (30 to 60 minutes), the client should come to the emergency room for evaluation and treatment.

*Catheter Embolus.*   This uncommon but life-threatening emergency requires immediate intervention. This complication occurs most frequently with the needle catheters. The tip of the catheter breaks off in the patient's vein and may migrate to the chest and lodge in the pulmonary artery or right ventricle. This can lead to pulmonary embolism, sepsis, thrombosis, endocarditis, cardiac tamponade, or ventricular dysrhythmias and may result in death. In some instances, the catheter tip may migrate throughout the circulatory system, resulting in little or no damage, and can be surgically removed. If the catheter tip is confined to the extremity, it can usually be removed with endoscopy forceps or by cut-down with a local anesthetic. If the catheter traveled to the chest, a thoracotomy or mediastinotomy may be necessary.

Signs and symptoms of catheter embolus include sudden onset of sharp pain at the IV site. Pain, inflammation, and swelling may also be present. When the IV is removed, the catheter will appear shorter, uneven, and rough. Cyanosis, dyspnea, chest pain, hypotension, or tachycardia indicates that the catheter migrated to the chest, causing impaired gas exchange, ventricular dysrhythmias, or pulmonary artery obstruction. Catheter embolus is a medical emergency, and the client and/or care provider needs to know that the client must be transported to the emergency room immediately.

Pressure is applied on the vein just above the tourniquet site to prevent, if possible, further migration of the catheter. A tourniquet applied above the insertion site but not tightly enough to obstruct the arterial pulse in the affected extremity may help to prevent further migration of the catheter. The affected extremity is immobilized, and, if possible, the catheter segment is brought to the emergency room to determine the length of the embolized segment. Catheter position is determined by x-ray, and a decision is made as to how to locate and remove the remaining segment of the catheter.

## Care of External Venous Access Devices

### Care of Client With Hickman Catheter

If the client has a double-lumen catheter, it will be necessary to differentiate each lumen. For example, at the external end of the lumens of the Hickman/Broviac catheter, the Hickman lumen is labeled "H." The Hickman catheter is larger (1.6 mm inside diameter) and is usually the preferred lumen for drawing blood specimens or administering chemotherapy or blood products. The "B" or Broviac lumen is also labeled at the external end of the catheter and has an internal diameter of 1.0 mm. Keep in mind that the Hickman/Broviac or any double-lumen catheter is two individual catheters fused together, which must be flushed separately to maintain patency. In addition, when using *any* dual-lumen catheter, it is important to identify which lumen is larger, because that is usually the preferred lumen for withdrawing blood samples and administering blood products and chemotherapy, although this may vary according to institution policy.

Since it is more common to have catheters inserted under local anesthesia on an outpatient basis, responsibility for catheter care instruction and maintenance will be a major responsibility for the home care nurse and client.

**Insertion Site Care.** The insertion site can be cleansed daily with hydrogen peroxide, which can be applied with sterile cotton-tipped applicators. The site is then dried, and a topical ointment such as bacitracin may be applied. The site can then be covered with a sterile sponge and tape applied. After 2 to 3 days, the insertion site wound may be left open to the air. Stitches or staples will be removed by the surgeon approximately 1 week to 10 days postoperatively. If after 10 days the incision is not completely healed, Steristrips may be applied.

*Exit Site Care.* Postoperatively, the exit site is covered with a sterile dressing. It is not unusual to observe a moderate to large amount of serosanguinous drainage from the exit site incision for the first 2 to 3 days. This occurs as a result of the subcutaneous tunnel that has been created, allowing drainage to flow by gravity downward through the exit site incision. Site care includes daily cleansing of the exit site with hydrogen peroxide and topical application of Betadine and/or an antibiotic ointment (e.g., neosporin or bacitracin). It is not uncommon for a scab or crust to form periodically at the exit site incision; this can be removed with gentle application of hydrogen peroxide using sterile cotton-tipped applicators.

Clean technique may be used with dressing changes after the first 24 hours *if* the patient is not immunosuppressed. If redness, swelling, tenderness, fever, and/or change in the nature and amount of drainage occur, the physician should be notified. Approximately 2 to 3 weeks postoperatively, the catheter is usually anchored by surrounding subcutaneous tissue, and the exit site drainage may be minimal; a dressing may not be necessary. However, some patients still prefer to wear a Band-Aid or small dressing.

A more recent development in exit site care includes the use of sterile transparent occlusive or semipermeable dressings (e.g., Op-site or Tegaderm), which can be applied directly over the exit site and the catheter. Direct visualization of the site provides convenient site assessment and still keeps water and bacteria out, while allowing water vapor to escape. In addition, this dressing can be left on a site up to 72 hours before being changed (barring any complications).

*Catheter Position.* The catheter is never allowed to hang loose. The catheter is looped and secured to the chest wall (See Fig. 7-1). Some patients have been very creative and innovative in developing necklaces and other devices to secure their catheters to prevent dislodgement or severing of the catheter. Often, women find that they are able to loop or tuck the end of the catheter inside their bra.

In addition to securing the catheter to the chest, the use of a cannula (bulldog) clamp may act as an added safeguard. The clamp is positioned over a piece of tape or a Band-Aid that is wrapped around the catheter to provide protection against breakage. The tabs of the tape may then be used to secure the catheter to the patient's clothing, and/or a safety pin may be looped through the clamps and attached to the tape tab. It is advised to *avoid* clamps with teeth or prongs, because they may cause abrasion or severing. Routine clamping between catheter use and with irrigation is not necessary. It is generally recommended, however, that the individual carry a clamp to be used in case of accidental breakage or severing of the catheter cap or disconnection of the Luer-Lok cap.

Some catheters, such as the Corcath, have a protective sheath or sleeve that covers the catheter and a clamp that provides minimal tension when clamped. The sheath or sleeve can also be repositioned on the catheter so that the same area of the catheter is not always occluded by the clamp, thereby reducing the risk of weakening or severing the catheter.

*Maintaining Catheter Patency.* To maintain patency, the catheter should be routinely irrigated. There is wide discrepancy and considerable controversy among health care professionals regarding the type, concentration, strength, and amount of solution to be used and the frequency of irrigations. Recommendations for irrigation most often include the use of a heparinized saline solution (with concentration strength varying from 10 units of heparin/ml to 100 units of heparin/ml to 1000 units of heparin/ml). Most heparinized saline solutions are now pre-mixed in 10 ml of multidose vials and can be purchased through pharmacies, vendors, and surgical supply companies. In some instances, normal saline has been used in place of heparinized saline solution with no adverse effects. The recommended frequency interval for irrigating/flushing the catheter varies in the literature from once every 12 hours to once a week. The intervals most frequently mentioned recommend flushing b.i.d. in the immediate postoperative period for 3 to 4 days and then once a day or at least three times a week.

The amount of solution used to flush the catheter also remains a controversial issue. The standard Hickman catheter volume capacity, for example, is less than 2 ml, and the Broviac catheter capacity is only about 1 ml. Recommendations for flushing have varied from 3 ml to 10 ml, with 3 ml to 5 ml most frequently recommended. It is important to remember that the length of the catheter is tailored to the person's body size and structure and is cut to fit by the surgeon at the time of catheter insertion, so that, in many instances, the total volume capacity will be even less. It is, however, important to establish a consistent program of care and maintenance to be followed by the patient and family at home.

The questions and issues raised reflect a vital need for nurses to pursue research in this area of care. There are implications for cost-effectiveness of amount and frequency of equipment and solution use and the time interval between catheter maintenance and flushing. Results of nursing research will provide documentation for guidelines for recommendation for catheter maintenance and care.

## Complications

Potential problems that can occur with the catheter include infection, malfunction (i.e., obstruction), and severing.

*Local Infection.*   Local infection will manifest symptoms of redness, pain, swelling, and exudate confined to the immediate area of the exit site incision. (Keep in mind, however, that neutropenic patients may not produce an exudate, even in the presence of an infectious process.) Initial management may include topical application (e.g., neosporin, bacitracin) to the exit site, with systemic antibiotics added if indicated. Removal of the catheter, however, is usually not warranted. The Dacron cuff of the catheter may prevent further penetration of infection-causing microorganisms. More serious infections may colonize the catheter tract, and the patient may exhibit a fever and complain of pain and tenderness, with visible redness and swelling along the catheter pathway and in the shoulder region. With systemic infections, oral or intravenous broad-spectrum antibiotics will be initiated, and cultures will be obtained, and, if the infection is not resolved, the catheter may have to be removed. Other criteria indicative of catheter removal usually include an organism cultured from the exit site consistent with an organism cultured from the blood and a positive blood culture drawn from the catheter while a peripheral blood smear is negative (Johnstone, 1982). Documented infection rates in patients with atrial catheters appear to be very low, with rates varying from approximately 3% to 4%. Common organisms that have been isolated include *Staphylococcus coagulase* negative and positive, *Candida albicans*, and *Pseudomonas aeruginosa*. Another organism, *Corynebacterium*, colonizes the skin. This organism is resistant to most antibiotics except vancomycin. Cellulitis, although not always yielding positive cultures, may be very painful and necessitate catheter removal. When catheters are removed, the tips will be cultured for evaluation and follow-up.

*Catheter Malfunction.*   Catheter malfunction can result from obstruction or blockage within the catheter. If the catheter is not placed near the junction of the superior vena cava and the right atrium, or if the catheter extends too far into the atrium, the tip may rest on the surface of the endocardium, resulting in catheter outflow obstruction (Goodman and Wickham, 1984). Also, fibrin sheath formation at the tip of the catheter may lead to a blockage. Usually, fibrin sheath formation is suspected if fluids or blood cannot be aspirated, even though the catheter flushes with no difficulty. The fibrin sheath is pushed away from the tip of the catheter when pressure is applied during aspiration. However, when there is an attempt to aspirate blood, the negative pressure causes the fibrin sheath to obstruct the tip of the lumen and block any fluid entering the catheter.

Intervention is directed toward an attempt to aspirate the fibrin sheath and prevent further fibrin sheath formation. Catheter removal may be necessary, however, with the insertion of a new catheter. Some catheters are now beveled at the tip to reduce the risk of clot formation, although there is question as to whether this may actually enhance sheath formation.

**Blockage of the Catheter.** Blockage of the catheter may also occur owing to clot formation from drug precipitation or inadequate irrigation. If fluid cannot be instilled or aspirated, it is recommended that a tuberculin syringe be filled with 1 ml of heparin (1:1000 units). Tuberculin syringes may provide extra pressure needed to inject the heparin into the catheter. The heparin is injected, followed by either one additional milliliter of heparin or normal saline if it can be instilled. The catheter is clamped for 1 hour. After 1 hour, aspiration is attempted with a 5-ml to 10-ml syringe. If the catheter still appears blocked, repeat the procedure and try again. If the second attempt is unsuccessful, it is imperative to notify the physician immediately. However, it is extremely important to remember that forcefully irrigating a catheter that is clotted may result in an aneurysm or tear at a previously weakened point in the catheter (Gray et al, 1982).

A fibrinolytic agent such as streptokinase may then be used to attempt to dissolve the clot. Streptokinase (10,000 units in 3 ml of saline) is injected into the catheter and clamped for 60 minutes. After 60 minutes, the catheter is unclamped, the streptokinase is aspirated, and the catheter is irrigated (Rubin, 1983).

Discussion regarding irrigation procedures actually contributing to aneurysm formation and silastic fatigue remains controversial. It has been recommended that by clamping the catheter during the injection of the last ½ ml of solution of a catheter, irrigation may prevent fibrin sheath formation; others contend that this procedure may actually contribute to aneurysm formation and silastic fatigue (Reed et al, 1983; Riella and Scribner, 1976).

Catheter irrigation is occasionally impaired by patient position. The tip of the catheter may rest against the surface of the endocardium (as discussed previously). Altering the intrathoracic pressure may reposition the catheter tip. This is best achieved by having the patient breathe deeply; change positions, such as lying flat, sitting up, turning to one side, or raising or lowering the arm or both arms; or performing the Valsalva maneuver. Some patients find that lying flat and raising the lower extremity (lifting their legs for 20 to 30 seconds) facilitates catheter irrigation.

**Severed Catheter.** If a catheter is severed or cut, the line is immediately clamped. A No. 14 blunt end needle of a No. 14-gauge 2-inch angiocath (with the stylus removed) is inserted into the severed end of the catheter and taped securely. The line should remain clamped, and the physician should be notified. The temporary measure is effective until a repair kit can be obtained from the manufacturer. If the catheter is severed and the client has no equipment available even for temporary measures, instruct the client to use pressure to clamp the catheter until medical assistance is available. Simply pinching the catheter together with finger pressure or the use of a rubber band twisted around the end of the catheter to occlude the lumen can be temporarily effective.

Infrequently, additional serious complications occur, including pneumothorax, embolization of catheter fragments, or catheter-related thrombi, superior vena cava or subclavian vein occlusion, and bleeding in thrombocytopenic patients (Anderson et al, 1982).

**Activity Restrictions.** The catheter should not restrict routine activities; however, it is necessary to check with the surgeon before showering or bathing (usually when the exit site is healed). After the exit site is healed, patients may swim; however, it may be recommended that they wear an occlusive or semipermeable dressing (Op-site or Tegaderm) while swimming. This can then be removed after swimming if the client is not routinely using a dressing. Involvement in strenuous activity such as lifting, aerobic dancing, and contact sports should be discussed with the physician. With normal activity, the patient is merely reminded to check that the catheter is secure and not kinked or hanging freely and that the Luer-Lok caps are secure. As mentioned previously, if clamps are not routinely used, it is advised that patients at least carry the clamps with them. It has not been unusual for thin patients to occasionally experience a rubbing sensation where the catheter "rides" over the clavicle in the subcutaneous pocket created on the chest wall. It may reassure the patient if he or she is informed that this is a normal sensation.

## Care of Client With Groshong Catheter

As mentioned previously, catheters with a two-way valve design eliminate the need for heparin locks and routine flushes. Catheter maintenance and care is greatly reduced, thereby decreasing the risk of potential damage to the external segment. In addition, even though the size of the catheter is considerably smaller, ranging in gauge from 3.5 to 8, high flow is permitted. (No. 7 French Groshong catheter with an inside diameter of 1.3 mm has an infusion rate of 3500 ml/hour of a saline solution or 2600 ml/hour of a solution similar in viscosity to TPN).

Any isotonic fluid may be used to maintain patency of the catheter without risk of clot formation in the lumen of the catheter. Routine irrigation generally includes once a month flushing with 5 ml of normal saline. In addition, clamping of the catheter is unnecessary, because the valve remains closed when fluids are not being infused or when blood is not being withdrawn.

Management of the external catheter may include the attachment of an IV extension set. This permits the catheter connector to be secured underneath the dressing, especially if a transparent air occlusive dressing is used, and results in less direct manipulation of the external end of the catheter (Cath-Tech, 1985).

Irrigation is recommended after administration of medication, infusion of TPN, or withdrawal of blood. After infusion of medication or TPN, routine irrigation of the catheter should be performed using 5 ml of normal saline. Prior to blood sampling, if the catheter is being used to infuse TPN or hyperalimentation, the catheter should be thoroughly flushed with 30 ml of normal saline.

Catheter function can also be impaired by clots formed from residual blood in the lumen if the catheter is not adequately flushed after aspiration of a blood sample. After blood sampling, irrigation should be performed with a syringe attached directly to the Luer connector of the catheter, because this allows for more vigorous irrigation using at least 20 ml of normal saline (Cath-Tech, 1985).

Other catheter care measures are similar to previously mentioned problems, including infection, blockage, and obstruction and severing of the catheter. In addition, however, it has been determined that if infusion pumps are used with an occlusion setting greater than 15 PSI, separation of the catheter and its connector may occur. This is why it is extremely important that individuals be closely monitored during pump infusions.

## Care of the Internal (Implanted) Vascular Access Device

Once the venous access device is surgically implanted subcutaneously, the skin surrounding the port may be edematous and sensitive to manipulation for about 1 week, until the incison is healed. Local injections of Xylocaine subcutaneously or topical anesthetic spray over the port may be used temporarily or at patient request prior to needle insertion to reduce discomfort. However, once implanted, the port can be accessed immediately.

***Using or Accessing the Port.*** To use the port, the skin should be prepped using sterile technique with a solution such as povidone-iodine. As mentioned previously, prior to inserting the needle in the port, a local anesthetic may be used. Only a special needle (e.g., a Huber needle) should be used to puncture the port; a conventional needle will "Core" holes in the septum and damage the septum's self-sealing capability (Wilkes et al, 1985). The Huber needle tears or slices the septum on entry, and the septum then reseals when the needle is removed. Port septums are guaranteed for a finite number of punctures and will vary from 500 to 1000 punctures depending upon the port used.

After the skin over the septum has been cleansed with povidone-iodine, a straight Huber needle or a 90-degree Huber needle should be attached to the Luer-Lok end of the extension tubing, which is filled with normal saline and connected to a 5-ml to 6-ml syringe that is also filled with normal saline. The port should be stabilized with one hand, and the septum should be palpated and located with the other hand. (The use of sterile gloves has been recommended during this procedure.) Insert the Huber needle into the port, and traverse the septum until the needle is felt to "touch" the posterior side of the port. To confirm needle placement and catheter patency, gently aspirate and observe for a blood return. (Keep in mind, however, that the narrow internal diameter of the catheter portion of the venous access device may collapse with aspiration, and a blood return may not be observed.) If blood is aspirated, flush the port with 5 ml to 6 ml of normal saline to assess catheter patency, and observe for any signs and symptoms of tissue infiltration. If blood is not aspirated or resistance is met when trying to flush the port with normal saline, try to advance the needle, as the bevel of the needle may be occluded by the port septum (Wilkes, 1985). Do *not* twist or angle the needle and syringe once in the septum; this may cut the septum and create a leakage. If the needle cannot be further advanced into the port and/or blood cannot be aspirated, the needle should be withdrawn from the port, and a new sterile Huber needle should be used to re-enter the port (Figure 7-4).

To maintain patency, the port is flushed with 3 ml to 5 ml of a heparinized solution (100 U/ml) after each use or a minimum of every 4 weeks using a straight Huber needle. As mentioned previously with other central line catheters, when instilling the heparinized solution, inject all the fluid except the last 0.5 ml. As the needle is withdrawn, instill the remaining 0.5 ml of the heparinized solution, which will create a positive pressure and prevent retrograde blood flow in the tip of the catheter.

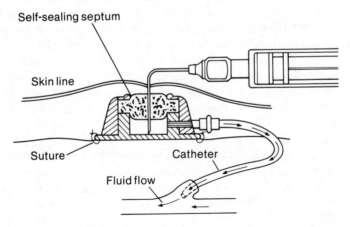

Figure 7-4. Accessing the implanted port.

***Bolus Drug Administration by Vascular Access Device.*** Prior to any drug administration, determine catheter patency and then flush the port with 3 ml to 5 ml of normal saline. Use of IV Luer-Lok extension tubing with a three-way stopcock attached to the syringe and Huber needle will allow manipulation of the tubing rather than the needle and reduce the chance of displacement of the needle and the risk of air embolism while administering the drug(s). After flushing the port with normal saline, inject the drug. If more than one drug is to be injected, it is suggested that the port be flushed with 5 ml to 6 ml of normal saline after each drug to prevent complications of drug incompatibilities. Most references suggest following the normal saline flush with 3 ml to 5 ml of a heparinized flush (100 U/ml). The needle is then removed by stabilizing the port between two fingers and withdrawing the needle straight out while maintaining a slight positive pressure on the syringe plunger.

***Continuous Infusions by Vascular Access Device.*** Continuous administration of fluids, medications, blood, and blood components will require the use of a right-angled (90°) Huber needle attached to Luer-Lok extension tubing, and a three-way stopcock. Currently, there are several lengths of right-angled Huber needles. For correct placement, the right angle of the needle should be positioned slightly above the skin surface. The needle can then be stabilized with gauze placed under the needle and the use of Steristrips and a dry sterile dressing or a transparent dressing such as Op-Site or Tegaderm. The benefit of antibiotic ointment at the needle injection site remains controversial, but it may provide some protection against local skin infections with infusions longer than 72 hours.

Infusion pumps may be used to deliver the prescribed fluid. Pump settings should generally not be higher than 40 psi, because, in some models, higher pressure may cause rupture or separation of the catheter (e.g., Port-a-Cath).

After the infusion has been completed, the system needs to be flushed with 5 ml to 6 ml of normal saline, and then 5 ml to 6 ml of the heparinized solution (100 U/ml). The needle is withdrawn in the same manner as discussed previously, and, initially, a small sterile dressing may be applied for several hours, because it is not uncommon for a small amount of serosanguinous drainage to be present. The Huber needle and extension tubing and dressing have been left in position up to 7 days before being changed, but the IV tubing is usually changed every 24 hours.

***Obtaining Blood Samples.*** To obtain a blood sample, withdraw 5 ml of blood from the port and discard. Then obtain the blood specimen using another syringe. After aspiration of the blood sample, flush with 20 ml of normal saline and resume the infusion, or, if the infusion is completed, flush with 5 ml to 6 ml of the heparinized solution (100 U/ml).

If blood cannot be aspirated, try the suggestions previously mentioned for Hickman catheters—change the patient's position (sit up or lay down or raise or lower head). Instillation of a fibrinolytic agent such as streptokinase or urokinase for 10 minutes may dissolve the fibrin sheath or cap.

## Complications

Potential complications of venous access devices include infection, extravasation of fluid, discomfort with repeated needle insertions, catheter occlusion and/or vein thrombosis, fibrin sheath formation, and "Twiddler's syndrome."

*Infection.*    Observe the site for swelling, warmth, redness, tenderness, increased skin temperature, and presence of drainage. Initial treatment may include topical antibiotics; however, if a systemic infection is suspected, and/or extrusion of the port through the skin is present, the venous access device is removed and another site is selected for reinsertion if necessary to continue therapy.

*Extravasation of Fluid.*    Improper position of the needle may cause extravasation of fluid. If the client complains of pain and/or a burning sensation, and if swelling occurs surrounding the injection port, stop the infusion and notify a physician. The site should be observed for 24 to 48 hours, and a decision should be made as to whether to use the venous access device again or replace it.

*Discomfort With Insertion.*    Repeated needle insertions may become very uncomfortable for patients. Use of a local anesthetic such as 2% lidocaine injected subcutaneously before insertion of the Huber needle may reduce discomfort.

*Catheter Occlusion and/or Vein Thrombosis.*    Blood clots can occur in, on, or around the catheter. Frequent blood sampling and infusion of packed red cells increase the risk of catheter occlusion. This complication can be reduced by flushing the catheter thoroughly and vigorously with 20 ml of normal saline immediately after aspiration of a blood sample. (Sometimes changing the Huber needle may prevent a catheter occlusion. Fibrin particles may have been drawn into the needle during aspiration of a blood sample, causing the occlusion.) In addition, packed cells should be infused "piggyback" with normal saline, using an infusion pump. Between units of packed cells, the line should be flushed with a bolus of 20 ml to 25 ml of normal saline.

If the catheter does not flush after changing the needle, attempt alternating gentle aspiration and irrigation using a half-full 50-ml syringe. (This will prevent exceeding the recommended pressure of 40 psi, which could result in a ruptured or separated catheter.) If this method is not successful, fibrinolytic agents such as streptokinase (0.5 ml to 1 ml [80,000 U/ml]) or urokinase (1 ml [5000 U/ml]) may be injected with a tuberculin syringe. After 10 to 15 minutes, an attempt should be made to aspirate the clot. This procedure can be repeated several times until the clot has been aspirated. If this is not successful, the physician will need to make a decision regarding the removal and reinsertion of another venous access device.

**Fibrin Sheath (Sleeve) Formation.** Platelets may adhere to the catheter and form a fibrin sheath or sleeve. When there is an attempt to aspirate blood from the implanted port, the fibrin sheath or sleeve is drawn into the lumen of the catheter causing an occlusion. This can be confirmed under fluoroscopy. The venous access device can still be used to infuse fluids but cannot be used to aspirate blood samples. The device may remain in place for infusions, but blood samples must be drawn peripherally.

**"Twiddler's Syndrome."** Patient manipulation of the venous access port may result in displacement or separation of the catheter, which can be determined by site assessment and confirmed on x-ray.

## Evaluation

The outcome criteria presented at the beginning of this section are used to evaluate the client's progress, make recommendations, and revise the contract (prescription). Criteria are also reviewed in relation to client/family satisfaction and standards of home health care.

## ‖ Peritoneal Dialysis

The patient with chronic renal failure or end-stage renal disease is dialyzed at regular intervals to sustain life. With the introduction of the Tenckhoff peritoneal catheter in 1972, long-term peritoneal dialysis became a viable alternative or option to hemodialysis. Medicare provides financial coverage for peritoneal dialysis for end-stage renal disease, and, in some states, catastrophic illness programs provide financial assistance.

This section focuses on the principles and concepts of peritoneal dialysis, with emphasis on continuous ambulatory peritoneal dialysis. Suggested outcome criteria with specific interventions are included for the person, family, and/or health care provider in the home care setting.

## Selected Diagnoses

Comfort, alterations in
Fluid volume, excess
Knowledge deficit, related to peritoneal dialysis management of renal
  disease

Peritoneal dialysis has several advantages over hemodialysis. It is cheaper, requires less equipment and space, and is easier for the individual to manage independently. Dietary modifications are less strict for the individual on peritoneal dialysis, and there is minimal hypotension, blood loss, and chemical disequilibrium (urea, creatinine, glucose, electrolytes). In addition, peritoneal dialysis offers an option to the individual who has poor vascular access and in whom further shunt or fistula sites may not be available for hemodialysis (Table 7-2).

Peritoneal dialysis involves the instillation of a dialysate through a catheter placed in the peritoneal cavity for the purpose of removing fluid and toxic wastes that have accumulated in the body. The peritoneum serves as

**Table 7-2.** *A Comparison of Peritoneal Dialysis and Hemodialysis*

| Peritoneal Dialysis | Hemodialysis |
|---|---|
| **Advantages** | |
| Less expensive | Less time-consuming |
| Less equipment for procedure | Less protein loss |
| Easier to manage unassisted | Lower level of triglycerides |
| Greater client mobility | |
| Less hypotension, blood loss, and metabolic imbalances | |
| Less restricted diet | |
| **Disadvantages** | |
| Increased time commitment | Increased cost |
| Abdominal pain | Vascular access |
| Peritonitis | Shunt/fistula clotting |
| Increased protein loss | Hypotension |
| Weight gain | Abrupt volume, metabolic and electrolyte changes (urea, creatinine, glucose, $K^+$, etc.) |
| Peritoneal catheter complications (outflow failure, displacement) | |
| | Risk of hepatitis |
| | Heparin use increases risk of retinal hemorrhage in diabetic clients |

a semipermeable membrane through which solutes (uremic wastes) diffuse. Factors that affect peritoneal dialysis include flow rate, temperature, pH, and osmolality of the dialysate.

An increase in the flow rate will increase fluid loss but will generally not increase solute (uremic wastes) loss. Solute removal (uremic wastes) can be increased by warming the dialysate to body temperature. A dialysate with a low pH can cause abdominal pain on inflow. Adding dextrose to the dialysate increases solute and water removal owing to the osmotic "pull" of dextrose (Binkley, 1984). The dialysate solution generally contains between 1.5% and 4.5% dextrose. If the dextrose concentration of the dialysate is increased, the individual is at risk for rapid fluid loss, hypernatremia, and hypovolemic shock (Fig. 7-5).

There are three variations of peritoneal dialysis:

1. *Continuous cycler peritoneal dialysis (CCPD)* is designed for use usually overnight while the patient sleeps and is about an 8- to 10-hour process. A cycling machine is attached to the peritoneal catheter, which continuously fills and drains the dialysate from the peritoneal cavity throughout the night (usually three exchanges). The final exchange is left in the peritoneum through the day. The individual is then free to resume activities during the day and then reconnects the peritoneal catheter to the cycler when he or she retires.

2. *Intermittent peritoneal dialysis (IPD)* is also called automated peritoneal dialysis (APD). Dialysis usually takes place several times a week for a period of 10 to 14 hours in a dialysis center or occasionally at home. The same type of cycling machine used in CCPD is used to add and drain the dialysate.

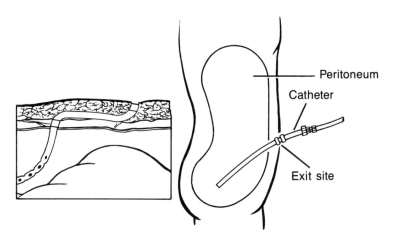

Figure 7-5. Insertion of peritoneal catheter and position of Tenckhoff catheter.

3. *Continuous ambulatory peritoneal dialysis (CAPD)* involves no machinery, electrical outlets, or water sources. Dialysate is instilled into the peritoneal cavity by the peritoneal catheter by gravity drainage. The empty dialysate bag is left attached to the catheter but is folded and concealed in the individual's clothing. After the dialysate has remained in the peritoneum for 4 to 8 hours (called "dwell time"), the dialysate bag is unfolded, the clamp is released, and the dialysate from the peritoneal cavity drains into the bag by gravity. The full bag is removed, a new bag of dialysate is attached, and the procedure begins again (Fig. 7-6).

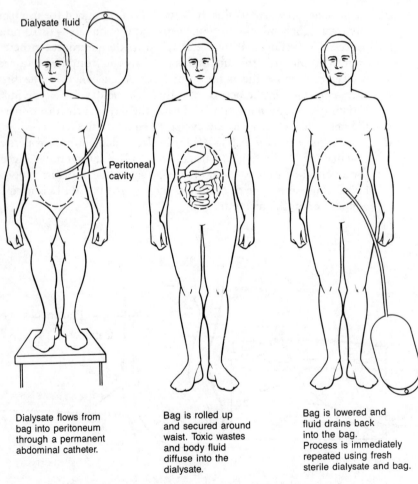

Dialysate fluid

Peritoneal cavity

Dialysate flows from bag into peritoneum through a permanent abdominal catheter.

Bag is rolled up and secured around waist. Toxic wastes and body fluid diffuse into the dialysate.

Bag is lowered and fluid drains back into the bag. Process is immediately repeated using fresh sterile dialysate and bag.

Figure 7-6. Continuous ambulatory peritoneal dialysis.

## Etiology and Defining Characteristics

Fluid volume excess as defined by Carpenito (1983) is "the state in which the individual experiences or is at risk of experiencing vascular, cellular, or extracellular overload" (p 196). Etiologic and contributing medical factors may include acute or chronic renal failure. CAPD provides the individual diagnosed with renal failure a viable alternative to hemodialysis.

Knowledge deficit, as defined by Carpenito (1983) is "the state in which the individual experiences a deficiency in cognitive knowledge or psycho-motor skills that alters or may alter health maintenance" (p 254). Etiologic and contributing medical factors may include any existing or new medical condition such as chronic renal failure. Learning to perform CAPD at home promotes self-care, increases independence, and decreases anxiety related to fear of the unknown.

## Focus of Nursing Care

Continuous Ambulatory Peritoneal Dialysis (CAPD)

## Outcome Criteria

The client and/or family member will

Demonstrate methods to reduce edema
Exhibit decreased edema
Demonstrate understanding of principles and concepts of peritoneal dialysis
Perform peritoneal dialysis (CAPD) competently and confidently
Identify complications of peritoneal dialysis and appropriate interventions
Demonstrate reduced anxiety and fear related to loss of control and fear of the unknown
Demonstrate reduced anxiety and fear related to change in self-concept and lifestyle

## Application of the Nursing Process

### Assessment

The individual with chronic renal disease or end-stage renal disease who decides to perform CAPD at home needs detailed and comprehensive information. Many hospitals and health care agencies provide at least a week's orientation program, presenting specific information regarding principles of CAPD, treatment regimen, specific procedures, and many hours of return demonstration and "hands on" practice. Individuals must demonstrate aseptic technique in performing the solution exchange procedure correctly prior to initiation at home.

The nurse in the home health care setting collaborates with the client and family and the referring agency to assess, monitor, and evaluate the plan of care (contract). The nurse or client in the home health care setting assesses:

1. Use of strict aseptic technique throughout the entire CAPD procedure
2. Suitability of home environment where the procedure is performed
3. Preparation, handling, storage, and disposal of sterile, clean, and contaminated (used) equipment
4. Ability of the client and/or family to explain "what they are doing" and "why" during the procedure
5. Ability of the client to recognize potential complications and react knowledgeably
6. Impact of CAPD on the client's and famiily's lifestyle, interactions with others, and coping strategies used
7. Ability of the other care providers to assist the client in performing CAPD
8. Availability of "back-up person" to assist when needed
9. Literacy skills, availability of telephone, and transportation

## Planning and Implementation

From the assessment data, the nurse determines which aspects of the CAPD procedure need reinforcement and review and what additional information needs to be discussed with the patient and family. Short-term goals will form the basis for the prescription for the nursing care plan.

The nurse, client, and family (if indicated) will implement the prescription (care plan), troubleshoot, and revise the care plan accordingly (Display 7-3).

### Monitoring of Client Status

Potential complications of CAPD can be avoided if the client or significant other and nurse systematically monitor the following assessment parameters routinely. Any abnormal signs or symptoms should be reported immediately to the appropriate health care provider and/or agency.

1. Weight
2. T.P.R. and B.P.
3. Lung auscultation
4. Skin turgor

(*Text continues on p. 229*)

*Display 7-3*
**Sample Care Plan: CAPD in the Home Setting**
*Long-Term Goals (Outcomes)*

At the end of 4 weeks, the client (individual and/or family member, significant other) will:

* Demonstrate understanding of principles and concepts of CAPD
* Demonstrate the ability to perform CAPD correctly
* Identify complications of CAPD and appropriate interventions
* Maintain positive nitrogen balance, and electrolyte balance
* Demonstrate measures to reduce fluid and weight gain
* Exhibit reduced edema
* Demonstrate reduced or minimal discomfort during CAPD
* Demonstrate or verbalize reduced anxiety and fear related to loss of control, change in lifestyle, and self-concept

*Short-Term Goals (Objectives) for Priority Problems*

Asterisk (*) indicates priority problems selected for this sample care plan but will vary according to each client/family and information elicited during assessment. It is also obvious when the client is *ready* to learn; nutrition is also very important, but, in this sample situation, it was not selected as a priority problem.

**Week I**

1. The client will verbalize to the nurse the major principles and concepts of CAPD.
2. The client will demonstrate the ability to perform CAPD correctly.

**Week II**

1. the client will verbalize signs and symptoms associated with complications of CAPD.
2. The client will verbalize interventions to treat complications of CAPD.
3. The patient will experience minimal pain from the CAPD procedure.

**Week III**

1. The client's peritoneal drainage will remain clear, with no evidence of infection.

*continued*

*Display 7-3 (Continued)*
## Sample Care Plan: CAPD in the Home Setting

*Short-Term Goals (Objectives) for Priority Problems*

2. The client's peritoneal catheter will remain intact, with no evidence of infection or catheter-related complications.
3. The client will verbalize understanding of dietary management to maintain positive nitrogen and electrolyte balance.

*Nursing Care Plan (Prescription)*

**Week I**

1. In the home, the nurse will review with the client and family the principles and concepts related to CAPD management, including:
   a. A diagram and discussion of peritoneal dialysis
   b. A list of equipment and supplies that will be needed (including what, where to order, approximate price)
   c. Review of aseptic technique with application to CAPD
   d. A step-by-step procedure, including preparation of equipment, CAPD procedure, disposal and storage of equipment
2. In the home, the nurse will demonstrate to the client and family member or significant other:

   * Step-by-step procedure of how to perform CAPD
3. In the home, the client and family member and/or significant other will demonstrate the entire CAPD procedure and will verbalize to the nurse "what" he or she is doing.

**Week II**

1. In the home, the nurse will review with the client and family member and/or significant other potential complications of CAPD and signs and symptoms, including:
   a. Peritonitis
   b. Catheter pain and/or displacement
   c. Infection of catheter and/or tunnel
   d. Negative nitrogen balance
   e. Bloody effluent
2. The nurse will provide the client , family, and/or significant other with a list of suggested interventions for the client to follow if he or she suspects any complication.
3. The nurse will provide the client, family, and/or significant

*continued*

*Display 7-3 (Continued)*

*Nursing Care Plan (Prescription)*

other with a list of dietary suggestions to prevent negative nitrogen balance and electrolyte imbalance and explain and answer any questions.

4. At the end of the session, the client, family, and/or significant other will verbalize:
    a. Signs and symptoms of CAPD-related complications
    b. Suggested interventions they can follow, including
    c. When and who they need to contact
    d. Suggested foods to include in their diet to prevent negative nitrogen balance and electrolyte imbalance

**Week III**

1. The client will review diet and discuss what protein sources are included on a regular basis.
2. The client, family member, and/or significant other will review and perform the CAPD procedure.
3. The peritoneal drainage will be clear and free of infection and the skin area around the peritoneal catheter will be free of infection.
4. The client will verbalize any new or continued concern related to CAPD managment, including anxieties and fears regarding self-concept, lifestyle, etc.
5. Evaluation will be made by the nurse and client/family, and/or significant other regarding continued visits based on
    a. Patient's needs and ability to perform CAPD
    b. Other related health/illness concerns
    c. Availability of insurance coverage
6. The client will verbalize what community resources he or she can use and what assistance can be offered.

5. Peripheral circulation
6. Abdominal pain
7. Catheter patency
8. Inflow and outflow totals through the peritoneal catheter
9. Cloudy or bloody drainage from the peritoneum
10. Catheter site inflammation
11. Electrolyte imbalances (confusion, nausea, tinnitus)

## Complications

Complications can include peritonitis, catheter site and/or tunnel infection, inflow and outflow problems, abdominal discomfort, and nutritional and electrolyte imbalances. Complications and interventions with implications for clients in the home setting are given below.

**Peritonitis.**   The most common complication of peritoneal dialysis is peritonitis. Potential sources include contamination during catheter insertion, introduction of pathogens by the dialysate or tubing, and break in sterile technique by client or significant other (i.e., spike technique) during CAPD procedure.

The best strategy is prevention. Strict aseptic technique must be followed by *all* individuals participating in the care of the client performing peritoneal dialysis. Equipment may vary, but it is essential that the entire procedure be followed in a systematic manner, with no short cuts taken, or equipment recycled and reused. If the nurse is not familiar with the equipment and/or procedure, in-service programming by qualified personnel is mandatory. The representatives of the manufacturer that produces the dialysate and equipment (e.g., Travenol) and nurses familiar with the equipment are available to discuss, review, and demonstrate step-by-step procedures.

To reduce the risk of infection, the individual should wear a mask throughout the procedure and use povidone-iodine swabs or soaks around or at connection sites. Some agencies and personnel recommend the use of gloves and in-line filters.

Signs and symptoms of peritonitis include fever, abdominal pain with rebound tenderness, nausea, malaise, and cloudy outflow. The physician should be notified immediately. Cultures of the catheter may be obtained, and cell counts of the peritoneal drainage (PD effluent) must be obtained. White cells are normally *not* present in the PD effluent; therefore, a white cell count above 100 with more than 50% neutrophils usually indicates peritonitis.

Treatment for peritonitis includes the administration of antibiotics added to the dialysate, which is then instilled into the peritoneum through the peritoneal catheter. (*Note*: Decreased renal function is considered in the choice of antibiotic administration, so the client's current BUN and Cr levels are evaluated.) CAPD can continue at home; the client and/or family is instructed to administer the antibiotics by way of the dialysate, to monitor the outflow drainage, to take body temperature daily, to monitor abdominal pain, and to communicate with the nurse or physician daily regarding progress. Usually, the infection is be resolved with antibiotics and rarely necessitates removal and replacement of the catheter.

Occasionally, bloody effluent is observed. The nurse should be notified, and a sample obtained to assess the hematocrit level. If the hematocrit of the outflow drainage (effluent) is higher than 1%, the individual is observed very closely. Treatment ranges from observation only to blood transfusions or surgery if necessary.

*Catheter-Related Complications.* Catheter-related complications can include catheter obstruction or occlusion, kinking or migration of catheter tip, and/or infection around the subcutaneous segment of the implanted catheter, and catheter leakage. Daily catheter care is minimal and requires only cleansing the catheter and catheter site with a mild soap and water. Some patients may also cleanse the area around the catheter and catheter site with Betadine daily. Routine use of topical antibiotics is not recommended. Patients usually shower to avoid submerging the catheter tip. A catheter site dressing is *not* required, although some clients prefer to use a dry sterile dressing or semipermeable dressing (e.g., Tegaderm or Op-site).

The client should report any localized redness, inflammation, fever, catheter site drainage, and abdominal tenderness immediately. Topical and systemic antibiotics are prescribed, and, if the infection does not clear, the catheter may be replaced.

Catheter obstruction or occlusion can occur if the patient has had previous abdominal surgery and there are adhesions, if the omentum has wrapped itself around a segment of the catheter, or if fibrin clot formation has occurred. Body weight, and inflow and outflow should be calculated every 6 to 10 exchanges to monitor for positive fluid changes.

A full colon can also affect outflow drainage; thus, a high-fiber diet, increased ambulation, stool softeners, suppositories, and/or enemas are suggested to the client. Teaching measures needing reinforcement include keeping the drainage or collection bag lower than the abdomen during outflow and hanging the dialysate to be infused a minimum of 4 feet above the client. Instruct the client to shift positions from side to side or sit up and press against the retroperitoneal spaces to enhance fluid drainage. Finally, if there is no evidence to indicate peritonitis or catheter obstruction, waiting 12 to 24 hours before resuming peritoneal dialysis may produce a delayed outflow (Binkley, 1984). The physician may increase the glucose concentration of the dialysate, which will create a higher osmotic gradient and promote increased drainage from the peritoneal cavity. X-rays may be indicated if no cause can be related to lack of drainage or outflow.

Catheter leakage is more common after initial placement. The client's peritoneal cavity must gradually adjust to the dialysate, so that small volume exchanges are used initially for 3 to 5 days, with the client's tolerance being increased gradually to 2-liter exchanges. If leakage around the catheter does occur, it is important to notify the nurse or physician. It may be recommended that the client drain most of the dialysate from the abdomen, leaving enough fluid to cushion the catheter and withhold further dialysis for 24 to 48 hours until leakage subsides (Binkley, 1984). Leakage around the catheter also warrants the use of a dressing and necessitates frequent observation to prevent skin irritation and breakdown from the dialysate outflow.

**Pain.**   Pain is caused by several factors. Abdominal discomfort may be present on inflow after initial catheter placement owing to intraperitoneal irritation. The client may even complain of referred pain between the shoulder blades caused by stretching and irritation of the diaphgram. It should be recommended to the client to use a smaller volume exchange until he or she adjusts to the sensation of the dialysate fluid in the peritoneal cavity (Binkley, 1984). It usually takes a week or two for the patient to adjust. The pain can be further irritated if the catheter comes to rest on the bladder or vaginal wall or root of the penis. If the pain or irritation persists, the client should consult with the physician for further evaluation.

Peritoneal dialysate that is cold or acidic may cause pain on inflow. The client can reduce some of this discomfort by warming the dialysate. Some clients use a heating pad, and some creative individuals have actually slept with one or two dialysate bags to warm the solution. Most dialysate has a $pH$ range of 5.5 to 5.7, but an alkaline substance such as bicarbonate or procaine may be added to reduce pain on inflow.

Pain is also associated with peritonitis; thus, other factors must be considered when the client complains of abdominal discomfort (e.g., cloudy outflow drainage, fever, and malaise). In addition, pain may also be caused by the introduction of air during the CAPD procedure into the peritoneal cavity. Air can sometimes be aspirated from the peritoneal catheter with the patient in the knee-chest or Trendelenburg position (Doenges et al, 1984).

**Alterations in Nutrition.**   Good nutrition is important to maintain positive nitrogen balance and prevent muscle wasting. Individuals on CAPD often experience anorexia, nausea, vomiting, stomatitis, and decreased absorption of calcium and iron. In addition, protein is lost across the peritoneal membrane with each exchange, and the presence of an infection or peritonitis can lead to further protein loss.

A high protein diet (100–120 g) is usually recommended. Calcium, iron, and vitamin supplements may be added. Sodium restriction will depend upon blood pressure, fluid weight gains, and serum sodium levels. Potassium restrictions are usually minimal, because the dialysate is potassium-free; however, routine serum levels will usually be ordered to monitor the client's serum potassium.

Diabetic clients will need to follow their recommended diet. Regular insulin can be added to the dialysate to cover blood sugar levels.

Assistive services such as occupational therapy may be needed (i.e., to assist individuals to spike their bags if they have some physical limitations and restricted mobility and vision. Some individuals have found the use of ultraviolet light technique for spiking to be most effective.) Meals-on-Wheels or the use of home health aides for meal preparation may help the home-bound client who is learning the "ropes" of CAPD.

## Evaluation

Progress is measured by meeting the short-term goals (objectives). Outcomes are measured according to the long-term goals and client and family satisfaction.

# Ostomy Management

Creation of an ostomy is a commonly used surgical procedure in the treatment of a variety of conditions, including inflammatory bowel syndrome, neoplasms, and/or trauma. Earlier discharge from the acute care setting, coupled with the myriad of equipment available often presents an overwhelming situation to the new ostomate and his or her family. Crucial to the rehabilitation of the individual with an ostomy is the ability to care for the stoma, including peristomal skin care and knowledge concerning appliances and prevention of complications.

This section focuses on the principles and concepts of ostomy management and suggested outcome criteria, with specific interventions included for the person, family, and/or health care provider in the home environment.

## Selected Diagnoses

> Skin integrity related to stoma problems
> Knowledge deficit related to stoma management
> Skin integrity, impairment of
> Sexual dysfunction

Ostomies are artificial openings to either the gastrointestinal or urinary tract. Treatment may be curative or palliative but involves a major lifestyle change for the individual. Placement and construction of the stoma are major considerations in the prevention of postoperative peristomal skin problems. If the stoma is placed in close proximity to a bony prominence, the umbilicus, skin folds, previous scars, or other skin surface irregularities, it will be extremely difficult to fit the appliance and may lead to complications of mechanical irritation from the appliance or excess skin exposure to fecal or urinary drainage. In addition, if the stoma is flush with the skin, it may be difficult to form an effective seal with the appliance and skin surface surrounding the stoma, and fecal or urine skin contact will increase peristomal skin complications. A protruding stoma may also prevent proper appliance fit and lead to mechanical irritation (Rothstein, 1985).

Colostomies involving the removal of the distal or descending colon (i.e., rectum, sigmoid colon) may still have a solid or semisolid stool. Ascending and transverse colostomies will have an increase in liquid stool content and an increase in stool frequency. Ileostomies (which include the removal of entire colon and/or large intestine) produce a constant, alkaline liquid fecal flow that contains pancreatic enzymes and is extremely irritating to the peristomal region (Fig. 7-7).

Urinary diversions can also create some problems, especially infection and urinary stasis around the stoma. These conditions result in an alkaline urine and irritate the stoma and peristomal region. The stoma may also undergo some thickening of the mucosal tissue (Rothstein, 1985).

The ostomy collection systems available today are numerous, and, with so many options to choose from, the client may be overwhelmed as to what products to select. The nurse and the client need to determine which system will best meet the needs of the client and also be cost-effective.

Generally, the ostomy collection system consists of a faceplate, skin barrier, pouch, closure (for drainable pouches), and accesories such as belts, cleansers, and wipes. The faceplate supports the pouch and is cut to fit around the stoma and attaches to the body. The skin barrier or "gasket" provides a leakproof seal between the faceplate and the skin. The pouch is the receptacle that holds the drainage (Fig. 7-8). The closure is the clamp

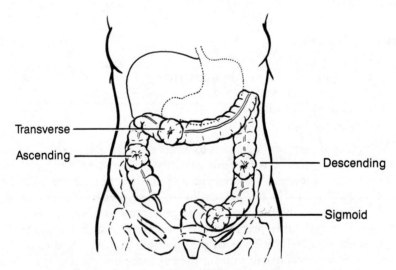

Figure 7-7. Anatomical position of ostomies on abdominal wall.

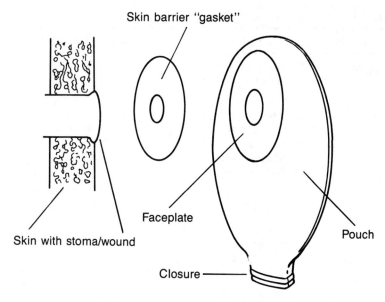

Figure 7-8. Ostomy collection system.

or clip that opens and closes the bottom of the drainable pouch (Felice, 1985).

The client should experiment with different equipment and mix and match parts, even from different manufacturers, until he or she is satisfied with all components of the system. For example, the client may find it more effective and cheaper to use a pouch from one manufacturer and a skin barrier and faceplate from another. Table 7-3 more fully describes the parts of the ostomy collection system with implications for the client.

## Etiology and Defining Characteristics

Impairment of skin integrity as defined by Carpenito (1983) is "a state in which the individual's skin is altered or is at risk of becoming altered," (p 436). Ostomies are created to treat and manage inflammatory bowel syndrome, neoplasms, and trauma. Etiologic and contributing factors related to stoma problems may include improper fitting appliances, mechanical and chemical irritation, and fungal or bacterial infections.

Knowledge deficit, as defined by Carpenito (1983), is "the state in which the individual experiences a deficiency in cognitive knowledge or psychomotor skills that alters or may alter health maintenance," (p 254). Etiologic and contributing factors related to stoma problems may include the inability to care for the stoma and lack of knowledge regarding stoma management.

**Table 7-3** *Ostomy Collection Systems*

| Components | Description/Types | Client Implications |
| --- | --- | --- |
| Faceplate | Mounting area that supports pouch and attaches pouch to body<br><br>Available as flexible or firm discs that are plastic, paper, metal, rubber, or adhesive, with center cut to fit around stoma. | Consider stoma factors of size, shape, location.<br><br>Flexible faceplates may fit a stoma located in a crease and also conform more readily to body contour.<br><br>A firmer faceplate may also be used if a stoma is in a crease to keep the stoma open. |
| Pouch | Collects and holds the drainage<br><br>Available as plastic, rubber or vinyl<br><br>Ostomy pouches are also available as closed, drainable, disposable, reusable one- and two-piece, and transparent or opaque | Client should consider if he or she wants reusable or disposable pouch, and/ or odorproof. (Disposable pouches can be washed and reused.)<br><br>Closed pouches are usually recommended for sigmoid or descending colostomies only, because they must be removed each time to dispose of contents.<br><br>Drainable pouches have a wide opening for thick drainage, such as feces, and narrow valve openings for urostomies for connection to straight drainage that can be used at night.<br><br>One-piece pouches contain all major parts of ostomy collection system and may be easier for client to manipulate. Precut openings can also be cut to fit. |
| Skin Barrier | Acts as a "gasket" to provide a leakproof seal between the faceplate and skin | The additional use of Gelatin-pectin or Karaya paste as a "caulk" to seal barrier around stoma |

*(continued)*

**Table 7-3** *Ostomy Collection Systems (Continued)*

| Components | Description/Types | Client Implications |
|---|---|---|
| **Skin Barrier** | Available as discs, paste, rings, or wafers | between the faceplate and the skin prolongs use of the skin barrier. Paste also fills in gaps around stoma, builds up skin surfaces, and improves the seal. |
| **Accessories** | | |
| Closure Clips | Open and secure the bottom of drainable pouch<br><br>Available as a clip, clamp, or valve | If drainable pouch and straight drainage system are used, connection can be made with adaptor or small piece of rubber tubing. |
| Straight Drainage | Used with drainable pouch and adaptor to collect drainage while patient rests | Straight drainage allows the patient to rest and avoids having to get up to empty the appliance during the night. |
| Belts | Assist in securing pouch system | Individuals wearing slacks may find use of ostomy belt bulky and awkward |
| Skin Products<br><br>Preparations<br>Cleansers<br>Deodorants<br>Ointments<br>Creams | Assists in cleansing, deodorizing, and prepping skin; may also protect, minimize, and reduce skin irritation | Use as directed. Some products may irritate sensitive skin. If signs of irritation occur, discontinue use. |

## Focus of Nursing Care

Ostomy Care

## Outcome Criteria

The person and/or family member or health care provider will

Demonstrate understanding of principles and concepts of ostomy care and related skin care

Demonstrate the ability to correctly change and secure an ostomy appliance

Demonstrate the ability to perform stoma skin care

Identify factors that may increase the risk of stoma-related complications

Demonstrate understanding of appropriate interventions for stoma-related complications

Demonstrate reduced anxiety and fear related to loss of control and fear of the unknown regarding ostomy management

Demonstrate reduced anxiety and fear related to change in body image, sexuality, and lifestyle

Manage dietary needs for odor, gas, constipation, and diarrhea problems

## Application of the Nursing Process

### Assessment

The client who has had surgery for the construction of a stoma faces the reality of a new situation that will be with him or her (usually) for the rest of his or her life. The initial management strategies must focus on the client's and/or significant other's or care provider's ability to manage to care for the ostomy and develop an optimal level of functioning. The home care nurse should assess the client and/or family's

1.  Interest and potential ability to perform ostomy care and management (Is the client ready to learn?)
2.  Ability to empty the pouch, perform peristomal skin care, and apply a new pouch
3.  Ability to explain "what they are doing" and "why" during the procedure
4.  Ability to safely irrigate a colostomy (if indicated)
5.  Ability of the client to recognize potential complications and react knowledgeably
6.  Knowledge of dietary principles for optimal ostomy management
7.  Knowledge of available community resources (i.e., ostomy supplies and equipment, United Ostomy Association, American Cancer Society)
8.  Reaction to an ostomy and the impact on the client's lifestyle, sexuality, interactions with others, and coping strategies used

### Planning and Implementation

The nurse will use the information obtained from assessing the client in the home environment to determine which aspects of ostomy management need reinforcement or review and what additional information needs to be discussed with the client and family. Short-term goals will then form the basis for the prescription for the nursing care plan. The nurse will implement the care plan (prescription), monitor the client's progress, and revise the care plan accordingly (Display 7-4).

(*Text continues on p. 242*)

---

## Display 7-4
### Sample Care Plan—Ostomy/Stoma Management

*Long-Term Goals (Outcomes)*

At the end of 4 weeks, the client (includes individual and/or family member, significant other) will:

* Demonstrate understanding of principles and concepts of ostomy and related skin care
* Demonstrate the ability to correctly change, secure an ostomy appliance, and perform stoma skin care
* Demonstrate knowledge of dietary management for odor-, gas-, constipation-, and diarrhea-related problems
* Identify factors that may increase stoma-related complications
* Demonstrate understanding of appropriate interventions for stoma-related complications
* Demonstrate reduced anxiety and fear related to loss of control and fear of the unknown regarding ostomy management
* Demonstrate reduced anxiety and fear related to change in body image, sexuality, and lifestyle

*Short-Term Goals (Objectives) for Priority Problems*

Asterisks (*) indicate priority problems selected for this sample care plan, but this may vary depending upon client and information elicited from assessment. It is also obvious from this plan that the client is *ready* to learn and does not demonstrate fear related to ostomy management.

### Week I

1. The client will verbalize the major principles and concepts of ostomy and related skin care.
2. The client will demonstrate the ability to empty, change, and secure an ostomy appliance.

*continued*

*Display 7-4 (Continued)*
**Sample Care Plan—Ostomy/Stoma Management**

*Short-Term Goals (Objectives) for Priority Problems*

3. The client will demonstrate the ability to perform stoma skin care.

**Week II**

1. The client will verbalize factors that may increase the risk of stoma-related complications.
2. The client will verbalize dietary factors that may affect ostomy management and suggested interventions.

**Week III**

1. The client will verbalize interventions to treat stoma-related problems.
2. The stoma and peritoneal area will be free of skin irritation and/or infection.

*Nursing Care Plan (Prescription)*

**Week I**

1. In the home, the nurse will review with the client and family the principles and concepts related to ostomy management, including:
   a. A diagram and discusion of the specific surgical procedure performed
   b. A list of equipment and supplies that will be needed (including what, where, approximate price, how to order and purchase)
   c. A list of community services available (i.e., American Cancer Society, United Ostomy Association) and specific assistance they offer.
   d. A step-by-step procedure of how to empty, remove, and apply a new pouch
   e. A step-by-step procedure of how to perform skin care
2. In the home, the nurse will demonstrate to the client and family member and/or significant other:
   a. Step-by-step procedure of how to empty, remove, and apply a new pouch
   b. A step-by-step procedure of how to perform skin care

*continued*

*Display 7-4 (Continued)*

*Nursing Care Plan (Prescription)*

3. In the home, the nurse will provide the client and family member and/or significant other with the opportunity to answer any questions they may have.
4. In the home, the client and family member and/or significant other will perform for the nurse:
    a. Correct procedure to empty, remove, and apply a new pouch
    b. Correct stoma and peristomal skin care

**Week II**

1. In the home, the nurse will review with the client and family member and/or significant other potential stoma-related complications and dietary factors that may affect ostomy management, including:
    a. List of stoma-related complications, including signs and symptoms
    b. List of dietary factors that may affect ostomy management and suggested interventions for the client
    c. An opportunity for the client to ask questions
2. At the end of the session, the client will verbalize:
    a. Signs and symptoms of stoma-related complications
    b. Signs and symptoms of dietary factors that may affect ostomy management and suggested interventions
3. At the end of the session, the client or family member and/or significant other will perform:
    a. Correct procedure to empty, remove, and apply a new pouch
    b. Correct procedure for stoma and peristomal skin care

**Week III**

1. In the home, the nurse will review with the client and family member and/or significant other:
    a. Specific interventions for stoma-related complications
    b. Written information provided to the client on products available and specific procedures for stoma and peristomal skin care–related procedures
2. The client's stoma and peristomal area will be free of skin irritation and/or infections.

*continued*

*Display 7-4 (Continued)*
**Sample Care Plan—Ostomy/Stoma Management**

*Nursing Care Plan (Prescription)*

3. At the end of the session, the client and family member and/or significant other will:
   a. Verbalize specific interventions for stoma-related complications
   b. Indicate specific community resources they can contact for questions

*Evaluation*

Progress will be measured by meeting of objectives
Outcomes as measured by meeting long-term goals

### Monitoring of Client Status

Potential complications of ostomy management can often be avoided or minimized if the client or significant other and nurse systematically monitor the following assessment parameters routinely as part of the prescription for the client who has an ostomy. Any abnormal signs or symptoms should be reported immediately to the appropriate health care individual and/or agency.

*Assessment Parameters*

1. Intact ostomy collection device with proper fit
2. Appearance of stoma and peristomal skin
3. Dietary management
4. Change in appearance, nature, and amount of ostomy drainage
5. Fever, abdominal distention, or pain
6. Sexual dysfunction

*Complications*

Complications may include a leaking or improper fitting ostomy collection device, skin and stoma complications, obstruction, and sexual dysfunction.

**Leaking or Improperly Fitting Ostomy Collection Device.** An ostomy collection device must be custom fit to the size and shape of the stoma, with no more than ⅛- to ¼-inch margin between the outer diameter of the stoma and the inner edge of the skin barrier disc.

If the margin is too small, mechanical irritation of the stoma mucosa can occur from the disc rubbing against the protruding mucosa. If the margin is too large, drainage will irritate the exposed skin. Leakage can also occur if the skin barrier disc or gasket is not secure and/or if the pouch is not drained frequently, thereby placing weight on the skin barrier disc, pulling it away from the skin.

Stomas with a normal round or oval shape can be measured using cards available with ostomy equipment and supplies. If the stoma is irregularly shaped, the stoma can be traced, and then the skin barrier disc or gasket can be cut according to the tracing (Rothstein, 1985). The client with a new stoma may require measurement of the stoma each time the ostomy disc and pouch are changed, as the stoma and surrounding skin become less edematous. In addition, slits cut ¼ inch through the discs will better accommodate an irregular skin surface contour.

The use of ostomy paste in combination with a skin barrier disc or "gasket" is very effective in forming a leak-resistant seal. Paste is spread around the inside opening of the skin barrier on the adhesive side; the skin barrier is applied to the stoma; and the "caulk" seals the opening edge. Ostomy paste is also very useful in building up skin or filling in gaps around irregularly shaped stomas when there are depressions, scars, and creases (Felice, 1985).

Other products that may improve the attachment of the skin barrier disc and/or pouch include double-backed adhesive rings, pectin products such as Karaya, adhesive sprays, and liquids. Table 7-4 provides a list of commonly used products and implications for their use.

***Stoma and Peristomal Skin Complications.*** Complications can result from mechanical irritation, reaction to certain product use (contact dermatitis), or infection. Skin irritation is more common with ileostomies and urinary ostomies because of increased frequency and type of drainage. This can lead to erythema, vesicles, ulcers, infections, and even abscesses. In addition, the warm, moist environment provided by the skin and occlusive appliance can cause folliculitis or bacterial or yeast infections.

Treatment includes reassessment of appliance seal and fit, discontinuation of any suspected irritating products, use of skin barriers, and keeping the involved site as clean and dry as possible. Bacterial and fungal infections need treatment with prescribed medication. Topical steroids may be helpful in reducing inflammation and discomfort from pruritus. The client should notify the nurse or physician if any suspected signs of infection are present and/or if skin irritation is not resolved within 24 to 48 hours.

***Dietary Complications.*** Diet can cause problems related to odor, gas, constipation, and diarrhea. Foods associated with increased odor include fish, eggs, spices such as garlic, peas, beans, cabbage, cucumber, turnips, broccoli, and asparagus.

**Table 7-4.** *Peristomal Skin Products*

| Product | Indications for Use | Implications for Nurse/Client |
|---|---|---|
| Skin Barriers (available in gels, wipes, and sprays) | Protects skin against mechanical irritation, and drainage<br><br>Promote adherence of appliance especially with moist or oily skin | Let dry 30–60 seconds after applying<br><br>Alcohol content stings irritated or broken skin<br><br>Cover stoma if using spray form |
| Gelatin-pectin and Karaya skin barriers (available as rings, wafers, pastes, and powders) | Protect skin, fill in gaps, crevices, and act as a gasket between skin and pouch<br><br>Promotes adherence or mounting area on faceplate or pouch | Gelatin-pectin is more water resistant than Karaya; suitable for urinary ostomies and will adhere even in the shower<br><br>Karaya melts at increased body temperature and in the presence of increased moisture. Not recommended for use with urinary osteomies. |
| Adhesives and adhesive removers (available as liquids or discs) | Generally not necessary, but may improve seal or may assist in removal | Apply lightly to skin surface or appliance. (Check product instructions, as this will vary.) |
| Ointments and creams | Ointments can be used as a protective barrier.<br><br>Creams are used for mild irritation and pruritis. | *Do not* use under appliances; interferes with seal and adhesion.<br><br>Use cautiously, notify physician if infection is suspected. |

To reduce odor, suggest that the client increase his or her intake of cranberry juice (most helpful for urostomies) and yogurt, buttermilk, and parsley (which are most helpful for bowel diversions). Some medications, such as antibiotics (especially penicillin), and vitamins may also be associated with increased odor.

There are also deodorant products that can be taken internally or used in the pouch to reduce odor. Products that contain chlorophyllin copper complex and bismuth subgallate have been determined to be safe and effective for use in reducing odor related to ostomies and incontinence. The drug is available without a prescription and is believed to reduce odor by interfering with the bacteria's ability to produce intestinal gas.

The client should try to identify which foods are associated with increased odor and then eliminate or reduce the associated food, increase fluid intake, eat or drink the recommended agents suggested for odor control, and use a deodorant preparation that can be ingested and/or placed in the pouch. If odor persists, this may indicate the presence of an infection, and the physician should be notified.

***Intestinal Gas or Flatulence.***   Large meals; carbonated beverages, including beer; foods from the cabbage family; and foods such as onions, beans, cucumbers, and radishes can aggravate flatulence. Chewing gum, smoking, and drinking liquids through a straw can also increase the amount of swallowed air.

The client should be encouraged to eat smaller meals at regular intervals and to chew food slowly with lips closed. Avoid "washing down" unchewed food; however, maintain an adequate fluid intake. Also encourage the client to avoid chewing gum or smoking.

Constipation can be caused by high-fiber foods such as nuts, coleslaw, corn, celery, raisins, grapefruit, and fried foods. Diarrhea can be caused by beer, raw fruits, and vegetables such as green beans, broccoli, spinach, and highly spiced foods. The client should be encouraged to determine which foods affect his or her system by trying one food at a time in small quantities, and gradually increasing the selection and amount of food.

***Sexual Dysfunction.***   Physiologic and psychological factors can cause sexual dysfunction. Extensive abdominal surgery can cause nerve damage that may affect a male's ability to achieve a full erection or impair a woman's vaginal sensations during intercourse. In addition, individuals may have difficulty accepting their altered body image and view themselves as unattractive. Self-esteem and self-confidence may be lacking, and the client may socially isolate himself from friends and family.

It will be most helpful if the client can identify his or her specific fears and concerns. This can sometimes be accomplished if the client is directly asked, "What concerns do you have since your surgery?" The client also needs accurate information about the specific type of surgery so he or she can understand what changes have occurred as a result of the operative procedure and what he or she can expect. It can also be reassuring for the client to know that it is not uncommon to feel the way he or she does, and that other clients experience similar fears and concerns.

***Other Complications.***   Change in appearance, nature, and amount of ostomy drainage; fever; abdominal pain; or distention may occur. These symptoms could be related to diet and fluid intake and may be easily managed, or they could indicate more serious complications such as infection or obstruction. The client should notify the nurse or appropriate health care provider if any of these symptoms persist for more that 24 hours.

## Evaluation

The outcome criteria presented at the beginning of this section are used to evaluate the client's progress, make recommendations, and revise the nursing care plan. Criteria are reviewed in relation to client and/or family satisfaction and standards of home health care.

## References

Anderson N, Aker S, Hickman R: The double-lumen Hickman catheter. *American Journal of Nursing* 82(2):272–274, 1982

Binkley L: Keeping up with peritoneal dialysis. *American Journal of Nursing* 84(6):729–733, 1984

Carpenito LJ: Nursing Diagnosis: Application to Clinical Practice. Philadelphia, JB Lippincott, 1983

Cath Tech Groshong CV Catheter: Technical Information Bulletin. No 6, November 14, 1985, Utah, Catheter Technology, 1985

Doenges M, Jeffries M, Moorhouse M: Nursing Care Plans: Nursing Diagnosis in Planning Patient Care. Philadelphia, FA Davis, 1984

Feldstein A: Detect phlebitis and infiltration before they harm your patient. *Nursing 86* 16(1):44–47, 1986

Felice P: The many parts of ostomy collection systems: What are your options? *Ostomy/Wound Management* 9:31–36, 1985

Goodman MS, Wickham R: Venous access devices: An overview. *Oncology Nursing Forum* 11(5):16–23, 1984

Gray G, Debonis D, Robinson G et al: Multiple use of TPN catheter is not heresy: Retrospective review and initial report of prospective study. *Nutritional Support Services* 2(9):18–21, 1982

Huey F: Setting up and troubleshooting. *American Journal of Nursing* 83(7):1026–1028, 1983

Johnstone J: Infrequent infections associated with Hickman catheters. *Cancer Nursing* 5(2):125–129, 1982

Koszuta L: Choosing the right infusion device for your patient. *Nursing 84* 14(3):55–56, 1984

Peck N: Perfecting your IV therapy techniques: Part II. *Nursing 85* 15(6):48–52, 1985

Phipps W, Long B, Woods N: Medical-Surgical Nursing: Concepts and Clinical Practice. St Louis, Mosby, 1979

Reed W, Newman K, deJongh C et al: Prolonged venous access for chemotherapy by means of the Hickman catheter. *Cancer* 52:185–192, 1983

Riella M, Scribner B: Five years experience with a right atrial catheter for prolonged parenteral nutrition at home. *Surgery, Gynecology and Obstetrics* 143:205–208, 1976

Rothstein M: Prevention and treatment of peristomal skin problems. *Ostomy/ Wound Management* 9:6–12, 1985

Rubin R: Local instillation of small doses of streptokinase for treatment of thrombotic occlusions of long term access catheters. *Journal of Clinical Oncology* 1(9):572–573, 1983

Wilkes G, Vannicola P, Starck P: Long-term venous access. *American Journal of Nursing* 85(7):793–795, 1985

Winters V: Implantable venous access devices. *Oncology Nursing Forum* 11(6):25–30, 1984

# Diagnostic Cluster: Activity Patterns (Self-Care, Integument, Exercise, Mobility, Sleep, Sex)

Six of the nursing diagnoses in the diagnostic cluster of activity patterns—self-care, integument, exercise, mobility, sleep, and sex—are discussed in this chapter within the context of a single medical diagnosis: acquired immunodeficiency syndrome (AIDS). In America and Western Europe, AIDS is a disease that affects homosexuals and intravenous drug users more than any other groups.

The first section of this chapter outlines home health care nursing interventions for the homosexual client, a man in a spousal relationship with a significant other of the same sex and with a circle of friends and family. The term *family* refers to the client's significant other, friends, and biological relatives. The term *spouse* refers to the client's significant other. The next section outlines home health care nursing interventions for the intravenous drug user client who is frequently alone and without friends or family. Infection control as it affects both groups is discussed in each section. Finally, trends in AIDS epidemiology and health care are discussed.

## Nursing Diagnoses

Activity intolerance
Diversional activity deficit
Family patterns, alterations in
Infection, potential for
Knowledge deficit
Mobility, impaired

Oral mucous membrane, alteration in
Self-care deficit
Sexual dysfunction
Skin integrity, impairment
Sleep pattern disturbance

The definition of acquired immunodeficiency syndrome (AIDS) in the United States is: A disease syndrome first recognized and reported by the Centers for Disease Control (CDC) in the summer of 1981, when 31 previously healthy homosexual men were diagnosed with Pneumocystis carinii pneumonia (PCP) and/or Kaposi's sarcoma (KS) (Centers for Disease Control, 1981). Since then, there has been an extraordinary escalation in the new case rate, with 27,704 adult and 394 pediatric cases reported nationally in December of 1986 (Centers for Disease Control, 1986). The mortality rate has remained at approximately 50%, 14,000 cases are still living. An AIDS-related complex (ARC) has also been identified, which accounts for many more thousands of patients not tracked by any reporting mechanism. ARC patients manifest a constellation of debilitating signs and symptoms, many of which require hospitalization for surgery or intravenous administration of medicines. Finally, there is a very large population of persons who are infected, shedding the virus, but who are asymptomatic. This population of seropositive individuals may already be as high as one and a half million.

AIDS is caused by infection with a retrovirus designated as human immunodeficiency virus (HIV). Previous and obsolete nomenclature included AIDS-related virus (ARV), Human T cell leukemia virus III (HTLV-III), and lymphadenopathy virus (LAV). Transmission is by inoculation with contaminated blood or semen. This mode of transmission has placed the homosexual community at greatest risk (73% of reported cases nationally) because of specific modalities of sexual expression (especially rectal intercourse). The next highest risk group in frequency of diagnosis is intravenous drug users, who account for 17% of reported cases nationally and whose vector for transmission is the sharing of contaminated needles. AIDS has a latency or incubation period of 18 months to 5 years, providing an insidiously long period of infectivity for those persons shedding the virus. AIDS is a terminal disease, with a mortality rate of greater than 95% at 2 years.

HIV infection attacks the body's cell-mediated immune system. Specifically, it destroys the body's T- and B-lymphocytes. AIDS does not destroy the entire immune system and is not similar to the "boy in the bubble" syndrome. AIDS patients are no more susceptible to common organisms than the general population, with a few important exceptions. These exceptions, for the most part, constitute the list of AIDS marker diseases, by which the diagnosis has historically been made. The diagnosis of AIDS is not made in the usual "recover an organism, prove the disease" manner of traditional medicine. Instead, because of the difficulty and expense of recovering the AIDS organism itself, the diagnosis is made on clinical criteria. The main factors in AIDS clinical diagnosis are that the patient (1) belongs to a high-risk group, (2) has a diagnosis that indicates that T cell or B cell immunity has been compromised, and (3) has no other apparent reason for such an immune compromise (e.g., undergoing cancer chemotherapy). With the increasing availability of HIV antibody and antigen testing, a more traditional approach to diagnosis is expected in the future.

A partial list of the symptoms and diseases that make up the Centers for Disease Control case definitions of AIDS and ARC are presented in Table 8-1. The specific markers for AIDS are organisms or neoplasms that

**Table 8-1.** *List of Most Frequent Infections and Neoplasms in Acquired Immunodeficiency Syndrome (AIDS)*

| Problem | Site |
| --- | --- |
| **AIDS-Related Complex** | |
| *Candida albicans* | Mouth (thrush) |
| Herpes simplex | Mucocutaneous; may be severe |
| Herpes zoster | Disseminated; may be severe |
| Lymphadenopathy | Generalized (always more than one lymph node) |
| Fevers | Usually greater than 100°F; persistent over months |
| Diarrhea | No organism recovered, or conventional organisms recovered |
| Weight loss | Progressive and sustained |
| Night sweats | Characteristically severe and drenching; persistent and sustained over months |
| Thrombocytopenia | Often accompanied by petechia; may be severe and life-threatening |
| **Infections** | |
| *Candida albicans* | Mouth (thrush); throat |
| *Cryptococcus neoformans* | Central nervous system (CNS); pulmonary; disseminated |
| *Pneumocystis carinii* | Pneumonia |
| *Toxoplasma gondii* | CNS |
| *Histoplasma gondii* | CNS |

*continued*

**Table 8-1.** *List of Most Frequent Infections and Neoplasms in Acquired Immunodeficiency Syndrome (AIDS) (Continued)*

| Problem | Site |
| --- | --- |
| Cryptosporidium | Intestine; diarrhea |
| Cytomegalovirus (CMV) | Retinas; intestine; pulmonary; disseminated |
| Herpes simplex | Mucocutaneous; severe |
| Herpes zoster | Disseminated; severe |
| Human immunodeficiency virus (HIV) | CNS, disseminated |
| Progressive multifocal leukoencephalopathy | CNS |
| *Mycobacterium avium-intracellulare* (MAI) | Disseminated |
| Mycobacterium tuberculosis | Pulmonary (TB) |
| **Neoplasms** | |
| Kaposi's sarcoma | Skin; disseminated |
| Burkitt's lymphoma | Lymphatic system |
| Non-Hodgkin's lymphoma | Lymphatic system |
| Mycosis fungoides | Skin (dermal lymphoma) |

are recoverable in diagnostic workup. ARC is mostly a collection of signs and symptoms designated as AIDS-related when seen (1) in a high-risk group member, or (2) in a person in whom HIV antibody is found. AIDS patients routinely have some or all of the symptoms of ARC. The list is not complete, but it may be seen that a sampling of AIDS diseases represents a remarkable number of medical and related nursing specialty areas, including neurology, neurosurgery, pulmonary, infectious disease, general medicine, general surgery, gastroenterology, opthamology, and urology.

The CDC has recently proposed a suggested revision of the case definition that (more accurately) describes AIDS as a disease with a spectrum of severity from ARC to frank AIDS (Centers for Disease Control, 1986a). If the revision is widely accepted, it will promote understanding and reduce problems in defining the disease for health and social service agencies.

The first of several identifiable periods in the AIDS disease process is a "honeymoon" period, which typically follows the first hospitalization for an opportunistic infection. Other periods that are not discussed in this chapter are typified by degrees of morbidity and, at the last, mortality. A typical history for the AIDS client is first time Pneumocystis carinii pneumonia (PCP) treated with trimethoprin/sulfa or pentamidine isethionate, administered intravenously in the acute care setting. It is during this "honeymoon" period, which may last for several months or longer, that the home health care nurse may first be referred to the client. This stage is an ideal point of entry for the home health care nurse because of the newness of the client's problems.

Initially, the client or family may expect the nurse to provide all care and direction. An early goal of care must therefore be to encourage as active a participation in health maintenance as the client and family can manage. The nurse must plan for frequent alterations in the level of participation on the part of both the client and the family owing to changes in the client's condition and alterations in family coping. Although discussion of it is beyond the scope of this chapter, spouse burnout syndrome has been observed in AIDS. The nurse has a responsibility to diagnose, plan, and intervene to ameliorate its effects. The reader is referred to the literature on this subject, especially to Ekberg, 1986.

Modes for transmission of the Human Immunodeficiency Virus (HIV) are of concern to the nurse both in teaching low-risk behaviors between the client and others, and in protecting him/herself. The reader is referred to Lusby, Martin, and Scheitinger (1986) for an example of infection control protocols to protect the health care worker.

# The Homosexual Client with AIDS

## Selected Diagnoses From Activity Patterns Related to Self-Care and Sex Pattern

Infection, Potential for
Oral Mucous Membrane, alteration in
Sexual dysfunction

## Etiology and Defining Characteristics

In the following section of this chapter, activity patterns related to self-care and sex patterns are discussed as they affect the homosexual client with a diagnosis of AIDS. A knowledge of the pathophysiology of AIDS is crucial to intervening effectively in the nursing diagnoses as well as the remainder of the cluster's diagnoses. The reader is referred to the current medical and nursing literature for the most current information. No citations are presented here because of the advancing understanding of AIDS pathophysiology.

Carpentio (1983) defines alterations in oral mucous membrane as "The state in which an individual experiences or is at risk of experiencing disruptions in the oral cavity" (p 307). Sexual dysfunction is defined as "The state in which the individual experiences or is at risk of experiencing a change in sexual health or sexual function that is viewed as unrewarding or inadequate" (p 407).

Oral candidiasis (thrush) is a common feature of AIDS, requiring topical and occasionally systemic chemotherapy to maintain remission. Alterations in white cell counts and composition as a result of AIDS or medications constitute a threat to the client's ability to cope with ubiquitous bacteria and fungi. Alterations in sexual function may be produced by viral infection or emotional disturbance.

## Focus of Nursing Care: The Homosexual Client with AIDS

The focus of nursing care for the homosexual client with AIDS is reviewed according to the selected nursing diagnoses of alterations in oral mucous membrane, potential for infection, and sexual dysfunction. Discussion includes care for the client and spouse's physiologic and psychosocial responses to AIDS as well as behaviors for promoting and maintaining health.

## Outcome Criteria

The following client-centered outcome criteria are specific to the selected nursing diagnoses and focus of nursing care:

1. The client will experience reduced incidence and/or severity of candidiasis infection and alterations in taste and appetite.
2. The client will verbalize and/or demonstrate ways to reduce risk of infection.
3. The client will verbalize and/or demonstrate effective coping strategies for managing changing sexuality.

## Application of the Nursing Process

### Assessment

The nurse applies knowledge of normal and altered anatomy to examine the oral cavity for signs of candidiasis, Kaposi's sarcoma, and other pathologic findings. Medications that the client is currently taking and their effects and side-effects are solicited and noted during the client history and physical. In addition, any medications that the client has taken in the past for the same complaint and their effects, side-effects, and reason for discontinuance are also noted. Altered taste as a side-effect caused by the infection or medication is of special importance, because it directly impacts on client nutrition.

The nurse assesses changes in white cell counts provided by laboratory documentation and their implication for the client's potential for infection. Neutropenia may be defined as a neutrophil count of less than 1000 per ml of whole blood. Profound neutropenia is usually defined as a neutrophil count of less than 500 per ml of whole blood. Whether neutrophil deficits are moderate or profound, the nurse's knowledge of AIDS and hematology will lead to some interventions in the form of infection precautions. Routes of possible entry for infection are assessed and noted (See Chapter 10). These routes may include open lesions, conjunctiva, the respiratory tract, and the rectal mucosa. Environmental infection hazards are also assessed and noted. Specifically, these hazards include dark, warm, and wet areas where fungi may grow, especially in bathrooms and kitchens, and also areas where dust and dirt may accumulate.

The nurse uses knowledge of pathophysiology, AIDS epidemiology, and human sexuality to assess changes in sexual function created by viral infection or emotional disturbance. HIV and cytomegalovirus (CMV) are suspect organisms in the cause of testicular atrophy and disturbances in adrenal function. Both the finding of passive disinterest in sexuality owing to physiologic alterations and aversion behaviors as a result of moral self-judgments and ineffective coping with AIDS as a sexually transmitted disease primarily affecting homosexuals (in the United States) are common features of the epidemic.

## Planning and Implementation

The nurse uses the assessment information gathered and his or her knowledge of nursing, microbiology, pharmacology, hematology, environmental health, human sexuality, and counseling strategies to develop goals and interventions to maximize the client and family's health. Following thorough history-taking and examination of the oral and oropharyngeal mucosa for signs of candidiasis, the nurse plans for effective intervention using a few important decision nodes (Fig. 8-1).

The process of nursing problem identification may move freely through this decision tree, both forward and backward. For example, a candidiasis infection may be out of control because of client noncompliance with the required frequency of medication administration, which, in turn, was caused by alterations in taste experienced when the medications were taken before meals. During assessment, the home health care nurse finds that the client thinks that he or she is required to take the medication just before meals because it was administered at those times in the hospital.

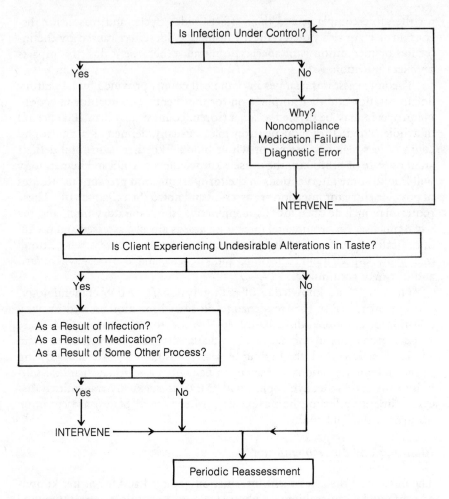

Figure 8-1.  Decision tree for intervention in oral/pharyngeal candidiasis.

Intervention takes the form of teaching the client the correct use of the medication, changing the medication administration times so that they do not coincide with meals, and following up serially to ensure that the medication and regimen are adequate to suppress signs of infection without causing alterations in taste. The home health care nurse also plans with the client and family for a diet to increase the appeal of food and eating. Fried foods, fatty meats, and acid foods should be avoided. Meal times should be regular, and the meal should be an event for interaction and enjoyment. Meals should not be rushed, served in front of the television, or composed of packaged processed food when it can be avoided.

Follow-up includes asking the client or family to inspect the oral mucosa daily and to note what foods or types of food preparation are most likely to cause alterations in taste and appetite. Brushing the tongue with a toothbrush helps to resolve infections more quickly.

The report that a home health care nurse receives from an inpatient facility may include information that the client's white blood cell count, especially the neutrophil count, is mildly depressed. If the home care agency does not have nursing protocols for neutropenia, the nurse can use those of the inpatient facility to ensure his or her client's safety. If the current deficit is not profound, the nurse's intervention takes the form of teaching the client to avoid such vectors for bacteria as raw food. This means teaching the client to avoid sushi, steak tartare, or any other raw meat and that all vegetables and fruits are thoroughly washed under running water.

Protocols for profound neutropenia are available in the literature and in hospital nursing and dietary policies. However, those policies generally do not address the possibility of bacterial entry through the rectal mucosa except to exclude the practice of taking rectal temperatures. When the client's sexual expression includes rectal intercourse he or she must be warned that engaging in rectal intercourse during profound neutropenic periods may represent a significant risk for bacteremia. If the client then decides to take the risk, a bacteriostatic lubricant (and of course a prophylactic) is recommended.

As previously mentioned, CMV and HIV have been theoretically implicated in testicular atrophy and adrenocortical changes commonly seen in AIDS. The behavioral result of such physiologic and anatomical changes includes decreased interest in sexuality and the inability to erect. Concurrently, the moral self-judgement of a client dying of a sexually transmitted disease—the symbolic "sex is death" message of AIDS—frequently creates an emotional ambivalence or aversion to sexuality.

Sensitivity to homosexual issues is demanded of the nurse who intervenes in this complicated problem of human sexuality. The nurse may find little personal identification with the client's sexuality or may have an aversion to discussing homosexuality. In situations in which a nurse is available who can empathize more effectively with the client, that nurse is the preferred care provider to approach these subjects. If such a nurse is not available and appropriate professional counseling is easily accessed, referral is another possible intervention. However, suburban and rural areas generally do not have these luxuries, and the home health care nurse is the sole resource. The nurse then must put aside personal prejudices and make himself or herself available to the needs of the client.

Intervention in sexuality issues of AIDS takes the form of gently helping the client and his or her significant other to extricate the physiologic from the emotional. The nurse teaches the physical changes that the disease creates while suggesting alternate, safer, and clearly caring sexual behaviors. These alternate behaviors include massage, frottage, change from penetrative to receptive roles (when client is unable to erect), and so on. Safer sex literature now includes detailed suggestions for alternative, non-orgasmic expressions. The nurse also listens patiently for pieces of the emotional picture to emerge. These emotional issues may include low self-esteem, stigmatization, anti-homosexual attitudes, blaming behaviors, grief, and so on. The issues are discussed one by one at the client's own pace. It is of crucial importance that the process not be deliberately hurried. The unfolding of the emotional issues of AIDS must assume its own natural rhythm.

The client is not alone in facing issues of changing sexual expressions and attitudes. The concerns of the spouse must also be addressed. If possible, the home health care nurse teaches and counsels both together. In situations in which counseling such couples is not possible or appropriate because of scheduling or reticence on the part of the client or spouse, separate teaching and counseling must take place. The home health care nurse's intervention can be helpful in healing the strained relationships between the client and his or her family by providing a forum for nonthreatening communication. Several organizations now offer individual, couples, and group counseling to persons affected by AIDS. Organizations listed at the end of this text will know of resources available in different geographic areas.

The home health care nurse also teaches the client and his or her significant other the concepts of low-risk sex and the use of prophylactics. If the client and his or her significant other have not yet begun low-risk sex practices, the home health care nurse encourages the couple to begin immediately. Repeated exposures may play a role in infection by the virus, and previous exposures should not promote either an attitude of immunity, nor one of fatalism. The following discussion presents suggestions for safer sex practices.

The home health care nurse has an absolute responsibility to teach the AIDS client how to decrease the risk of transmitting the virus to others. Educational materials have been created and are available to teach low-risk practice. Addresses of organizations from which more information can be gathered are listed in Appendix H.

"Safe Sex = Latex" has become a teaching mneumonic popular in San Francisco. Safe sex equals the use of prophylactics. Anal intercourse is the primary mode of virus transmission among homosexuals. When teaching low-risk sex, the home health care nurse must emphasize the point that propylactics break when incorrectly applied, when insufficient lubrication is used, or when sex is rough. A prophylactic may break even when low-risk sex maneuvers are carefully adhered to; thus, low-risk sex is really *safer* sex, rather than "safe", and depends upon proper choice and application of both prophylactics and lubricants, gentleness, and even a little luck. Table 8-2 outlines low-risk sex guidelines.

The use of water-based lubricants must be stressed by the home health care nurse. Petroleum-based lubricants such as Vaseline will dissolve latex,

***Table 8-2.*** *Low-Risk Sexual Behaviors*

| Behavior | Risk |
| --- | --- |
| Mutual masturbation | Safe |
| Massage | Safe |
| Frottage (body-to-body rubbing) | Safe |
| Use of unshared sexual toys | Safe |
| Vaginal intercourse with condom | Probably safe (condoms may break) |
| Anal intercourse with condom | Probably safe (condoms may break) |
| Cunnilingus (oral-vaginal contact) | Probably safe if skin and mucous membranes intact (plastic wrap will increase safety) |
| Fellatio (oral-penile contact) | Probably safe as long as no pre-ejaculate or ejaculate contacts broken skin or mucous membranes (plastic wrap or condoms will increase safety) |
| Analingus (oral-anal contact, "rimming") | Probably safe if plastic wrap or other barrier used; otherwise unsafe |
| French kissing (wet kissing) | Probably safe if skin and mucous membranes intact |

causing the prophylactic to break. If the client prefers the use of a petroleum-based lubricant, the more expensive "natural" prophylactics (usually made of lamb gut) may be safely used. Water-based lubricants include KY Jelly and a number of new products now marketed under such names as "Astroglide" and "ForePlay."* The home health care nurse cautions the client and significant other to examine the contents listing on the back of lubrication products to be sure of appropriate purchasing.

The use of lubricants containing spermicidals in low-risk sex between men and women is also not recommended. Unfortunately, because one can never be sure of coating all surfaces that may come in contact with infected ejaculate, spermicidals can never be advised as more than an adjunct to low-risk sex. However, greater lubrication will reduce the risk of vaginal laceration, which might lead to infection if the prophylactic were to break. And, in the event of a broken prophylactic, the use of a spermicidal might help to decrease the number of viable HIV particles that might migrate to the uterus and cross the tissue barrier there. The use of spermicidals in low-risk homosexual sex is also recommended with the caveat that the effect of the spermicidal on rectal tissue is unknown. Rectal tissue is substantially more fragile than vaginal tissue, and, conceivably, a chemical irritation

* The use of trade names is not meant in any way to be an endorsement of a product.

could result. Any sign or symptom of a contact dermatitis or burn should be reported to the physician, and use of the product should be discontinued at least temporarily.

### Monitoring of Client Status

Returning to the specific nursing diagnoses, the status of oral candidiasis is monitored by physical examination during each visit or as frequently as necessary. A rating scale of 1 to 4 (where 4 is the greatest) is used for severity. Documentation of changes in infection over time is of critical importance. Oral candidiasis always exists even if it is in remission; whether the infection is the same, better, or worse must be documented in hopes of identifying an optimal regimen for the individual client.

The absence or presence of infection is noted on progress records. High fevers are a feature of HIV infection, are usually short-lived, and are generally amenable to treatment with antipyretics. HIV fevers, which may be as high as 39°C to 40°C (102°F to 104°F), are also remarkable for causing little malaise in patients (with the exception of short-term rigors during temperature rise, and diaphoresis on temperature fall). When fevers of 38.5°C (101.5°F) or greater are accompanied by malaise or other signs of sepsis, or when the patient reports a difference in symptoms associated with more usual fevers, the nurse considers the possibility of bacteremia and consults with the client's physician.

Process evaluation of the nursing care plan associated with changing sexuality is approached with sensitivity. Impressions of client ease in discussing these issues is documented. Increasing ease of discussion indicates successful coping, even if no behavioral change occurs. The nurse must frequently take the initiative to introduce the subject because of client unease with verbalizing sexual matters. It is reasonable and appropriate for the nurse to say, "We talked last week about how difficult it is for you to talk with your lover about not wanting sex right now and we came up with some ideas for how to start the conversation. Did any of those work?" Sensitivity and a good will go a long way in bringing out these difficult problems and promoting successful coping.

### Evaluation

The success of nursing intervention is measured by the degree to which the previously established outcome criteria are met. For just this reason, goals should be established with some flexibility: the rigid form of goal writing, for example, "the patient will experience *no*" is not appropriate to nursing the AIDS client and has little value in setting outcome criteria for any nursing diagnosis.

Improved health status, the goal of so many nursing diagnoses, may not be attainable in nursing the client with AIDS. AIDS is a chronic/terminal disease characterized by physical wasting despite best nursing and medical efforts. The nurse must acknowledge the professional-emotional crisis that this represents in his or her practice. It is emotionally difficult to nurse the patient who fails to improve even with the best nursing care. It is imperative that the nurse acknowledge his or her feelings in this setting and have the empathetic support of peers and supervisors.

# The Intravenous Drug User With AIDS

## Selected Diagnoses from Activity Patterns Related to Integumentary and Exercise Patterns

Skin integrity, impairment of
Infection, potential for
Diversional activity deficit

The following section focuses on activity integumentary and exercise patterns as they affect the intravenous drug user client with a diagnosis of AIDS. The issue of diverting the intravenous drug user from illegal drug use is a critical one. Certainly it is ideal that the client should stop the practice of intravenous drug use immediately, but often such an ideal is impractical. The home care nurse is responsible for continually assessing the client's willingness to join a diversionary program (e.g., Methadone Maintenance, Narcotics Anonymous). However, it is as important that the home health care nurse intervene to decrease the effects of intravenous drug use in the client who will not stop the practice. The scenario that follows is typical for the intravenous drug user who has no significant other or family and who has no current intention of surrendering the "habit."

## Etiology and Defining Characteristics

Carpenito (1983) defines Skin integrity, impairment of as "A state in which the individual's skin is altered or is at risk of becoming altered" (p 422). Diversional activity deficit is defined as "The state in which the individual experiences or is at risk of experiencing an environment that is devoid of stimulation or interest" (p 160).

Intravenous drug use implies special nursing problems for this high-risk group. Skin integrity may be impaired by the sequelae of AIDS through a number of different mechanisms, a few of which are Kaposi's sarcoma and mycosis fungoides (two dermal neoplasms), *Trichophyton* sp. (tinea corporis/pedis or athelete's foot), and *Cryptococcus neoformans* (a fungus more frequently manifested as a meningitis but which may appear on the skin and mimic Kaposi's sarcoma or infection with *Pseudomonas aeruginosa*). For the intravenous drug user with AIDS, the potential for infection is greater because of local abscesses and systemic infections caused by substances used and contaminated "works," that is, the needle and syringe, which are frequently shared and inadequately cleaned.

The AIDS client who uses intravenous drugs is also at risk for developing systemic health problems associated with intravenous drug use (e.g., endocarditis). Finally, a severe diversional activity deficit occurs in this population when the ability to maintain the intravenous drug user's lifestyle is impaired by the disease.

## Focus of Nursing Care: The Intravenous Drug User With AIDS

The focus of the nursing care discussion in this section relates to the intravenous drug user client with AIDS. It addresses some of the problems that this client group experiences by exposure to infectious processes and having to cope with changes in lifestyle.

## Outcome Criteria

The following outcome criteria apply to the intravenous drug user client with AIDS and nursing diagnoses of skin integrity impairment, potential for infection, and diversional activity deficit.

1. The client will experience a reduced incidence of skin integrity impairment.
2. The client will verbalize and/or demonstrate ways to prevent infections by contaminated "works."
3. The client will verbalize and/or demonstrate effective coping strategies for dealing with a changing lifestyle.

## Application of the Nursing Process

### Assessment

The home health care nurse uses knowledge of normal and altered anatomy to examine the body surface for signs of infection, lesions, and trauma. Common to all AIDS clients are the problems of weakness, debilitation, and poor nutrition, which contribute to increased friability of skin; pressure sores are an almost certain outcome of AIDS. However, in the intravenous drug-using client, a special history of substances used, frequency, duration of use, and preparation technique is solicited in a supportive and nonjudgmental manner so that the nurse can plan for the special problems of the intravenous drug-using client. The nurse may take the opportunity to touch the patient during examination in a way that indicates support and reassurance. A hand on the shoulder while listening to breath sounds can help to increase provider credibility and establish a teaching–learning relationship between the client and the home health care nurse.

The home health care nurse uses knowledge of microbiology, physical assessment skills, and infectious disease to assess the potential for infections specific to the intravenous drug-using client. Complaints of chest pain are carefully documented as to frequency, duration, character, and precipitating factors. The home health care nurse also solicits from the client what behaviors, medications, and licit and illicit drugs relieve or decrease pain. The intravenous drug user, like the alcoholic, will frequently increase his or her substance use in response to anxiety or pain, even though the net effect is to further undermine personal health. Physical assessment includes careful documentation of adventitious heart sounds suggestive of valvulitis.

The home health care nurse uses knowledge of counseling strategies and substance abuse to assess the client's desire and ability to maintain the present lifestyle, discuss alternatives to the lifestyle, and change the lifestyle. The intravenous drug-using client is often harshly judgmental of his or her lifestyle and the home health care nurse's motivations. A firm, supportive, and slightly humorous effect from the nurse—the so-called hard love response found in half-way houses and drug abuse counselors—is usually more effective than most approaches.

## Planning and Implementation

The home health care nurse uses the assessment information gathered and his or her knowledge of nursing, microbiology, pharmacology, infectious disease, oncology, substance abuse, and counseling strategies to develop goals and interventions to maximize the client's and his or her family's health. Intravenous drug use and lifestyle issues are among the most difficult for health care providers to address. The home health care nurse's primary weapons are information and teaching, and realistic outcome criteria are imperative. The home health care nurse must constantly reassess the client and adjust the health care goals appropriately.

Following thorough history taking and examination, the home health care nurse plans a strategy and content for teaching the client how to avoid pressure sores. Of particular concern with the intravenous drug-using client is that if the client continues to "use," long periods of immobility may ensue during times when the client is "stoned." The home health care nurse suggests that the client reduce his or her dosages because of the general debilitation and and increased sensitivity to drugs (substance) produced by AIDS.

So called "shooting abscesses" are of prime concern to the home health care nurse. Some substances (e.g., Ritalin) cause worse-than-usual sequelae for the user, usually because they are compounded with silica or some other nondegradable substance. The home health care nurse collaborates with local substance abuse programs and the client's physician to identify these problematic substances and counsels the client to avoid them.

The intravenous drug-using client is at greater than normal risk of infection. Subacute bacterial endocarditis (SBE) and "cotton fever" are frequent outcomes of intravenous drug use. Endocarditis is most frequently caused by equipment contaminated with *Staphylococcus* strains. Onset of SBE is insidious and may mimic other complaints. Fevers are commonplace, as they are to AIDS. The chills, malaise, and arthralgia are also common to both diseases. Janeway lesions (erythematous macules on soles and palms) and Osler's nodes (tender nodules on the tips of fingers) may appear and are a highly significant finding. Comparative physical assessment findings are important, because a murmur not heard on initial examination, then heard subsequently in or out of the setting of other symptoms, is highly suggestive of endocarditis. Nephritis may develop as a consequence of SBE.

Cotton fever is a generalized inflammatory response caused by fragments of cotton, through which the injected substance was filtered, being injected into the vein and finding its way to pulmonary vasculature. Cotton fever is characterized by fever, chills, malaise, and pleuritic chest pain. Onset is rapid following injection, usually within several hours. In the non-AIDS intravenous drug-using client, cotton fever rarely progresses beyond the inconveniences listed. However, insufficient experience with the AIDS population should lead one to be cautious; each old syndrome manifests itself in this new disease. Complaints of pleuritic or cardiac chest pain, fevers, malaise, arthralgia, and similar symptoms are reported to the attending physician together with physical assessment findings and nursing opinions. Nursing intervention in this problem area takes the form of education on maintaining the intravenous drug user's equipment in the most sanitary condition. "Safer shooting" techniques are discussed in the following paragraph.

Ideal safer shooting facts for the client are: (1) always use new "works" (equipment) and (2) never share. Since the cost of new equipment may be prohibitive, and what is sold as new often is not, such advice is usually unrealistic. An alternative is to teach the client to wash his or her works thoroughly under running water, then draw household bleach through the needle and into the barrel until full, repeat the procedure, and finally rinse thoroughly with water. The home health care nurse teaches the client to clean his or her works before sharing and to teach the technique to other intravenous drug users (Fig. 8-2). The home health care nurse also teaches safer sexual behavior to the intravenous drug user.

In planning and intervening for diversional activity deficits, the home health care nurse takes a careful history of those activities of the client that have been successful in the past. Included among such activities most cer-

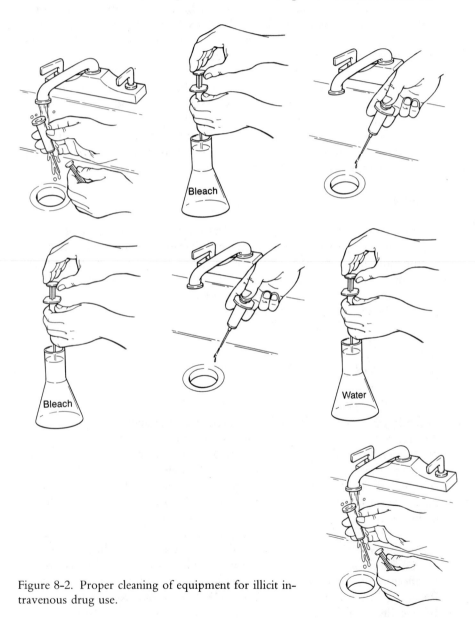

Figure 8-2. Proper cleaning of equipment for illicit intravenous drug use.

tainly is intravenous drug use. When the nurse identifies behaviors that are life and health promotive, those behaviors are reinforced by discussion and approval. With the exception of practical intervention similar to those just listed, intravenous drug use is better *not* discussed. The home health care nurse's time is more advantageously spent supporting those diversional activities that will contribute to the client's health. Supportive diversional activities include group and individual counseling programs, religious and other spiritual activities, and alternative health modalities that do not interfere with current therapy, meditation, and so on.

Intervention in the nursing diagnoses of skin integrity, impaired, and infection, potential for, take the form of education on (1) pressure sore control, (2) substances to avoid and dosing sensitivities, and (3) "safer shooting" techniques of cleaning and not sharing equipment (works). Interventions for diversional deficits are behavioral reinforcement of health- and life-promoting alternatives and de-emphasis on intravenous drug use and any other diversions that are not positive in nature.

### Evaluation

The previously listed outcome criteria serve to measure the degree of success of the nursing care plan and the client's health status. Reducing the incidence of infection in this high-risk population group is critical. The nurse must be realistic in helping the client to cope with lifestyle changes. Flexible, individualized, and realistic outcomes for nursing care are vital components of the nursing process for these clients.

## The Future of AIDS

Recently, the CDC released figures predicting the epidemiologic trend of the AIDS epidemic (Cimons, 1986). Using the CDC model, as many as 91,000 persons will be seeking care for AIDS in the year 1991, one in every 933 Americans will have the disease, 74,000 new cases will be diagnosed, and 54,000 people will die. AIDS will then become the seventh leading cause of death in America, at a cost of $8.5 billion per year (Harris, 1986)— higher even than the annual cost of automobile accidents.

At the current state of research, the only obstacle to realizing these predictions is low-risk sex and safer shooting education to the general public. Of paramount importance is that this education reach adolescents and preadolescents before they begin experimentation with high-risk behaviors. Recently, Admiral C. Everett Koop (1986), the Surgeon General of the United States, made education to the youth of America a strong recommendation in his report on AIDS. There can be no higher education priority in the epidemic than to reach those who are currently seronegative (have not been exposed). Even if a vaccine were ready tomorrow, it would not substantially affect the numbers of new cases until 1992 or later. The home health care nurse, as well as other health care providers, must take a central role in AIDS education.

The relative percentages of homosexuals, intravenous drug users, and heterosexuals who develop the disease have remained stable over the past 5 years, but many authorities believe that the distribution will change. The distribution of the AIDS epidemic in Central Africa has been 49% female in a setting where heterosexual transmission is clearly the efficient route for the disease. No currently used model explains the discrepancy between the Central African and the American manifestations. There is the possibility of co-factors for the disease that may exist in one place and not another; the leading candidate for such a co-factor would probably be poor nutrition—a surmise that might help to explain why AIDS more severely affects lower socioeconomic groups in this country. Nonetheless, the reality of heterosexual transmission of AIDS has begun to be realized. With the increase in heterosexual infection has come the stigmatization of AIDS by the disease's association with homosexuals and intravenous drug users. The home health care nurse must recognize and plan interventions for this psychosocial problem.

Babies born to intravenous drug-using women with AIDS are being seen with greater frequency in urban areas of America. Problems emerging are the different presentation, morbidity, and mortality of AIDS in newborns, maternal–child bonding, and medical foster parenting. Home health care nurses will be called upon to recognize and plan for the unique problems of the intravenous drug-using mother and newborn child. Among these problems are issues of infant drug withdrawal, fetal alcohol syndrome, breastfeeding and nurturing problems, and the fact that this is a child with a terminal disease. Additional issues include whether the child remains with the mother and, if not, finding foster parents who are willing to accept a child with AIDS. The medical contraindication of administering live-virus vaccines to persons with AIDS creates the possibility of increased incidence of previously controlled childhood diseases.

The number of black, brown and people of color with AIDS has been disproportionately higher than in the mainstream Caucasian population. The home health care nurse must recognize the unique psychosocial and health care problems of minorities and plan effectively to render care under conditions of different value systems and world views. In particular, the nurse must realize the psychopathologically potentiating nature of being both black and homosexual, or Latina and an intravenous drug user, with long-standing feelings of being "run over" by "white" middle-class American values. An "atmosphere of individual acceptance" (a phrase so common to nursing care plans and one that many nurses forget to implement) and a tolerance for social rage is prerequisite to care giving in this epidemic. Nurses must learn to work with and through the psychosocial problems of minorities and double minorities in this country.

Human experimentation in the epidemic has raised logistical and ethical problems in which nursing has become involved. The nurse with experience in AIDS will be called upon to answer questions about substances used in university studies and those used on the street. The public perceives a level of knowledge and information among AIDS nurses in excess of many other nursing subspecialties. Clients will ask nursing opinions before entering studies, and nurses will be called upon to advocate for clients who are involved in experimental protocols. Therefore, a potential for conflict exists between nursing and medicine over the issues of experimentation. If medicine and nursing are to collaborate in research issues, communication lines must stay open between the two disciplines.

A move is underway to discard pieces of traditional medical experimentation methods, especially double-blind, randomized protocols, and animal model protocols. Many of the approved and unapproved substances now being tested for AIDS are highly toxic, and, if advocates of modified methods succeed, substances tested could become even more toxic or lethal. The home health care nurse may find himself or herself monitoring signs for drug intolerance as well as changes in the disease state. The nurse must advocate for the patient by becoming familiar with the experimental protocol, including expected side-effects and criteria for discontinuing the study or breaking the code (determining what substance the patient is taking). The nurse must communicate signs of unacceptable levels of toxicity to the physician of record, the experimenter, his or her own supervisors, and, potentially, even the Institutional Review Board or Ethics Committees responsible for approving the research.

Finally, the need to network health care resources to provide comprehensive care to the AIDS client cannot be overstated. Social work will take a more prominent role in AIDS care in the future with the increasing problems of finances, income, residence, discrimination, and the need for practical help and supervision. The home health care nurse is in a unique position to manage the network of services to the client at home and to follow up as needed to ensure high-quality, comprehensive care.

## Conclusion

The importance of the AIDS epidemic to the future of home health care cannot be underestimated. The AIDS epidemic is challenging the health care professions in ways that have not been seen since the polio epidemic. The frequency with which home care is being used to support the patient outside the hospital setting has made home health care nursing a critical component in the management of this tragic disease.

The information in this chapter is not meant to be encyclopedic. The AIDS epidemic is too new for any author to speak ex cathedra on nursing practice. However, the author has furnished some scenarios from his own experience and hopes that readers will use their professional skills and imagination to enlarge the body of AIDS nursing knowledge. In addition, the names and addresses of a few organizations from which the reader can gain more information are found in Appendix H. The home health care nurse must remain current on recommendations for low-risk sex and safer shooting—client behaviors that are necessary if we are to reduce the risk of disease transmission.

## References

Carpenito LJ: Nursing Diagnosis: Application to Clinical Practice. Philadelphia, JB Lippincott, 1983

Centers for Disease Control: Follow-up on Koposi's sarcoma and pneumocystis pneumonia. Morbidity and Mortality Weekly Reports. 30:409–410, 1981

Centers for Disease Control: Classification system for human T-lymphotrophic virus type III/lymphadenopathy-associated virus infection. Morbidity and Mortality Weekly Reports. 35:334–339, 1986

Centers for Disease Control: Update—Acquired immunodeficiency syndrome— United States. Morbidity and Mortality Weekly Reports. 35:757–766, 1986

Cimons M: "AIDS Shock Wave Due to Sweep U.S." *Los Angeles Times*, pp. 1, 35, December 7, 1986

Ekberg JY, Griffith N, Foxall JM: Spouse burnout syndrome. Journal of Advances in Nursing. 11(2):161–165, 1986

Harris S: "The Cost of Compassion Is Soaring." *Los Angeles Times*, pp. 1, 3, December 8, 1986

Lusby G, Martin J, Schietinger H: Infection control at home. American Journal of Hospice Care. 3(2):24–27, 1986

# 9

# Diagnostic Cluster: Interaction and Communication Patterns

Three of the nursing diagnoses in the diagnostic cluster of interaction and communication patterns are discussed in this chapter. There is a paucity of information in the literature relating to the impact of provision of long-term care to family members at home by relatives. The purpose of this section is to identify family members' needs when caring for the individual at home and to discuss implications for nursing from both the client and family perspectives.

## Nursing Diagnoses

Anxiety
Communication, impaired
Coping, ineffective, individual
Family processes, alterations in
Fear
Grieving
Knowledge deficit
Powerlessness
Self-concept, disturbance
Social interactions, impaired
Social isolation
Spiritual distress

## Selected Nursing Diagnoses: Coping, Ineffective; Grieving; and Self-Concept, Disturbance in

Nurses and health care providers need to assist families and significant others to understand the health care options (or lack of options) available to the terminally ill client. The growth of the hospice movement has been relatively slow in the United States. This may be related in part to the highly mobile nature of our society, where it is not unusual for the family to be geographically separated (Campbell, 1986).

Hospice programs that have evolved in North America and the United States are modeled after St. Christopher's Hospice in England. The goals of hospice are based on Dr. Cicely Saunder's palliative care philosophy, which emphasizes the maintenance of a comfortable, pain-free client, without diminished sensorium during the final stages of living (Campbell, 1986). In addition to pain control, there are other major components of hospice care (Petrosino, 1986; Garfield, 1978), which follow:

### Hospice Program Goals

Utilization and availability of interdisciplinary team
Symptom control (physical, psychological, spiritual, and social)
Utilization of volunteers as part of hospice team
Twenty-four-hour availability of health services
Central administration and coordination of services
Bereavement care and follow-up
Respite care
Family participation in care
Home care service in collaboration with inpatient facilities
Client and family together are unit of care

Family member needs of clients who are terminally ill have been identified in the literature. In a study conducted by Hampe (1975), interviews were conducted with 27 spouses of terminally ill adults. Of the 27 spouses, 25 identified the same eight needs:

1. To be with the dying individual
2. To be helpful to the dying individual
3. To receive assurance of the dying person's comfort
4. To be informed of the dying individual's condition
5. To be informed of impending death
6. To ventilate emotions

7. To receive comfort and support from family members
8. To receive acceptance, support, and comfort from health care professionals

It is interesting to point out that families also listed how often their needs had been met. Only three needs were reportedly met for at least half of the subjects:

1. The need to be with the dying person (63%)
2. The need to be helpful to the dying person (74%)
3. The need to be informed of the impending death (74%)

Although the sample is small, findings indicate that although some needs were met, *many* of the unperceived needs were unmet (Kirschling, 1985).

One study by Freihofer and Felton (1978) examined what family members perceive as the *most* desired nursing behaviors for the terminally ill client. These included

1. To keep the client well groomed
2. To allow the client to do as much for himself or herself as possible
3. To administer medication as often as possible
4. To keep the patient physically comfortable

The four *least* desired nursing behaviors were the following:

1. Encourage me to cry
2. Hold my hand
3. Cry with me
4. Remind me that the client's suffering will be over soon

One additional exploratory study with 20 nurses as subjects ranked 75 nursing behaviors according to their perceived helpfulness (Skorupka and Bohnet, 1982). The five *most* helpful behaviors identified by the nurses were

1. Provide emergency measures for the client when needed
2. Assure the client that nurses are available around the clock
3. Answer the care giver's questions honestly, openly, and willingly
4. Allow the client to do as much as possible
5. Teach the care giver how to maintain the client's physical comfort

The four *least* helpful nursing behaviors included

1. Pray with the care giver
2. Make plans with the care giver to talk with others experiencing similar problems
3. Help the care giver understand what the loss will mean
4. Cry with the care giver

Again the study sample was small, but the findings were similar to Freihofer and Felton's subjects, who tended to focus on the terminally ill person's needs rather than their own. These studies begin to provide some guidelines for working with families experiencing a terminal illness.

The dying individual has many needs and fears that need to be identified and resolved. Commonly expressed are fears of loneliness and the need to maintain control (Norton, 1985). Coping tasks of the client with a chronic or terminal illness aid the individual in regaining self-esteem and self-concept and in functioning effectively. Kiely (1972) categorizes three types of stress that initiate the coping response:

1. Loss or threat of loss of psychic "objects" (personal relationships, body function, image)
2. Injury or threat of injury to body
3. Frustration of biological drive satisfaction

Utilization of coping strategies can assist the client and/or family member to master, control, or resolve the tasks. If the nurse can facilitate coping, coping can facilitate client and/or family powerfulness (Miller, 1983).

## Etiology and Defining Characteristics

Ineffective individual coping as defined by Carpenito (1983) is "A state in which the individual experiences or is at risk of experiencing an inability to manage internal or environmental stressors adequately due to inadequate resources (physical, psychological, or behavioral)" (p 144). Contributing factors may include disruption of emotional bonds, lack of or inadequate support system, alteration or loss of body part, low self-esteem, and feelings of helplessness.

Grieving as defined by Carpenito is "A state in which an individual or family experiences an actual or perceived loss (person, object, function, status, relationship) or the state in which an individual or family responds to the realization of a future loss (anticipatory grieving)" (p 203). Etiologic and contributing factors may include actual or potential loss of body function, chronic illness, and inadequate or lack of social support.

Disturbance in self-concept as defined by Carpenito is "The state in which the individual experiences or is at risk of experiencing a negative state of change about the way he feels, thinks, or views himself. It may include a change in body image, self-esteem, role performance, or personal identity" (p 389). Etiologic and contributing factors may include loss of body part or function, loss of significant other, and chronic illness.

Caring for an individual with a chronic, debilitating/terminal illness at home can be an emotional rollercoaster for both the client and the care provider. Little attention has been given to the physical and psychological effects of care giving on family members. In addition, changes in health care funding indicate that diagnostic-related groupings (DRGs) and additional financial pressures will literally "drop" the client from the institutional setting into the community. Thus, community hospice programs will become one of the viable options of care in the United States for the terminally ill *if* the reimbursement issue can be resolved.

## Focus of Nursing Care

The focus of nursing care should be on coping strategies for clients and families experiencing a chronic/terminal illness with implications for the home setting.

## Outcome Criteria

The client and/or care provider will

1. Demonstrate behaviors that reflect adaptive/appropriate coping strategies
2. Recognize personal limitations and seek assistance/support when indicated
3. Verbalize and/or share grief feelings and meaning of loss with significant others
4. Demonstrate progress toward acceptance of altered body image
5. Maximize ability to achieve or maintain body control
6. Use pain relief and symptom control measures
7. Demonstrate increased comfort

## Application of the Nursing Process

### Assessment

The client with a chronic/terminal illness who chooses to return or remain in the home care setting will need continual nursing assessment, monitoring, and reassurance that he or she will not be left alone. The nurse in the home care setting assesses

1. Availability of 24-hour care and back-up in case of emergency
2. Client's comfort level
3. Family's knowledge, skill, and ability to provide quality care
4. Family's and client's previous coping strategies for loss, grief, and crisis
5. Client's and family's perception of illness experience and the meaning it holds for them

6. Family's attitude toward death and caring for a family member with a terminal illness
7. Support resources (e.g., respite, home health aides equipment, services, supplies)

## Planning and Implementation

The nurse will use the information obtained from assessing the client and family in the home environment to develop a comprehensive plan of care. Short-term goals will form the basis for the prescription or the care plan. The nurse, client, and family will implement the prescription (care plan) and revise the care plan accordingly (Display 9-1).

## Evaluation

The outcome criteria presented at the beginning of this section are used to evaluate the client's progress, make recommendations, and revise the contract (prescription). Criteria are also reviewed in relation to client and/or family satisfaction and standards of home health care.

## Conclusion

Assisting the client and family members to cope with chronic, debilitating, and end-stage diseases is a critical component of the role of the home health care nurse. It represents the caring element of the nursing process, which the authors of this text believe is the connecting link between the nurse and the client and/or family in the home setting as they move toward an improved health status. The nursing diagnoses closely related to the stresses of chronic illness and the death and dying process were listed in the beginning of this chapter, with an emphasis on the nursing diagnoses of coping, ineffective, individual; grieving; and self-concept disturbance.

An unfortunate aspect of the current home health care arena and the health care system in which it functions is the lack of financial support for assisting clients with the psychosocial aspects of chronic disease and terminal illness. There are reimbursement systems for treating physiologic problems such as medications, assistive devices, high-tech therapies, and personal care, but there are no financial support systems for the counseling, sympathetic listening, health guidance, and referral for the nursing diagnoses of spiritual distress, anxiety, fear, powerlessness, and grieving, which are also closely related to chronic and terminal illnesses.

The authors have observed that the nursing diagnoses listed in the preceding paragraph are not documented in client health records, yet nurses report that they are meeting these types of needs for clients during home visits. The written record documents "skilled nursing care" and special

## Display 9-1.
### Sample Care Plan for Client with Chronic/Terminal Illness at Home

*Long-Term goals (outcomes)*

At the end of 3 weeks, the client will:

1. Demonstrate behaviors that reflect adaptive/appropriate coping strategies
2. Recognize personal limitations and seek assistance/support when indicated
3. Verbalize/share grief feelings and meaning of loss with significant others
4. Demonstrate progress toward acceptance of altered body image
5. Maximize ability to achieve or maintain body control
6. Use pain relief and other additional symptom control measures
7. Demonstrate increased comfort

*Short-Term Goals (Objectives)*

**Week I**

1. The client and/or care provider will verbalize to the nurse correct information regarding disease condition and present health status.
2. The client and/or care provider will review specific procedures for symptom control measures with the nurse:
   Pain/discomfort
   Feeding, elimination

**Week II**

1. The client and/or care provider will demonstrate positioning techniques and use of assistive devices.
2. The client will verbalize increased comfort.

**Week III**

1. The client and/or care provider will instill realistic hope and increase client self-esteem and control.
2. The client will express concerns and feelings about illness and dying.

*Nursing Care Plan (Prescription)*

**Week I**

1. In the home, the nurse will review with the client and family the specific disease process, including:

*continued*

*Display 9-1. (Continued)*
**Sample Care Plan for Client with Chronic/Terminal Illness at Home**

*Nursing Care Plan (Prescription)*

    *a.* A diagram and discussion of disease-related concepts
    *b.* A list of equipment/supplies/assistive devices needed by client
    *c.* A step-by-step procedure of any specified technique
2. The nurse will encourage the family and client to ask questions and express concerns. Ask them, "What do you want to know about your illness that will help you to better understand and cope?"
3. The nurse will review any potential equipment that could malfunction and the implications for its management.
4. The nurse will ask the client and/or care provider to draw a picture depicting the meaning that their present illness has and ask if they are willing to share this with the rest of the family and client.

*Week II*

1. The client and/or care provider will demonstrate procedures and techniques to the care provider that were learned last week. The nurse will encourage any questions.
2. The family, client, and nurse will re-evaluate the situation and determine whether additional support is needed.

*Week III*

1. The nurse will encourage a discussion of the client's and family's meaning of loss or death and attempt to encourage "grief work" discussion again.
2. Role-play with the client and family to explore feelings of self-esteem (use the role-playing situation).
3. Review and revise the client's care plan based on the client's progress, stabilization, or deterioration.

therapy interventions for financial reimbursement, yet the equally important phases of nursing care that provide the psychological comfort measures and the social support for the client and family are usually not credited in the record or to nursing. It is hoped that in the future, the interventions to support the client and family as part of the holistic approach to home health care will be valued by the health care financial system and that the intervention strategies and subsequent client outcomes will gain equal attention.

Although the present health care financial system does not adequately support hospice care, the hospice concept serves as a model of care for clients who are terminally ill or experiencing chronic, debilitating health problems. Many home health care agencies choose not to provide hospice services because of the financial constraints and lack of adequate and qualified staff. Communities are beginning to establish hospice services through privately funded organizations and local general funds (city, county, and town governments). The hospice model demonstrates the myriad of services necessary to assist the client and family through the terminal illness. Volunteer groups are an invaluable part of the model, and their visits to the home provide direct care and respite for clients and their families. They also help to relieve some of the costs to agencies and their clients who participate in the program by supplementing professional services.

Providing direct care, teaching strategies for moving through the grieving process, and ensuring follow-up care for the bereaved assist the client and family in maintaining as high a level of health as possible. As further research is conducted and findings demonstrate the positive outcomes for clients and families, the hospice model should gain momentum and receive the needed financial support it requires. The quality of life and the ability to allow dying at home are essential components of the model. At the same time, it is important to demonstrate the cost savings to the health care system if society expects to institutionalize the model in the community.

The hospice concept began with the humane provision of care for the dying person (particularly those diagnosed with cancer and the aged in terminal stages of chronic disease) and their families. Clients and families could choose to have the patient stay at home as long as possible and thus maintained control over their situation. The hospice concept assists families and their ill member through times of great stress, and it is applicable to all ill people who choose to remain at home for as long as possible.

The current epidemic of AIDS and its manifestations has created another population group desiring hospice services whose demographic characteristics differ from the original hospice aggregate. The clients are mostly young adults with the accompanying lifestyle, developmental needs for maintaining an income and self-identity through an occupation or schooling, need to support family and significant others, and the ability to make independent decisions in an illness situation that limits autonomy and places them in a dependent role with little assistance from a caring society. Society is beginning to assume care for these clients and to offer specialized services for AIDS clients. However, most of the support groups come from the private sector with limited resources.

The needs of the chronically ill and dying who choose to spend their remaining days at home and the needs of their families require bereavement support, respite for the primary care provider of the ill client, and day care for those clients who can be maintained at home for limited hours of the day or night. These needs transcend all health care settings and are not unique to home health care. They should be of concern to health care professionals in acute care settings when planning for the discharge of clients, in long-term care facilities to meet rehabilitation and end stages of disease if indicated, in day care centers for providing quality care and for providing respite for care givers, and in the home setting for maximal client and family comfort. The hospice concept and the comprehensive, multilevel models for care have no boundaries. They are the forecasters of a cost-effective health care system that provides quality care for the total (biopsychosocial-cultural) needs of clients and their families or significant others.

## References

Campbell L: History of the hospice movement. Cancer Nursing 9(6):333–338, 1986

Carpenito L: Nursing Diagnosis: Application to Clinical Practice. Philadelphia, JB Lippincott, 1983

Freihofer P, Felton G: Nursing behaviors in bereavement: An exploratory study. Nursing Research 25:333–337, 1978

Garfield C: Psychosocial Care of the Dying Patient. New York, McGraw-Hill, 1978

Hampe S: Needs of the grieving spouse in a hospital setting. Nursing Research 24(2):113–119, 1975

Kiely WF: Coping with severe illness. Advances in Psychosomatic Medicine 8:105, 1972

Kirschling JM: Support utilized by caregivers of terminally ill family members clinical implications for hospice team members. American Journal of Hospice Care 2(2):27–31, 1985

Miller J: Coping with Chronic Illness: Overcoming Powerlessness. Philadelphia, FA Davis, 1983

Norton MA: Daring to care. American Journal of Nursing 85:1098–1099, 1985

Petrosino B (ed): Nursing in hospice and terminal care. The Hospice Journal 1(2):1–9, 1986

Skorupka P, Bohnet N: Primary caregiver's perceptions of nursing behaviors that best meet their needs in a home care hospice setting. Cancer Nursing 5(5):371–374, 1982

# 10

# Diagnostic Cluster: Health Promotion, Maintenance/Management, and Safety Patterns

Chapter 10 summarizes diagnostic clusters and their related nursing diagnoses as they apply to the major domain of nursing practice in the home setting, the environment. It is divided into three major sections:

1. Health promotion and maintenance/management patterns in the home environment
2. Safety patterns: Prevention of injury
3. Safety patterns: Control of infection

The control of the physical environment as it relates to the prevention of infection and injury for families and their ill members is of special concern. These clients are vulnerable to secondary health problems owing to their debilitating physical conditions and the required changes in the home environment for providing care. They are often members of high-risk age groups such as the frail elderly and chronically ill young. The home health care nurse becomes a role model for preventing infection through aseptic technique and assessing and maintaining a safe home environment free of hazards.

Major health problems affecting home health care clients, such as arthritis, cancer, cardiovascular disease, congenital defects, cystic fibrosis, diabetes, and respiratory problems, require the services of various health care team members with the client and family. The nurse acts as advocate for the clients by identifying collaborative health problems requiring the expertise of other health professionals. The processes of referral, coordination of care, and counseling are critical components of nursing practice in home health care. Knowledge of community resources and reimbursement systems is essential to the nurses's ability to provide appropriate services for clients at the right time and to continue care when financial support for home visits discontinue. The final section of Chapter 10 discusses some of these aspects as they apply to home health care nursing practice.

## Nursing Diagnoses

Coping, ineffective, family
Coping, ineffective, individual
Family processes, alterations in
Health maintenance, alterations in
Home maintenance management, impaired
Infection, potential for
Injury, potential for
Knowledge deficit
Mobility impaired, physical
Self-care deficit

# Health Promotion and Maintenance/Management Patterns in the Home Environment

## Selected Diagnoses

Coping, ineffective, family
Coping, ineffective, individual
Family processes, alterations in
Health maintenance, alterations in
Home maintenance management, impaired
Knowledge deficit
Self-care deficit, total or partial

Many of the diagnoses in this cluster are generic to other diagnoses. For example, a client with congestive heart failure will require nursing care related to the diagnoses of cardiac output, alterations in; respiratory function, alterations in; and tissue perfusion. At the same time, the family has to cope with the ill client, provide a safe home environment, and adjust their lifestyle.

Today's home health care clients are frequently referred from hospitals to agencies and providers in high-acuity stages of illness (National League for Nursing, 1986). The focus of services to clients in the home is to assist them to recover, promote them to their optimal level of health and functioning, and prevent complications, disability, unwarranted death, and new illnesses. Many times, clients are referred for a knowledge deficit related to a newly diagnosed illness that will affect the family and/or significant others' lifestyles as well as the client's. The selected diagnoses for this diagnostic cluster in the nursing practice domain of environment are considered and ruled out or verified. The particular diagnoses that need primary attention will depend upon the health condition, the home environment, and the judgment of the nurse, client, and family.

## Etiology and Defining Characteristics

Carpenito (1983) defined ineffective individual coping as "a state in which the individual experiences or is at risk of experiencing an inability to manage internal or environmental stressors adequately due to inadequate resources (physical, psychological, or behavioral)" (p 144). Ineffective family coping is defined as "the state in which a family demonstrates destructive behavior in response to an inability to manage internal or external stressors due to inadequate resources (physical, psychological, cognitive, and/or behavioral)" (p 153). Alterations in family processes is "the state in which a normally supportive family experiences a stressor that challenges its previously effective functioning ability" (p 167).

Alteration in health maintenance management is defined as "states in which the individual experiences or is at risk of experiencing a disruption in his present state of wellness because of inadequate preventive measures or an unhealthy life style" (p 215). Impaired home maintenance management is defined as "the state in which an individual or family experiences or is at risk to experience a difficulty in maintaining self or family in a safe home environment" (p 230). Self-care deficit is defined as "the state in which the individual experiences an impaired motor function or cognitive function, causing a decreased ability to feed, bathe, dress, or toilet oneself" (p 374).

Newly diagnosed chronic diseases such as cancer, cardiac problems, cerebral vascular accidents, diabetes, hypertension, and rheumatoid arthritis contribute to the etiology of the nursing diagnoses of health maintenance and promotion and home management patterns. Other illnesses in acute stages, such as chronic obstructive pulmonary disease, congestive heart failure, endocrine disorders, and exacerbations of leukemia, lymphoma, multiple sclerosis, and so on, can also contribute to the nursing diagnoses. Hemapoietic diseases and trauma are additional etiologic factors leading to these diagnoses. The diagnoses affect the individual client and the family and/or significant others to the extent of their ability to adjust their activities of daily living, the home environment, and family functioning.

The medical problem has a far-reaching impact on the health of the client and family. The availability of family members to provide care to the ill person will influence other family functions such as continuation of work, attendance at school, maintenance of the home environment, provision of basic necessities, preparation of meals, and rest and relaxation. Financial resources and knowledge of community resources for providing care, equipment, and supplies are necessary to the support of the ill client at home. The members of the family and their roles and functions influence how the client and others will cope with the illness situation.

## Focus of Nursing Care

Chapter 8 discusses in detail knowledge deficit and the teaching plan as the intervention of choice for the diagnosis. Other interventions pertaining to the diagnostic cluster include counseling of the client and family, consulting with other health care providers, and referring to other agencies or professionals.

## Outcome Criteria

Suggested goals for the diagnoses from the diagnostic cluster related to health promotion and maintenance/management patterns are listed below.

The person and family member and/or health care provider will

1. Demonstrate appropriate coping strategies for managing stressful situations
2. Verbalize a knowledge of the disease by describing the characteristics of the disease process
3. Achieve an optimal level of health
4. Provide care for the ill family member at home
5. Maintain wellness by periodic checkups with care providers
6. Provide the basic necessities for its members

## Application of the Nursing Process

### Assessment

A review and physical assessment of the client's health status and reason for referral help to measure the impact of the illness on the client and family. A profile of family members' roles and functions provides additional data for analysis of family needs. A survey of the home environment reveals the milieu and resources available for providing basic necessities for the client and family.

Nursing diagnoses are identified after the data are analyzed. They are listed and reviewed by the nurse, client, and family. Those most pertinent to the situation and amenable to nursing/client action are chosen as the primary diagnoses. Client-centered outcomes are developed for each diagnosis and can be similar to those listed above as outcome criteria for this component of the diagnostic cluster.

## Planning and Implementation

The methods for reaching the goals are listed and agreed upon by the client, family, and care provider. Objectives for the nursing care plan are formulated, and plans are written, including the where, when, how, by whom, and method of documentation. For example, if the nurse and client and family decide that the newly diagnosed diabetic, blind grandmother needs to have insulin administered each day by her daughter who works, the diagnosis might be: family processes, alterations in; or coping, ineffective, family.

Another nursing diagnosis is knowledge deficit relating to the daughter's need to gain knowledge and technical skills to administer the insulin and to monitor her mother's condition. Thus, a teaching plan becomes the procedure of choice. At the same time, certain family adjustments must take place so that the daughter may continue to work and care for her mother. Another family member may have to assist in the morning activities to prepare the younger members for school to allow time for the daughter to care for her mother. The procedure of choice in this instance would be counseling the family or perhaps referral for a temporary housekeeper.

Planning and implementation include short-term, intensive nursing home visits to provide direct care, to teach the client and family about the illness and its control, to facilitate their assumption of care, to counsel family members on their changing health care needs, and to prevent negative outcomes affecting the health status of the client and family.

If the nurse is limited in time and unable to assist the family to develop coping skills, a consultation with a social worker or specialist may be indicated (e.g., a medical social worker for interpersonal relationship problems or social agency referrals and a nutritionist in the case of a diabetic's dietary needs). Complex problems not in the domain of nursing or requiring intensive time commitments may be referred to other agencies or professionals if agreed upon by the family.

The Meals on Wheels nutritional program is an example of a community-based agency providing low-cost services and a basic necessity for home health care that helps to maintain the client at home. Reimbursable professional services in addition to nursing include the therapies (physical, occupational, and speech) and social work.

Nutritionist and health educator services are not reimbursable, however, both professional groups are involved in the political action arena for recognition by Medicare and other third-party payors. Home health care nursing strategies include a multidisciplinary health team approach to caring for clients. Although the nurse may often make solo visits, it is common for other care providers to be involved in the complex and specialized care of home health care clients.

Coordination of care is essential, and, because nursing usually has responsibility for the majority of visits, it becomes the nurse's function to coordinate and collaborate client services with the other team members. A strong working relationship and communication system must be established between the nurse and physician to maintain therapies appropriate to the client's condition. Planning with the other team members for visits at critical stages of the client's illness and for the family's care providing needs is essential to effectively use the limited number of visits for which the specialists can be reimbursed.

### Monitoring of Client Status

Process evaluation is measured periodically by checking the client and family's progress in carrying out the objectives of the nursing care plan. The written documentation of the care giving activities and the client and family's reports of satisfaction provide data for evaluating the progress.

### Evaluation

When the client and family are discharged from service or when a nursing diagnosis is resolved, the overall goals serve as the criteria for measuring the extent of the outcome in terms of the achievement of the predetermined goals. The sample goals listed previously are suggested as outcome criteria for the diagnoses in this cluster. As the nursing diagnostic classification systems become more sophisticated and as research is conducted, additional diagnoses will be identified, and present diagnoses will be combined or refined.

## Safety Patterns: Prevention of Injury

### Selected Diagnoses

Family processes, alterations in
Health maintenance, alterations in

Home maintenance management, impaired
Injury, potential for
Knowledge deficit
Mobility, impaired, physical
Self-care deficit

These nursing diagnoses are included in the diagnostic cluster of safety patterns according to etiology, defining characteristics, and client and family needs and priorities. Maintaining a safe physical environment in the home setting is essential to the recovery of the ill client and the maintenance of the health of other family members.

## *Focus of Nursing Care*

Nursing interventions related to the selected diagnoses will vary according to the client's medical diagnoses, rehabilitation status, activities of daily living abilities, and potential of the family for the care of the client. Interventions could include ambulation, transfer techniques, positioning and body alignment, range-of-motion techniques, activities of daily living exercises, and the creation of a therapeutic and rehabilitative environment in the home.

Clients with deficits in self-care need certain appliances and equipment that facilitate their activities of daily living. Examples of appliances in the home setting are raised toilet seats, shower bars and stools, handrails and ramps for mobility throughout the home, hoyer lifts if indicated for transfer from bed to chair to tub to commode, wheeelchairs, and other assistive devices.

Clients with limited mobility will need appliances and equipment that facilitate the movement of the client in the home for care giving activities, feeding, rest, and relaxation. Appliances and equipment include grab bars, handrails, wheelchairs, walkers, tripods, crutches, and canes.

Safe techniques on the part of the client and care provider(s) for utilization and maintenance of the equipment and appliances are essential to care. Proper crutch walking, including the appropriate positioning of crutches against the chest wall and correct length of crutches, using a cane on the unaffected side to assist ambulation, and placing the walker in front of the client and stepping into but not up to the front of the cage are examples of safe techniques with assistive devices in the home. Review of basic nursing and rehabilitation texts such as Brunner and Suddarth (1986); Lewis (1984); Patrick, Woods, Craven, Roksoky, and Bruno (1986); Potter and Perry (1985); Smith and Duell (1985); and Swearington (1984) will help the nurse and family with procedures for specific equipment and assistive devices.

Techniques for ambulation and transfer of the client are reviewed with the client and family prior to discharge from the acute care facility and again at home on the first visit by the home health care nurse. The nurse, client, and family consult with physicians, physical therapists, occupational therapists, and durable medical supplies specialists as necessary.

## Etiology and Defining Characteristics

Carpenito (1983) defines potential for injury as "the state in which the individual is at risk for injury because of a perceptual or physiological deficit, a lack of awareness, or maturational age" (p 238). Impaired physical mobility is defined as "a state in which the individual experiences or is at risk of experiencing limitation of physical movement" (p 264).

There is a myriad of health problems leading to the seven potential nursing diagnoses listed earlier in this section. Medical diagnoses related to the nursing diagnoses include

Arthritis
Cerebral vascular accident
Chronic and debilitating diseases
Congestive heart disease
Injuries
Neuromuscular disorders
Orthopaedic conditions
Surgical procedures (and so on)

Other etiologic factors include the ability and availability of the client and family to learn new techniques, care of the client, and manipulation of necessary equipment. The conduciveness of the home environment to change in interior and external features to accommodate the equipment is essential to the maintenance of the home for the ill client. For example, a second-story apartment with a narrow stairway is not readily adjusted to wheelchairs and hoyer lifts, thus alternate plans are indicated.

Defining characteristics for the nursing diagnoses include an inadequately furnished home environment for client care, a family or primary care provider with limited knowledge in the care of the client and the use and maintenance of the necessary equipment, clients with health problems that limit their mobility and activities of daily living, clients who are at risk for injury owing to perceptual system deficits, advanced age frailties, maturational crises, and interruptions in cognitive processes.

## Outcome Criteria

The following outcome criteria are client- and family-centered. The client, family, and/or care provider will:

1. Provide a safe home environment for the ill client and family
2. Create a home environment conducive to client mobility, comfort, rest, rehabilitation, and growth and development

3. Have access to basic necessities in the home and diversional activities
4. Experience no injuries

## Application of the Nursing Process

### Assessment

The nurse, client, and family identify major problems that they must confront to assist the ill client in reaching the highest possible level of health. Factors to consider include the home environment and its physical characteristics that help or hinder the recovery process, the client's physical condition (including present health status and prognosis), the client and family member's age and developmental level, and the assistive devices and equipment necessary for client care. As the data are collected and analyzed, the potential nursing diagnoses are listed, refined, and ruled out to identify those applying specifically to the client and family's situation.

#### Life Cycle Assessment

The majority of home health care clients are elderly, and many are classified in the frail elderly category. The chronic diseases of arthritis, cancer, and heart disease are common to this population and have implications for the diagnostic clusters within the functional patterns of health promotion, health maintenance, and safety (Hogstel, 1985). Infants, children, and adolescent home health care clients continue to grow and develop in spite of their acute or chronic illnesses that require home health care. All these factors are part of the assessment activities for identifying existing and potential threats to health and their related nursing diagnoses.

Many of the nursing texts on aging and home health care discuss in detail factors rendering the elderly vulnerable to injury or immobility, strategies for improving and/or maintaining their functional levels, and some of the major problems facing care providers in delivering home health care services to the elderly (Pelham and Clark, 1986; Steffl, 1984).

Nurses providing home health care services for the young should conduct frequent growth and development assessments in addition to monitoring the child's health condition status. Growth and developmental milestones are discussed with the parents, and anticipatory guidance for expected age or developmental changes in behavior are reviewed. Teaching this knowledge to parents provides them with anticipatory health guidance to prevent injuries and to promote health specific to the child's increased physiologic, neuromuscular, social, and cognitive development.

#### Home Environment Assessment

One of the nurse's activities during the initial home visit is an assessment of the physical home environment. The nurse explains to the family the purpose of the assessment and how it relates to the recovery of the sick member and maintenance of other members' health. The nurse requests a tour of the home, particularly with the member of the family who is the primary care provider. The nurse and family member assess the physical environment for existing or potential hazards affecting the health status of the family. Cultural factors and value systems of the family and nurse are considered, because they may be at variance from one another. The nurse judges the situation according to actual hazards in the home and not according to aesthetics, which are subject to the nurse's personal opinion.

The room or site where the family has decided to place the ill client or where most of the physical care will be provided is surveyed. The location is assessed for its heat, lighting, accessibility to water, electrical outlets, equipment, disposal of wastes, and room for maneuvering if procedures such as medication administration, irrigation, dressing changes, physical therapy, or other treatments are ordered. Rugs, furniture, steps, and widths of doorways are inspected for possible access interference. Equipment such as the bed, walking aids, chairs, electrical appliances, and so on are inspected for their working condition and for any potential hazards arising from their use.

Rails placed at strategic sites in the bathroom for showering and toileting are installed if long-term disability is anticipated. Raised toilet seats and over-the-tub seats assist in the transfer of the client from a wheelchair or walker and can offer some measure of independence to the client in carrying out activities of daily living. There must be ample room for the manipulation of such equipment as Hoyer lifts. These appliances are stored out of the way of other family members who could injure themselves. Clients with visual or hearing deficits can have braille-assisted devices or signal lights installed to assist them for moving about the home. Ramps or lifts both inside and out of the home are desirable for clients confined to wheelchairs or requiring ambulation devices.

The nurse and family member(s) tour the home to gather data related to its adequacy for providing home health care. Included in the data are

Access of the home environment to health care providers
Emergency exits
Potential fire hazards
Easy and safe routes for client mobility
Sanitary and adequate facilities for care of equipment
Areas and equipment for food preparation and disposal
A safe water supply
A disposal site for wastes that will not harm the family's or community's
    health
Clean air
Adequate lighting
Adequate heat/ventilation

Pleasant surroundings that do not overload perceptual systems

An environment that will provide stimulation, comfort, promote recovery, and prevent infection and injury

After the initial assessment activities, the nurse and family review the data gathered and list any actual or potential problems that can affect the recuperation period of the ill family member or the health of the family. The appropriate nursing diagnoses are identified and could include

Family processes, alterations in

Potential for injury

Potential for infection

Mobility, impaired

Health maintenance, alterations in

Home maintenance management, impaired

Self-care deficit

Relevant goals for each of the diagnoses are set by the family and nurse and could include the outcome criteria listed previously.

## Planning and Implementation

Plans for eliminating the potential hazards for injury are developed. The nurse considers the economic situation of the family and does not propose plans that are impossible to complete owing to financial constraints. If problems exist in a rented home or are due to inadequate community services, the nurse can act as advocate for the family in contacting the landlord or appropriate agency to rectify the situation. These plans are agreed upon by the family and are incorporated into the plan. At no time should the nurse contact other people or agencies in the community without the family's consent, because such action can be detrimental to the family's relationships in the community.

Each problem and its etiologic or contributing factors are listed with the related goals and objectives. The plan for each problem is written, and the nurse and family decide who will be responsible for carrying out the objectives, the methods, and the expected dates that the goals and objectives will be met.

### Monitoring of Client Status

The nurse monitors the progress toward problem resolution during each subsequent visit. The Home Environment Assessment Guide serves as an outline for collecting data to identify actual or potential health hazards related to the safety of the home environment. It can also be used for recording the problem, its plan of care, and documentation of the progress toward resolution. The Guide can be found in Appendix G.

## Evaluation

The long-term goals and objectives for each diagnosis serve as the criteria for measuring the final outcome of nursing care. Improved client and family health status and their satisfaction with the nursing care provided serve as the overall outcome criteria.

## Safety Patterns in the Control of Infection

## Selected Diagnoses

The major selected diagnosis for this safety pattern is infection, potential for. However, there are several diagnoses that closely relate to the client and family's needs as they seek to prevent infection in the home setting. The related diagnoses are:

> Family processes, alterations in
> Health maintenance, alterations in
> Home maintenance management, impaired
> Knowledge deficit

These selected nursing diagnoses focus on the client's and family's and/or significant others' functional safety patterns as they relate to the control of infection. The nurse identifies possible infectious threats to the client and family and relates them to appropriate nursing diagnoses. The nursing process specific to the diagnoses begins with the initial visit and continues throughout the nurse–client–family interaction.

A knowledge of the infection cycle is fundamental to nursing care and is directed toward breaking the chain of events in the cycle to prevent infections and/or complications of illness. The classic agent, host, and environmental approach to epidemiology is useful as a model for examining potential causes of infection in the client at home.

Lillienfeld and Lillienfeld (1980) discuss major agent, host, and environmental factors and the mode of transmission of disease. Home health care clients are more susceptible to bacterial, viral, and fungal agents. Host factors are multiple and include the specific nursing and medical diagnoses or health problems of the client, age, sex, ethnic group, physiologic state, immunologic state, intercurrent or pre-existing disease, and behavioral factors. Environmental factors include physical, biological, and socioeconomic environments (pp 47 and 48).

The modes of transmission in the home setting are the dynamics of

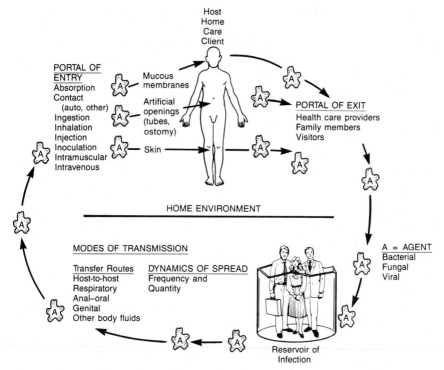

**Figure 10-1.** Infection chain applied to home health care. (In collaboration with William Bigler, Ph.D., Chairman, Center for Advanced Medical Technology, San Francisco State University)

spread (contact, ingestion, inhalation, injection, inoculation, intramuscular, and intravenous) and transfer routes (host-to-host, respiratory, anal-oral, genital, and other body fluids routes). The portals of entry and exit for the host are important factors to consider and include open body systems such as conjunctiva, skin, mucous membranes, and artificial openings (tubes, ostomies) (Lillienfeld and Lillienfeld, 1980, p 49).

The principle danger of infection for home health clients is in other people—care providers, family members, and visitors to the home—becoming potential carriers of infection both to and from the client. The nurse analyzes the cycle of infection and aims intervention strategies at breaking into the cycle of events to prevent disease. Figure 10-1 illustrates an adaptation of the infection chain applied to home health care.

## Etiology and Defining Characteristics

Usually family members in close contact with one another and confined to the home environment are less likely to develop infections because of their previously established compatibility with one another and the environment. However, the ill client at home is more susceptible to infection because of the body's lowered resistance from the disease process and the interplay of physiologic, sociologic, and psychological factors.

Other factors external to the individual client leading to possible infection include previous exposure to infective organisms in the health care institution during the acute phase of illness, increased contact with health care providers and equipment that enters the home environment, and lack of knowledge relating to aseptic techniques on the part of the family or other care providers. Preventive measures are essential because of the effects of illness and the associated stresses on the client who is less able to cope with infectious processes.

## Focus of Nursing Care: The Control of Infection in the Home

The selected basic intervention relating to the control of infection in the home environment is aseptic technique through application of the traditional community health nursing "bag technique." Aseptic technique as a nursing procedure and demonstrated to the family as a safe health practice is critical to the promotion of healing and the prevention of infection. Many community/public health nursing and home health care agencies continue to use the traditional method of bag technique. Other agencies and nursing personnel choose to adapt the technique by practicing medical asepsis (handwashing is of priority) and adapting to existing facilities and equipment in the home.

### Outcome Criteria

The practice of home health care nursing requires the use of vigilant aseptic technique on the part of the professional. The nurse must also demonstrate aseptic technique to the client and family in the control of infection. The following outcome criteria apply to the client and family. By practicing aseptic technique in the home setting, the client and/or family will

1.  Experience no secondary infections
2.  Experience no newly diagnosed communicable disease

### Application of the Nursing Process

#### Assessment

The nurse uses the infection chain components as guides for collecting data and assessing the client at risk for infection. The ill client in the home is a susceptible host who is experiencing both physiologic and psychological stresses. The nature of the client's illness will determine the potential portal of entry into the body, including the skin, conjunctiva, mucous membrane, and respiratory, genitourinary, and gastrointestinal systems. When assessing the client, specific variables that render body systems open to infection are noted, that is, open wounds, urinary catheters, indwelling circulation catheters, respiratory appliances, ostomies, and so on. The factors related to the body systems are assessed in light of their portal of exits and the potential for autonomous transmission of infection to other members of the family, visitors to the home, or health care providers.

The mode of transmission is analyzed according to the involved body system(s) and the nature of the agent—bacterial, viral, or fungal. A knowledge of microbiology is necessary to understand how the microbe lives, its usual habitat or reservoir, and its methods of transport from one site to another. All these factors—host, agent, portals of entry and exit, and mode of transmission—are considered within the context of the physical, biological, and socioeconomic environment of the home. The client and family's knowledge of infection control; home facilities, including water, food, and waste handling; and resources for providing home care are included in the assessment for the diagnosis of potential for infection.

## Planning and Implementation

The factors listed under assessment are reviewed, and relevant findings are listed as etiologic or contributing factors to the diagnosis. Based on these factors, client outcomes or goals are developed to improve the health status of client and maintain the health of the family. Aseptic technique is essential to planning and providing nursing care for the prevention of infection in the client and family. Clients receiving home health care are ill and vulnerable to infection and must be protected from microbes that invade the home.

The following steps outline bag technique for the implementation of medical aseptic technique in the home setting. Independent nurse clinicians, nurse practitioners, and nurses in home health care agencies may use different bag designs and basic equipment according to specific practice needs. Nurses should follow agency bag technique policies and procedures or may adapt the following procedures according to their client's needs and the type of services provided. The nursing bag is always carried in case of unanticipated situations calling for assessment or nursing care.

### The Nursing Bag

Most nursing bags have the same basic equipment, with supplemental items for specific procedures carried in either the bag or separate containers. Basic equipment includes:

## Basic Equipment

1. Paper towels are used to dry hands and create an area to protect the family's environment from the "dirty" outside of the bag and to protect the bag from home environment microorganisms and/ or allergens. Placing the bag on a paper towel helps to prevent cross-contamination from one client and/or nurse to another. It may be necessary to establish one area near the bag and running water for handwashing purposes and another near the client's bedside or location where care is provided.
2. Soap in container (cleansing agent). Each agency has its own preference for type of soap, or the nurse may use soap in the client's home, although bar soap can harbor organisms. In some instances, disposable pre-treated soap pads or cloths may be used if there are no running water facilities in the home.
3. Aprons (optional and are usually disposable)
4. Antiseptic wipes are used as a disinfectant for procedures and cleaning items returned to the nursing bag.
5. Paper or plastic bags are used for disposal of waste materials and to return used equipment to the agency for disposal or processing. The nurse may use her or his judgment in disposing of materials into suitable waste containers in the home as an alternate method. Any infectious materials such as old dressings, disposable catheters, syringes, irrigation bags, and plastic tubing are handled carefully, double-bagged, and discarded in outside containers. The family is educated about the handling of infectious materials. If there is potential or actual threat to waste handlers, the material is returned to the agency for proper disposal.

## Assessment Equipment

1. Thermometers with Disposable sheaths (It is preferred to use the client's own thermometer in the home.)
2. Sphygmomanometer with several sized cuffs for measuring the blood pressure of clients of varying age and size
3. Stethoscope with bell and diaphragm for measuring blood pressure and auscultation of respiratory, circulatory, and other appropriate systems
4. Plastic-coated or metal tape measure for assessment of head, chest, and length measurements in children and assessment of limbs and joints
5. Penlight for assessing presence of light reflex in eyes, mouth, and nasopharynx; in special instances, transillumination
6. Otoscope, ophthalmoscope, and tongue blades for assessing head and neck

## Emergency Equipment

1. Benadryl or other antihistamine and sterile tuberculin syringe with prescribed amount of adrenalin according to agency policy; used in cases of urticaria, extreme allergic reactions, and/or anaphylactic shock
2. Band-Aids, antiseptic solution, ace bandages, slings, splints, and so on

## Special Procedure Sets (usually disposable)

These depend upon the client's condition, needs, present health status, and plan of care. It is advisable to carry extra sets in case of contamination or defect in the equipment. Examples of sets include

Catheterization sets (straight and indwelling type)
Irrigation sets
Intravenous therapy equipment
Suctioning catheters
Enema sets

## Setting Up

### Step 1
The nursing bag is placed on a flat, open, and clean as possible surface (paper towel, optional). It should be near a sink and kept out of the reach of children and pets. The outside and inner top of the standard nursing bag are considered unclean, whereas the inside and contents (equipment) of the bag are considered clean. Other types of bags are treated as though the inside is clean, with outside pockets containing paper towels and soap for setting up.

### Step 2
If an apron is used, it is put on prior to handwashing. The soap container and several extra paper towels are then removed and placed on the work area. If a paper or plastic bag is to serve for waste, it is opened and set up in a corner of the work area for disposal of used materials. A paper towel is tucked under the arm, and soap is placed in one hand. Hands are washed vigorously under running water, rinsed thoroughly, and wiped dry with two paper towels, which are then used to turn off the faucets. Figure 10-2 illustrates the correct handwashing technique in the home.

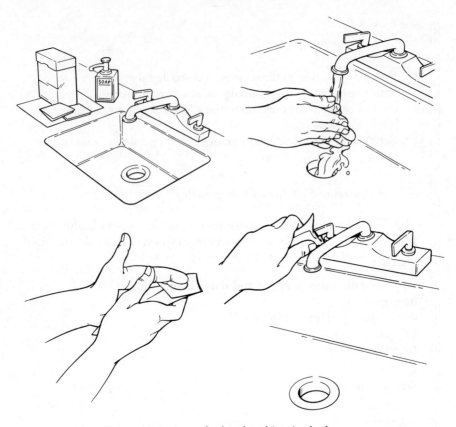

Figure 10-2. Steps for handwashing in the home.

### Step 3

After the hands are washed, any equipment that is necessary for providing care is removed from the bag. Special procedure sets are set up near the client, and appropriate medical or surgical aseptic techniques are instituted. The nurse serves as a role model for the client and family and uses the opportunity for teaching about the prevention of infection. Any time that additional equipment is needed from the nursing bag, hands must be washed again; thus, it is wise to have extra paper towels available on the clean work area in case they are needed.

### Step 4

Assessment and special procedure supplies are placed on the clean or sterile field work areas. After use, they are washed with soap and water, dried, wiped with a disinfectant such as alcohol, and returned to the nursing bag. Equipment in the home is cleaned, disinfected, and stored in closed, protected containers for future use. Materials that can be disinfected by soaking in antiseptic solution or boiled for at least 20 minutes in water can be processed in the home. Some materials can be sterilized by placing them in the oven at 350° for 30 minutes.

The type of equipment, its material, and its purpose define the procedure used for disinfection or sterilization. Glass and stainless steel can be sterilized by autoclaving. Disposable plastic and rubber materials can disintegrate and could produce toxic reactions when processed; thus, it is best to check the manufacturers' instructions and discard questionable disposable materials safely, that is, in the agency if necessary rather than in the home (Axnich and Yarborough, 1984). Some agencies have policies requiring the return of syringes and needles to the agency for syringe count and other safety factors.

Equipment such as stethoscopes, tape measures, soap containers, specula, and otoscopes are recycled for multiple client use. Before returning them to the bag, the items are cleaned and, if possible, washed and wiped with alcohol or other disinfectant. If there is suspicion of possible contamination, the item under question is placed in a separate paper or plastic bag and returned to the agency for proper processing, disinfection, and/or sterilization. If the nursing bag and its contents become contaminated, they are returned to the agency for disinfection.

### Monitoring Client Status

The nursing plan for preventing infection of the ill client at home and maintaining the family's health care through aseptic technique and home maintenance is monitored by the nurse during each visit to the home. An improved health status of the client is measured by the progress in attaining optimal health for the individual. For example, a client recovering from surgery will exhibit no secondary incision infections, respiratory illnesses, or other illnesses from exposure to infectious or communicable diseases. His or her family will maintain its health status throughout the client's illness, and, if other members have health problems, they will demonstrate improved health directly attributed to the health teaching and intervention of the home health care nurse.

## Evaluation

The outcome criteria developed as the long-term goals for the nursing care plan serve as measures of evaluation. Client and family satisfaction are additional measures for effectiveness of nursing care. Home health agencies should have monitoring systems for detecting unwarranted infections in their client population. Research activities are indicated for epidemiologic studies to correlate rates of nosocomial infections to shortened lengths of stay in the hospital. It is possible that fewer complications and secondary infections will be observed in the client population owing to the decreased exposure time in the acute care environment.

Additional research is recommended for study of the rates of recovery, numbers of complications, disabilities, and unwarranted deaths related to early discharge from the hospital and the possible lack of adequate support systems in the home and community. The changes in the health care system indicate a need to increase protective nursing behaviors to prevent the spread of infection in the home and to speed recovery time for clients experiencing episodes of illness.

## References

Axnich KJ, Yarborough M: Infection Control: An Integrated Approach. St Louis, Mosby, 1984

Brunner LS, Suddarth DS: The Lippincott Manual of Nursing Practice. Philadelphia, JB Lippincott, 1986

Carpenito LJ: Nursing Diagnosis: Application to Clinical Practice. Philadelphia, JB Lippincott, 1983

Hogstel M: Home Nursing Care for the Elderly. Bowie, MD, Brady Communications Co, 1985

Lewis LW: Fundamental Skills in Patient Care, 3rd ed. Philadelphia, JB Lippincott, 1984

Lillienfeld A, Lillienfeld D: Foundations of Epidemiology, 2nd ed. New York, Oxford University Press, 1980

National League for Nursing: The quest for quality. NLN Public Policy Bulletin. IV 2: Summer, 1986

Patricki ML, Woods SL, Craven RF, Rokosky JS, Bruno PM: Medical-surgical nursing: Pathophysiological Concepts. Philadelphia, JB Lippincott, 1986

Pelham A, Clark W (eds): Managing Home Care for the Elderly: Lessons from Community Based Agencies. New York, Springer, 1986

Potter PA, Perry AG: Fundamentals of Nursing: Concepts, Process, and Practice. St Louis, CV Mosby, 1985

Smith S, Duell D: Clinical Nursing Skills Presented in the Nursing Process Basic to Advanced Skills. Los Altos, California, National Nursing Review, 1985

Steffl B (ed): Handbook of Gerontological Nursing. New York, Van Norstrand-Reinholdt, 1984

Swearington PL: The Addison-Wesley Photo Atlas of Nursing Procedures. Menlo Park, Addison Wesley, 1984

# Home Health Care: Issues for Nursing

In Chapters 11 and 12, some of the professional issues confronting nurses who practice in home health care are presented. Quality assurance is a major responsibility of the nurse, other professionals, paraprofessionals, management and administrative staff, and home health care agencies. In Chapter 11, this concept is discussed on a macro level compared to the micro level of evaluation, which examines the direct delivery of care to the individual client and family and/or significant others. The latter form of quality assurance takes place during each encounter between the client and family and health care provider(s). It is an essential component of the nursing process.

Chapter 4, which deals with the nursing process discusses micro level evaluation as it applies to the individual client, family, and/or significant others. Included in the discussion is process evaluation, that is, the measuring of the progress of the client as he or she moves through the short-term goals (objectives) defined in the nursing care plan. Outcome evaluation takes place when the services are discontinued and is measured by the client and/or family's satisfaction with care and the extent to which the specified long-term goals of care were met. Each of the chapters focusing on diagnostic clusters frequently encountered in home health care nursing discusses the recommended evaluation activities according to the selected nursing diagnoses and individual client and family outcomes.

Common quality assurance conceptual models and frameworks applied to program development and evaluation activities are discussed in Chapter 11. Laws and regulations affecting practice and the delivery of services are discussed, as well as the professional standards of care that serve as criteria for measuring quality home health nursing care.

Application of quality assurance as part of program development and evaluation is introduced. Diagnosing community needs in terms of home health care and evaluating the programs that provide services to clients are part of the macro level of quality assurance. Nurses in all levels of practice are responsible for the delivery of quality professional services. The consumers of care, including the client, the family and/or significant others, and aggregate client groups expect accountability for services rendered. Practicing quality assurance through case review, record reviews (audits), program evaluation, staff evaluation, and community assessment is part of the analysis of the data that document safe, health-promoting services. Whether regulated by law, mandated as part of reimbursement, expected by professional standards, or self-imposed by professional ethics, quality assurance is a vital component of the practice of home health care nursing.

Chapter 12 briefly reviews the research process as it applies to home health care nursing. A sample study is used to demonstrate research applications to home health care. The study describes a pilot study of a tool to measure patient outcomes in home health care. The nursing diagnostic classification system served as the conceptual framework for the study. Goals or client outcomes related to each diagnosis served as the criteria to measure the client outcomes. Other researchable questions in the home health care field are posed.

Issues facing home health care providers are discussed, and there is an attempt to forecast trends in the health care system as they influence home health care. Home health care nursing with its rich history is a traditional service moving into a specialty of the current high-technology age. Nurses practicing in the field are urged to examine present and future issues confronting them and the clients they serve, the health care system that creates the milieu, and the professional issues influencing practice.

# 11

# *Program Evaluation and Quality Assurance*

## *Overview and Definitions of Terms Used in Evaluation*

Florence Nightingale was one of the first nurse evaluators, as demonstrated by her collection and analysis of data for epidemiologic studies and documentation of nursing care. The process of evaluation in nursing has many of its roots in program evaluation from public health and education theories. Terms such as *formative, summative, goal-based,* and *goal-free evaluation* are found in education literature. Application of quality assurance concepts to nursing relates to the consumer movement of the 1960s, the business world, and the manufacturing industry, where such terms as *quality control, audit,* and *structure, process,* and *product evaluation* are found.

Home health care agencies are involved in two major forms of evaluation activities: evaluation of nursing service and health care programs, and quality assurance as measured by client-centered outcomes. For the purposes of evaluation applied to home health care, the following terms are defined:

*Evaluation*—the process of assessing a program (or nursing care) by collecting and analyzing data; judging its worth according to standards; and making decisions concerning the program's future.

*Formative evaluation*—evaluation that takes place during the assessment, planning, and implementation stages of program development or patient care.

*Summative evaluation*—evaluation that measures the outcomes or product of the program or nursing care. For the nursing care of individual clients, it measures the success in reaching the predetermined goals of nursing care. Theoretically, summative evaluation judges the final product; thus, it should rarely occur for program evaluation activities, because home health care agency programs are ongoing.

*Goal-free evaluation*—a method of evaluation that is usually subjective in nature, that is, it is the observation of a program or service, and qualitative information is gathered. The evaluator usually has no prior knowledge of the goals or objectives of the program or service and has only a general knowledge of its purpose. Data are collected through direct and indirect observations and during interviews of program participants and consumers. It can be both formative and/or summative in nature.

*Goal-based evaluation*—a method of evaluation that is usually objective. Data are collected according to the predetermined purpose, goals, and objectives of the program. Data are analyzed, and judgments about the program are based on the progress of the program toward meeting its purpose, goals, and objectives.

The previous definitions were derived from Worthen and Sanders (1973).

*Quality assurance*—the monitoring of the activities of client care to determine the degree of excellence attained in the implementation of activities (Stanhope and Lancaster, 1984).

*Quality control*—the monitoring of the processes and outcomes of the program and its services according to its stated goals and objectives. This includes taking corrective measures to pilot the program through its intended course and outcomes.

The following three definitions are based on Donabedian's (1966) classic theories on evaluation as related to nursing:

*Structure framework for evaluation*—study of the systems within which the program or nursing care services operate. Included for home health care are agency organization, administration, physical facilities, staffing patterns, financial support, qualifications of the staff, and so on.

*Process framework for evaluation*—study of the implementation or means of delivery of the services of the home health care program or nursing care. It includes the actual delivery of care and how it is done.

*Product framework for evaluation*—study of the results or outcomes of the home health care program or nursing services.

*Quality care audit*—the evaluation of care delivered. It appraises all significant steps taken in the care of a client, with attention to the nature of, the rationale for, and the degree to which they help the patient reach specified and attainable goals. It may be accomplished through a concurrent or retrospective review of a random sample of clients' records (National League for Nursing, 1980, p 48).

## Models of Evaluation

Donabedian's (1966) model of evaluation includes structure, process, and product components and is frequently adopted as a framework for evaluation activities. It is not uncommon to see the process/product components of the model combined for judging the worth of programs and their activities. Such studies demonstrate the quality of the product or services and how well they are delivered.

## The Kessner and Kalk Model (1973)

Kessner and Kalk (1973) used another type of model for evaluating the quality of health care delivery to groups of people rather than to specific individuals. It is the Tracer model of evaluation and involves selecting one major health problem common to a group of clients. In order for it to succeed as a model, the health problem must be easily diagnosed and defined and prevalent, and it must have an effect on the health status of the aggregate. Based on overall analysis of data collected from this model of evaluation, the care provider sets certain criteria or standards of care for the specific health problem that will reduce the risk factors for the affected population (Stanhope and Lancaster, 1984).

The application of the Kessner and Kalk model to home health care has many possibilities. For example, a group of staff nurses could select one nursing diagnosis common to many of their clients that presents the agency with problems of quality of care, patient outcomes, frequency of visits, and cost-effectiveness. To apply the Tracer model to home health care, the evaluator collects data pertaining to

1. The etiologic factors leading to the diagnosis
2. Specific defining characteristics of the diagnosis
3. Assessment criteria
4. Specific nursing care
5. Client outcomes

Actual nursing care and patient outcomes are then measured against the predetermined goals.

The following sample case study illustrates the Tracer method applied to home health care:

> During a monthly staff meeting, several nurses noted that many of their clients were elderly and cared for at home by their spouses or adult children. The family members' care providing activities were supplemented by the professional services of the home health agency. A common problem for the clients and their primary care providers at home was the lack of interaction with people outside their home environment.
>
> Through discussion and record review, it was found that most of these families had a nursing diagnosis of social isolation related to multiple health problems requiring clients and their care providers to remain in the home. Common etiologic and contributing factors leading to the diagnosis included advanced age of the client and family members, ex-

tensive nursing care necessary for control of the other health problems, geographic location, isolation from extended families and friends, and numerous environmental and sociocultural factors associated with an aging population.

The nurses set the defining characteristics for the diagnosis as follows:

The family

1. Has limited social contact with people outside the home as measured by less than one contact per week
2. Verbalizes the need for contact with family, friends, and/or socializing agencies (e.g., senior citizens groups, church, clubs)
3. Demonstrates negative behavior such as frustration with care providers and each other, anger, and sadness

Assessment criteria for the aggregate included the observation and documentation of at least two of the three defining characteristics within the family as previously listed. The nurses set the following goals for client outcomes.

The family will

1. Have contact with selected people other than care providers at least once a week in or out of the home
2. Report having made social contacts
3. Demonstrate a change in behavior through increased positive attitudes

Planning took place through collaboration with churches and social organizations to provide social support to the families. Plans were made for increased visits to the clients and families through these organizations. It was agreed that each of the nurses would select the clients in her or his caseload with the diagnosis and, at the end of every 3-month period, prepare a report of the clients' progress toward the pre-set goals. The data from these reports would be analyzed and applied toward future plans in trying to prevent the occurrence of the problem in other families with similar predisposing factors.

## The Rutstein Model (1976)

The Rutstein (1976) sentinel method of evaluation is based on examination of the specific parameters of the outcomes of care. It adapts an epidemiologic approach to the study of the client's health status (Stanhope and Lancaster, 1984). Included in its measures are the negative aspects of a client's condition. These include three major negative outcomes: unwarranted death, disability, and complications. Carpenito's (1983) client-centered outcomes relating to specific nursing diagnoses include these as major classifications for negative outcomes of nursing care provided. These outcomes are easily measured.

Application of the Rutstein model to home health care settings has immense potential because of its efficiency and speedy access to the data. The three major classifications of client negative outcomes (complications, disability, and unwarranted death) are identified and used as the criteria for measuring negative outcomes. Data are collected through audits of client records. Findings of concern are then reviewed for evaluation of the structure or process factors that led to the negative outcomes. Examples include lack of financial support, incompetent staff, poor follow-up, and inappropriate plan of care.

To demonstrate the Sentinel model of evaluation, the following example presents the nursing diagnosis of potential for infection related to loss of skin integrity.

Fifty records of clients in a home health agency who had experienced loss of skin integrity owing to a variety of health problems such as surgery, injury, and lesions were randomly selected. A review of the records 2 months following admission to service revealed the following negative outcomes:

1. Complications: 13 cases (diagnosed infection)
2. Disability: 3 cases (scarring of skin, nonresolved infection, loss of normal body functioning owing to infectious process)
3. Unwarranted death: 1 case (treatment for infection was delayed)

Based on the findings, the staff reviewed the records of the clients, with negative outcomes. An epidemiologic approach revealed that 10 of the cases had been visited by the same home health aide. Nasopharyngeal cultures demonstrate this aide as a carrier of *beta streptococci*, the same organism found in the clients. Appropriate interventions took place to treat the aide and prevent recurrence of the problem.

## Licensure, Accreditation, and Certification

Other models of evaluation and quality assurance in nursing include individual and institutional licensure (one of the oldest methods of ensuring quality care), accreditation, professional standards of care such as the Joint Commission on Accreditation of Hospitals and the American Nurses Association, Divisions on Practice, and certification (Stanhope and Lancaster, 1984).

Licensure for the individual nurse in the United States arises from the various states' Nurse Practice Acts and their enforcement through regulations. The states may also require licensure or certification for the operation of health agencies. Nurse administrators in agencies must be knowledgeable about the laws that apply in their specific states.

Accreditation of an agency is usually voluntary and reflects a commitment on the part of the agency to quality care. The National League for Nursing and the Council of Home Health Agencies have developed criteria and standards for home health and community nursing services. Agencies who meet these criteria and standards are eligible for accreditation by the American Public Health Association and the National League for Nursing (National League for Nursing, 1980). Griffith (1986) discusses how one agency participated in accreditation for quality assurance purposes and the benefits to staff, agency, and clients.

Recently, the National League for Nursing (NLN) published a position paper on ensuring quality in home health care. NLN believes that nurses are the predominant providers in home health care and should assume the lead in protecting the consumer from fraud, abuse, and substandard care. NLN's position states:

> In light of these trends, NLN affirms our belief that it is the responsibility of the nursing profession, which historically has been the predominant home care provider group, to establish and to uphold standards of home health care. The quality of nursing care delivered in patients' homes should be monitored by nurses themselves through a self-regulatory process that relies on nursing expertise, augmented by the participation of professionals in other provider disciplines and representatives from the community (National League for Nursing, 1986).

The certification process can apply to an individual practitioner or to an agency and is used to demonstrate excellence in quality. Certification usually occurs, in the case of the individual, through continuing education, with a resulting issue of certification by the educational institution, state regulating body, or professional organization.

Examples of these three certification processes for the individual include:

1. Certificate in primary health care nursing issued by a university that does not necessarily indicate meeting certain degree requirements such as a master's degree in nursing
2. School nurse teachers receiving a certificate from their state boards of education or health departments indicating that they have met certain educational and/or experience requirements set by state regulations
3. The American Nurses Association certification examination for Community Health Nurses is an example of a professional organization certifying the competency of practitioners. Certified nurses pass an examination, meet specified educational requirements, and demonstrate a prerequisite level of experience.

## Mandated Evaluation Programs

The federal government and state regulating agencies have certain mandated quality assurance programs. They include evaluation of services rendered to recipients of certain government medical care benefits. Although these programs do not apply directly to individual consumers of care, especially in the private pay sector of the health care system, they do have an impact on the whole system. Federal and state rules and regulations contain specific standards of care and criteria that agencies must meet in order to be issued a certificate for operation. The federal regulations are enforced through the Health Care Financing Agency as part of the Social Security Act. It can delegate its functions to the various state regulating agencies.

In addition to federal law, the various states have codes and regulations that enforce state laws regulating home health care agencies. A variety of state agencies act in this role, including the state education department, state and local health departments, and the health systems agency (New York State, 1982; Health Care Financing Administration, 1981). Personnel in agencies should be familiar with the regulating bodies in order to operate legally and meet certification standards.

Examples of these types of quality assurance programs that are particularly appropriate to today's home care are described here. Utilization Review programs were part of the 1965 Medicare Law designed to evaluate care and demonstrate cost containment (Stanhope and Lancaster, 1984). The program is administered through the Health Care Financing Administration (HCFA); the guidelines for review may be found on the HCFA–1572 form (1972). The process focuses on the need for care and is usually carried out through record reviews. Agencies set up Utilization Review Committees comprised of the various health team members who review selected records to learn whether the delivery of care is appropriate to the level of need demonstrated by the client. There are three types of review processes:

1.  Prospective—an assessment of the necessity of care before giving service
2.  Concurrent—a review of the necessity of the services while the care is being given
3.  Retrospective—an analysis of the services received by the client after the care has been given (Stanhope and Lancaster, 1984, p 224).

The Professional Standards Review Organization (PSRO) of the 1972 Social Security Act and its more recent Professional Review Organization (PRO) were created as quality assurance methods for peer review. These models were established as peer evaluation tools for quality of care and cost containment purposes as they apply to individual practitioners. They consist of peer review processes, and, although they were originally intended to monitor medical care, nurses have become involved in their implementation (American Nurses' Association, 1976).

The Health Care Financing Administration of the federal government administers the PRO program. Although PROs are not used in home health care, there is the possibility that they eventually will apply. Quality assurance programs are indicated as a response to the effect of the diagnostic-related groupings (DRGs) and the prospective payment financial construct in the current health care system. The DRG system classifies clients' problems into medical diagnoses and the related factors that influence the length of stay in the hospital. Hospitals receive Medicare funding according to the projected budget derived from the previous year's costs and the DRG classification. The system replaces the reimbursement for services rendered mechanism of financing medical care.

The change in the health care system has brought about early discharge from the hospital, with patients in the home who are experiencing more acute care and high-technology nursing service needs. The change in the health care system has influenced certain regulatory evaluation requirements for home health care. For example, home health care agencies are required by the HCFA to provide a prospective summary of the services that the agency plans to provide for each patient upon his or her admission to service for 60 days thereafter. Follow-up reports to HCFA provide retrospective information on the services actually provided (HCFA, 1985).

## Methods and Tools for Evaluation and Quality Control

It is recommended that a master plan of evaluation be developed in each health agency or private practice. The model for evaluation includes the processes for data collection, analysis, decision–making, and implementation of changes that are recommended. To ensure that a comprehensive evaluation takes place, all components of the model are included (structure, process, and product).

Donabedian's (1966) structure, process, and outcome is a classic model of evaluation. Another model borrowed from education's evaluation theory is that of Stufflebeam (1974): the context, input, process, and product (CIPP) framework. It assists the evaluator in studying the situation and identifying its many parameters. An interpretation of this model defines the context component as the major objectives or goals of the program under evaluation, and the input becomes the identification of the "what" that is being evaluated. The process is the actual implementation of the design or program. The product is the attainment of the objectives or goals and the decisions for continuation, modifications, or termination of the program.

There are many models available in the literature, and agencies select that which best meets their individual needs and situation. *The Administra-*

*tor's Handbook for Community and Home Care Services* (Fish, 1984) has a section that offers such a model and provides specific examples for data collection and analysis. Management personnel, such as supervising nurses, need agency support time to review the literature to identify appropriate tools and to test and implement their application to practice and evaluation of nursing services.

Many forms, questionnaires, interview schedules, auditing tools, scales, and indices are available. Many have tested reliability and validity. Others need further refinement (see Chapter 12). Nurses are urged to review and evaluate existing tools, to use them to support nursing's claims for uniqueness of service, quality control, and professional accountability.

One of the earliest quality assurance tools developed for community health nursing is that of Phaneuf (1965). The purpose of this tool was to measure quality of care. It included an appraisal of deficiencies in doctor's orders, the health professional's identification of client health problems, and the remaining elements of the nursing process—planning, implementing, and evaluation of the care provided. Manfredi (1986) conducted reliability and validity studies on the Phaneuf tool and found it to be reliable for internal consistency; however, further studies for its construct validity are indicated.

Examples of such tools may be found in Ward and Lindeman (1978). A partial listing includes "Provider–Client Interaction: Client's Perception of Provider, Client Care, and Health Services" (Abdellah and Levine); "Patient Satisfaction Interview" (Collins); "Functioning Status Assessment Form" (Densen, Danhey, Flagle, and Katz); and "Geriatric Rating Scale" (Plutchik, Conte, Hope, Lieberman, Bakur, Marcella, Grossman, and Lehrman).

Examples of specific agencies throughout the country that have developed tools include *Patient Classification/Objectives System—What Is It?*, Albany Visiting Nurses Association, Albany, New York, 1982; *Quality Assurance Program*, Florida Association of Home Health Agencies, Inc., 1980; *Outcome Criteria Public Health Nursing Services and Home Health Care Services*, Public Health Nursing Section, Minnesota Department of Health, 1983; and *Quality Assurance in Home Health Care*, Pennsylvania Assembly of Home Health Agencies, 1975.

## Nursing Diagnosis Classification System as an Evaluation Tool

In Section II of this text, we discuss nursing diagnostic clusters relevant to the delivery of high-technology care in the home setting. The nursing classification system provides a tool for measuring process/product in the delivery of these services. Chapter 12 describes a study that pilot–tested a tool for using the system in measuring client outcomes. The nursing diagnosis classification system lends itself to interpretation of the processes or means of the delivery of nursing care and the client's health status as measured by the attainment of predetermined goals relating to the diagnoses.

## Data Collection and Analysis: Computer Technology Advances

Today's high technology and its utilization of both mainframe and personal computer systems has much to offer in the administration of home health agencies and the assurance of quality nursing care. Large agencies may have the financial resources to establish a centralized computer system that can provide budget and recordkeeping activities, quality assurance, and staff development services. In these instances, they are able to hire computer scientists and/or technicians to operate the system in a cost-effective manner. Eventually, as society continues to develop technologically, nurse computer scientists will offer the expertise necessary for applying computer science to the knowledge and practice of nursing.

Small agencies, corporations, or private nursing practices for home health care services can purchase personal computers that provide almost the same services provided by larger computer systems. Their utilization can help to organize the financial structure of the agency and to keep client and administrative records. The initial investment of money is minute when one considers the time saved and its streamlining of recordkeeping costs and delivery of care.

There are many software packages available to nurses that are appropriate to home health care. Mini courses and computer assisted instruction packages (CAI) are available to teach basic skills in programming. Having these skills allows the nurse to write her or his own programs specific to nurses' and clients' needs. Many of the nursing diagnostic categories are easily quantified and translated into computer programs. The Omaha Nursing Diagnosis Classification System is one example (United States Department of Health and Human Services, 1980). Romano (1986) discusses a computerized diagnostic classification system implemented in the hospital setting. A computerized system allows nurses to

1. Make diagnoses based on assessment data through the use of pre-defined defining characteristics and functional patterns
2. Identify client goals or patient care outcomes particular to each diagnosis
3. Utilize pre-set nursing care plans if appropriate for the individual client
4. Maintain flowsheets documenting the client's progress

One of the main stressors in community health nursing is the paperwork activities required. Data–based systems can alleviate this problem, as well as being a part of the quality control system and having cost-effective advantages.

Many large home health care agencies have data-based, computerized systems in place for collecting and analyzing data, particularly as they relate to the financial structure of the agency. As nurses become increasingly literate in computers, they are applying the tool to nursing services and quality assurance programs. The agency that has a well–developed evaluation or quality assurance program in place, with specified goals and objectives for agency services, will find that quantifying the data is relatively simple.

Existing administrative data-based management systems relate to budgets, reports of services delivered, and records of numbers and types of visits to clients. As mentioned previously, these data-based processes relate to the structure or administrative aspects of the agency. Examples of some software packages specific to administrative aspects include CareData (1985), Delta Computer Systems, Inc. (1985), Health Agency Management System (1985), Home Care Information Systems, Inc. (1985), Home Care Pac (1985), Home Health Care (ACPI Ltd, 1984), Home Health Care System (Fleet, 1985), HOMIS 80 (1985), InfoMed (1985), and MEDI/VISIT (1985).

McHugh (1986) discusses the use of computerized or data-based management systems for strategic planning in carrying out the mission of the agency. Administrative data-based management systems are vital to the efficiency and life of the agency. At the same time, nursing must concern itself with the quality of nursing services delivered to clients. The development of Nursing Information Systems (NIS) will help to extract nursing- and client-centered information, which will add to quality assurance and research activities.

In order to develop these systems, some knowledge of computer technology is necessary, or consultation from an expert is advised. A well-developed evaluation plan based on one of the theoretical models described earlier in the chapter is advised. Existing quality control systems can be quantified and adapted to the computer. Several examples of basic resources useful for developing computerized systems or finding existing software packages are the texts, *Using Computers in Nursing* by Ball and Hannah (1984) and *Essentials of Computers for Nurses* by Saba and McCormick (1986) and the journal *Computers in Nursing* published by J.B. Lippincott (1984+). The latter journal periodically carries a complete listing of the software applicable to nursing that is currently on the market. A non-nursing journal in the public market is *Personal Computing*, a valuable reference for software as it pertains to personal computers. This list is not intended to promote resources, nor is it comprehensive.

An example for collecting and analyzing data that relates to the structure of the agency is the "Overall Agency Evaluation Report" form in the *Administrator's Handbook for Community and Home Care Services* (Fish, 1984, p 334). Application of a computerized version of the Phaneuf "Nursing Audit" would assist in process/product evaluation. The Phaneuf form is presented in the same manual (Fish, 1984) starting on page 382. It is possible to adapt existing tools, or new tools specific to an agency's needs can be developed for computers. A word of caution: New instruments must be validated, and reliability studies must be conducted to verify their worth.

Personal computers (PCs) are readily available in today's market. The nurse consumer is urged to review the literature available concerning each product's advantages. If nurses are not knowledgeable in the field, they should seek consultation from competent users of the hardware (computers). The basic hardware necessary for setting up a system is as follows: a computer with a single- or double-disc drive, a monitor, and a printer. Usually, dot matrix printers are adequate for recordkeeping activities as contrasted to the more expensive letter-quality printers for business and professional correspondence.

Some of the factors to consider when purchasing a computer are cost; estimated return for investment, such as savings in time; accuracy of records, editing ability, and compatibility with other computers such as home computers and the mainframe that is used in another agency or system. In the latter case, a modem or the ability to communicate with other computers will be an additional piece of hardware. Part of the cost of this addition includes the installation of the modem and monthly phone charges for cable access to the mainframe.

The following considerations are offered when purchasing software for computers. There are many programs available that are compatible with other PCs in case there is need for interchange between staff members for recordkeeping purposes and quality control. The following is a list of software that are compatible with many PCs currently on the market and applicable to small agencies, nursing corporations, or private practices. The software packages are listed for purposes specific to home health care agencies. They are only suggestions susceptible to outdating and are not meant to be comprehensive. The reader is urged to read current literature listing the more recent programs available.

Budgets: Visicalc (Beil, 1984) allows budget management, planning, forecasting, budgeting, cash flow analysis, and other features. PFS File, Graph, and Report (Page, Mays, Mack, and Langworthy, Software Publishing Corporation, 1984) also have accounting possibilities. For setting up nursing diagnosis classification systems and their quality control activities, the various PCs have programs that teach how to write programs specific to the users' needs. An example is PC/PILOT by Washington Computer Services (Kheriaty, 1985).

The PFS Write, File, and Report systems are pre-packaged interactive systems that are "user friendly" and have possibilities for a quality control system. The Apple Works (Williams, 1984) is an interactive system that features word processing, file management, and report systems that can be used for multiple purposes and are purported to be user friendly.

It is possible to conduct epidemiologic studies with personal computer software. Although communicable disease and disease processes are the usual groups of health problems under study in epidemiology, nursing problems or diagnoses are also appropriate. There are many statistical packages available for data analysis. One of the most friendly packages, which also contains a file management system for recordkeeping purposes and statistical reporting, is Statistics with Finesse (Bolding, 1984). Other statistical packages with extensive methods available for analysis are Beta-STAT by Belanger (1984) and Crunch Interactive Statistical Package (CRISP) (CRUNCH, 1986).

For the small agency or for the individual staff nurse, several word processing packages are available that are extremely useful in writing progress notes, letters, and reports. Some of the user friendly packages include Apple Writer II (1984), PFS Write (Edwards, Leu, Crain, Doerr, and Varteressian, 1984), and WORDPERFECT (1985). Modern society and its computer technology offer much that can help to document nursing care and at the same time be cost-efficient. Staff development and patient education packages can be developed by nurses using personal computers. Examples of software authoring system programs to guide the user are PC/ PILOT (Kheriaty, 1985) and a graphics software package (CHART, 1985), which allow the user to create illustrations to enhance the learning materials.

## Program Planning and Evaluation as Part of Quality Control

Agency and private practice home health care services are classified as programs offered to the public. Previous discussion on evaluation in this chapter implies that quality assurance takes place on the individual patient, aggregate client, and agency service levels. Theories and models of evaluation were reviewed according to their application to agency or program assessment. The following discussion applies to the implementation of evaluation theories during the program planning, development, implementation, and outcome stages.

## Program Development, Planning, and Implementation

Overall purposes and goals of the agency or private practice serve as the organizing themes for programs, for example, nursing services, health education, and control of communicable disease. Specialized programs in home health care are part of the nursing services provided by a single-purpose agency, combined agency, hospital-based program, or private practice. Examples of specialized home health care programs include Application of High Technology to the Home Setting, Hospice Care, Respite Care, Long-Term Care, and Care of the Frail Elderly. Program planning for specialized services in the community takes into account population needs and community participation. The American Nurses Association (1985) has developed a guide for community-based services, and this model can assist program planners in developing a philosophy and purposes for the services, needs assessment, a working relationship with the population, a plan based on goals and objectives, and a quality assurance program.

## Program Development

Before a program is initiated, a needs assessment of the community in which the program is to be implemented is necessary. A needs assessment includes a diagnosis of the home health care problems within the community. Many programs in community settings fail because the problem and/or the aggregate client for which it is targeted does not exist, nor is it perceived as a problem by the population.

If an agency or health care provider plans to conduct a needs assessment of the community, the chosen methods for data collection should be subjected to reliability and validity analyses. Methods for analyses include, but are not confined to, interviews, questionnaires, check lists, and opinion surveys. A review of the literature may produce relevant instruments from past studies. These studies should include a discussion of the tools' reliability and validity, and, although time-consuming, if there are no reports of validity and reliability in the literature, the assessor should conduct pilot studies of the chosen tool.

Newly developed tools are subjected to reliability and validity analyses. Analyses include a review of the construct, content, and/or face validity by experts in the field. Reliability studies could include a small pilot study for test–retest reliabilities, inter- and intrarater reliabilities, and internal consistency, if indicated. Professionals interested in detailed descriptions of how to conduct these tests are directed to basic nursing research texts such as Polit and Hungler (1985) and Waltz, Strickland, and Lenz (1984). Utilization of reliable and valid tools for collecting data when assessing the community is essential to accurate needs identification and diagnoses.

The needs assessment team collects the data with the chosen instrument(s), quantifies it according to the type of data and statistical procedure planned, and carries out an analysis of the data. Results are summarized and directed toward the basic needs assessment questions. Examples of needs assessment questions include

> What are the demographic characteristics of the general population?
>
> How does the anticipated target population compare to the general population?
>
> What are the major health problems occurring in the community, and how do they relate to home health care?
>
> Who are the major home health care agencies and providers in the community?
>
> What are the types of home health care services provided?
>
> To what extent are present home health care needs met?

What are the financial resources for home health care in the community, for families, and for individuals?

To what extent does the population identify home health care as a need?

## Program Planning and Implementation

As the data answer the needs assessment questions, they are presented in report form to the community and program planners. Based on the responses to the questions, specific home health care problems are identified as they relate to possible programs of services to meet the needs. The community, as client, and the health professionals are involved in the assessment, needs identification and diagnosis, and formulation of the goals and objectives for the program. The groups meet to agree on priority of problems and the goals they hope to achieve through program development and implementation and to schedule events throughout the planning stages that will help to measure progress toward the establishment and maintenance of the program. Chapter 2 of this text provides samples of community diagnosis of home health care problems, development of long- and short-term goals, and methods for planning programs.

### Formative Evaluation

Models of formative and summative evaluation are applied to the new program according to its nature, its personnel, stage of planning or implementation, and specific environmental factors, including resources, finances, and people. The long-term goals provide the framework for summative evaluation, whereas formative evaluation of the program takes place by measuring for the short-term goals. The long-term goals are set in terms of what the program hopes to accomplish, the primary beneficiaries, the role of the health care providers, and the expected dates of achievement. Each short-term goal is a step toward achievement of the long-term goals and must include what is to be done, by whom, and the expected dates of completion.

Setting time parameters for both long- and short-term goals helps to measure the progress of program development and its outcomes. It gives the planners information on the realities of the plans and the implications for success. Program evaluation takes place throughout all phases of needs assessment, diagnosis of home health care problems, program planning and development, and implementation of the program. The reader is directed to the Program Evaluation Review Technique (PERT, Roman, 1969) for an excellent model of program planning and evaluation. PERT identifies the key components of the planning for a program. Schedules for completion of the activities related to the planning are set. Progress is measured by the completion of critical components of the program within the defined time frame.

Any model of evaluation appropriate to the situation may be applied to measure progress. It is important to carry out evaluation or quality control techniques as the program develops in order to take corrective action if problems occur, such as inadequate data, inappropriate diagnosis, or lack of community participation. An example of a model of formative evaluation as it applies to program development is that of goal-free evaluation as defined in the beginning of this chapter (Worthen and Sanders, 1973).

Data collection might consist of measurement of home health care indices, for example, numbers of referrals for home health care services, acuity levels of ill clients in the home, available home health care services with similar programs, and awareness of need for home health care on the part of the populace. An example of a specific tool for data-based program planning in home health care is *Use of Patient Statistics for Program Planning* (Levenson, 1979).

The data are analyzed according to the purpose of the evaluation, that is, relevance to home health care needs and progress toward specific program development. A report to the program planners by the evaluator or evaluation team compares the observed overall purposes and goals of the program to the intended objectives for program development.

### Summative Evaluation

The overall long-term goals of the program and standards of home health care by professionals, regulating agencies, and professional organizations provide the framework for summative evaluation activities. An example of a summative evaluation technique is the utilization of Worthen and Sanders (1973) goal-based model of evaluation. In contrast to goal-free evaluation, the evaluator or team uses the pre-defined purposes and goals of the program to measure outcomes.

Measurements according to the pre-set goals might include improved health status of the target population, increased caseload, a financially sound budget, satisfactory reports from regulating agencies, certification or accreditation by professional organizations and regulating agencies, satisfied clients and personnel, and indicators of the need for expansion of services. Failure to achieve the expected outcomes leads the evaluators and agency personnel toward process evaluation to identify the reasons for not meeting expectations. Decisions are made concerning the maintenance, expansion, or discontinuance of the program.

## Professional Accountability in Home Health Care

In this chapter, we have discussed the many facets of evaluation and quality assurance as they apply to the field of home health care. Each agency or nurse clinician in the specialty is accountable for her or his individual practice and the delivery of services and programs to the client. Home health care is becoming the arena for the delivery of care that once was traditionally placed in the hospital, and it provides a tremendous challenge for the nursing profession.

Recently, the American Nurses Association (1986) revised its standards for Community Health Nursing Practice. The standards apply to community health settings and to both generalists and specialists. Thus, some of the standards apply to home health care nursing practice, if nursing considers this area of nursing practice to be a subspecialty of community health nursing. Until home health care is defined as a specialty in its own right and its practitioners develop their own professional standards, the community health nursing standards can be adapted as one measure of professional accountability.

One of the strategies for coping with this challenge is through nurse-to-nurse collaboration. Traditional community/public health nurses may not have the experience and education for the skills associated with high-technology care for acutely ill clients. Adult and pediatric clinical specialists have these skills in their repertoire. At the same time, the latter groups of advanced nurse specialists may not have the expertise in family theory and assessment nor the necessary knowledge related to community action and its resources.

Collaboration between the various groups of nurses providing home health care services is indicated. Acute care setting nurses need to invite their community colleagues into the hospitals to meet potential clients, build a trust relationship, become competent in the technical aspects of care, and plan together for a smooth transition between acute care setting and the home. At the same time, community/home health care nurses can assist acute care colleagues in gaining knowledge of the available nursing services in the community. Community-based nurses can share information regarding home, family, and community assessment in order to facilitate an orderly transition from the varying levels of care, that is, home to acute care, acute care to home, or alternate care facilities. It is through such collaboration that the product of nursing care can be assured—quality care for the consumer of nursing care.

## References and Selected Readings

Albany Visiting Nurses Association: Patient Classification/Objectives System—What Is It? Orientation material, VNA #490, #491, #492, #493, #494, #495, 8/82, 9/82, 10/82

American Nurses Association: A Guide for Community-Based Nursing Services. Kansas City, ANA, Council of Community Health Nurses. ANA Publica, 1985

American Nurses Association: Standards of Community Health Nursing Practice. Kansas City, ANA, Council of Community Health Nurses. ANA Publica, 1986

American Nurses Association: Guidelines for Review of Nursing Care at the Local Level. Kansas City, ANA Publication Code: NP–54 3M, 12/76

Apple Writer II. A software package for personal computers. 1984

Ball MJ,Hannah KJ: Using Computers in Nursing. Reston, Virginia, Reston Publishing Company, 1984

Barkauskus V, Engle J: The evolution of a public health nursing performance evaluation tool. Journal of Nursing Administration 9: 8–16, 1979

Beil DH: The Visicalc Book. Reston, Virginia, Reston Publishing Company, 1984

Belanger RR: BetaSTAT. A software package for personal computers, 1984

Bly JL: Measuring productivity for home health care nurses. Home Health Care Service Quarterly 2: 23–29, 1981

Bolding J: Statistics with Finesse. A software package for personal computers, 1984

CareData: Indianapolis, CareData Systems, 1985

Carpenito LJ: Nursing Diagnosis Application to Clinical Practice, Philadelphia, JB Lippincott, 1983

Ceglarek JE, Rife JK: Developing a public health nursing audit. Journal of Nursing Administration 37–43, 1977

Computers in Nursing: A referred nursing journal. Philadelphia, JB Lippincott, 1984+

Crunch Interactive Statistical Package (CRISP): San Francisco, Crunch Software, 1986

Davidson SV: Community nursing care evaluation. Nursing Care Evaluation, 37–55, 1978

Daubert EA: A system to evaluate home health care services. Nursing Outlook 25: 168–171, 1977

Decker F, Stevens L, Vancin M, Wedeking L: Using patient outcomes to evaluate community health nursing. Nursing Outlook 27:650–653, 1979

Delta Computer Systems: Altoona, PA, 1985

Donabedian A: Evaluating the quality of medical care. Milbank Memorial Fund Quarterly 44:166, 1966

Edwards S, Leu C, Crain B, Doerr C, Varteressian L: PFS: Write. Mountain View, Software Publishing Corp, 1984

Fish CW: Administrator's Handbook for Community Health and Home Care Services. New York, Pub No 21–1943, NLN, 1984

Florida Association of Home Health Care Agencies, Inc: Quality Assurance Program, 2nd ed. Florida Association of Home Health Agencies, Inc, 1980

Flynn BC, Ray DR: Quality assurance in community health nursing. Nursing Outlook 650–653, October 1979

Graphics Package: Microsoft CHARTS: Bellevue, WA, Microsoft Corp, 1985

Griffith DG: Blending key ingredients to assure quality in home health care. Nursing and Health Care 7(6):300–302, 1986

Health Agency Management System: Springfield, MO, Management Software, 1985

Health Care Financing Administration: Medicare conditions of participation for home health agencies. Code of Federal Regulations, Chapter IV, 405.1201, Rev. Oct. 1, 1981

Health Care Financing Administration: Home health care agency information form and plan of treatment. Form HCFA–443. Washington, DC, Department of Health and Human Services, 8/85

Health Care Financing Administration: Home Health Agency Survey Report. Form HCFA–1572. Washington, DC, Department of Health and Human Services, 3/72

Home Care Information Systems: Totowa, NJ, 1985

Home Care Pac: Systems and Programming Resources. Oak Brook, IL, 1985

Home Health Care: Cable Place, NY, ACPI Ltd, 1985

Home Health Care System: Providence, RI, Fleet Information, 1985

HOMIS 80: Software Innovations. West Chester, PA, 1985

Hughes SL: Home health monitoring. Ensuring quality in home care services. Hospitals 74–84, November 1, 1982

InfoMed: Information systems for home care. Princeton, Research Park, 1985

Kheriaty L: PC/PILOT. Bellingham, WA, Washington Computer Services, 1985

Kessner DM, Kalk CE: Assessing health quality—The case for tracers. New England Journal of Medicine, 288:189, 1973

Levenson G: Use of Patient Statistics for Program Planning. New York, NLN, Pub No 21–1794, 1979

Manfredi C: Reliability and validity of the Phaneuf nursing audit. Western Journal of Nursing Research 8(2):168–180, 1986

McHugh ML: Information access: A basis for strategic planning and control of operations. Nursing Administration Quarterly. 10(2):10–20, 1986

MEDI/VISIT: Warwick, RI, IMI Health systems. Division of Information Management International, 1985

Minnesota Department of Health: Outcome Criteria Public Health Nursing Services and Home Health Care Services. Public health nursing section, 1983

National League for Nursing: Criteria and standards manual for NLN/APHA accreditation of home health agencies and community nursing services. New York, Pub No 21–1306, NLN, 1980

National League for Nursing: Position statement on ensuring quality in home health care. New York, NLN, Pub No 11–2166, 1986

New York State: Public Health Law, Amended L. Article 36–Home Care Services. Sec. 3600–3620, 1982

PFS Graph: A software package for personal computers. Mountain View, Software Publishing Corp, 1984

Page J, Mays M, Mack R, Langworthy B: Pfs: File and Pfs Report. Mountain View, Software Publishing Corp, 1984

Pennsylvania Assembly of Home Health Agencies: Quality Assurance in Home Health Care. Camp Hill, PA, 1975

Phaneuf M: A nursing audit method. Nursing Outlook 5:42–45, 1965

Phaneuf MC: Quality assurance: A nursing view. Hospitals 47:62–68, 1973

Polit DF, Hungler BP: Essentials of Nursing Research. Philadelphia, JB Lippincott, 1985

Roman D: The PERT system: An appraisal of program evaluation technique. In

Schulberg H et al (eds): Program Evaluation in the Health Fields. New York, Behavioral Publications, Inc, 1969

Romano CA: Development, implementation, and utilization of a computerized information system for nursing. Nursing Administration Quarterly 10(2):1–9, 1986

Rutstein DD et al: Measuring the quality of medical care—A clinical method. New England Journal of Medicine 294(11):528, 1976

Saba VK, McCormick KA: Essentials of Computers for Nurses. Philadelphia, JB Lippincott, 1986

Shamansky SL, Young KJ: Quality assurance in the community health care setting: Getting started. Washington State Journal of Nursing 53:33–37, 1981

Stanhope M, Lancaster J: Community Health Nursing Process and Practice for Promoting Health. St Louis, Mosby, 1984

Stufflebeam DL: In Popham WJ: Evaluation in Education. Los Angeles, McCutchen, 1974

United States Department of Health and Human Services: A classification system for client problems in community health nursing. DHHS Pub No HRA 80–16. Hyattsville, Bureau of Health Professions, 1980

Waltz CF, Strickland OL, Lenz ER: Measurement in Nursing Research. Philadelphia, FA Davis, 1984

Ward MJ, Lindeman C: Instruments for Measuring Nurse Practice and Other Health Care Variables, Vols 1 and 2. Western Interstate Commission for Higher Education, Washington, DC, USDHEW, 1978

Williams RE: The Power of Appleworks. Englewood, MIS Corp, 1984

WORDPERFECT: Orem, Utah, Satellite Software (SSI), 1985

Worthen BR, Sanders JR: Educational Evaluation: Theory and Practice. Belmont, CA, Wadsworth Publica, 1973

Zimmer MJ: Guidelines for development of outcome criteria. Nursing Clinics of North America 317–321, June 1974

Zimmer MJ: Quality assurance for outcomes of patient care. Nursing Clinics of North America 9:305–315, 1974

# 12

# Home Health Care Research—
# Implications and Issues:
# Meeting the Challenge

The rapidly changing health care system has had a tremendous impact on the acuity levels of patients discharged from hospital settings to home and on the numbers and types of home health care agencies. The practice of home health care nursing has also changed and is evolving into a clinical specialty. Research topics include demographics of the client population, organizational structure of agencies, types of client services, quality assurance issues, and the nature of nursing practice, including process and outcomes.

Research in nursing has come of age. Early studies concentrated on nursing education and the definition of nursing, whereas in the past two decades, we have seen an increase in clinical studies. One of the weaknesses in nursing research is the lack of studies verifying the reliability and validity of previous studies and their instruments. There are numerous pieces of nursing research needing replication. The Phaneuf tool used for quality assurance purposes in nursing care is an example of a tool used by nurses for years and only recently subjected to reliability and validity studies (Manfredi, 1986; Phaneuf, 1973). Nurse researchers exploring new problems are urged to search the literature, including unpublished master's theses and doctoral dissertations, for studies to replicate for reliability and validity purposes, especially those relating to home health care nursing.

The field of home health care offers numerous researchable problems. The previous chapter on program evaluation and quality assurance generates many questions that address administration and management issues in home health care. The questions include the following:

1. To what extent does a specific program provide for the needs of specialized client groups?
2. To what extent are the services provided cost-effective?
3. How do specific services demonstrate quality care and cost-effectiveness?
4. To what extent does a computerized system for recordkeeping improve cost-effectiveness, staff satisfaction, quality of care, and legal responsibilities?
5. To what extent does the organizational structure of the agency meet the needs of clients and staff?
6. What is the future administrative role for nurses in home health care?
7. To what extent are specific management philosophies, strategies, and styles effective?

The latter questions relate to the structure and organizational aspects of home health care agencies. Because the majority of home health care services focus on nursing, analyses of the nursing process and client outcomes are indicated. There are many existing tools to measure client satisfaction, nursing process, and client health condition. Many of these are used to measure the processes of delivering nursing care. The Phaneuf tool (1973) is a classic example of an instrument that measures nursing process and outcomes in community health nursing. Other tools for measuring quality assurance and nursing process are available and were reviewed in the literature (Ward and Lindeman, 1978). Reliability and validity studies for many of these instruments are included in the literature.

## Research Process

Nurses who do not have educational preparation or experience in research can still be a vital part of the research process through collaboration with nurse researchers. Many times it is the nurse in practice who generates the questions that are most important to clinical problems in nursing. Having a nurse researcher to collaborate with staff to conduct research is a luxury few health agencies currently experience because of the cost of an equitable salary for the researcher and the costs for proposing, conducting, and analyzing studies. Some agencies employ nurses who serve in multipurpose roles, that is, as educator/staff developer, researcher, quality control manager, and consultant. However, if the research outcomes relate to cost-effectiveness of programs or project trends for future services for strategic planning purposes, the agency may have good cause to plead for the support of a research position or project.

Grants to conduct research are available through the federal government, including the Division of Nursing, Health and Human Services, and the National Institute of Nursing. Other sources include short-term grants from state agencies and federal block grants to states for demonstration projects, professional organizations, and private foundations and endowments. Nurse researchers are available through educational institutions or large medical centers. If an agency provides student clinical experiences, the students' faculty supervisors are usually prepared in the research process. Nurse educators are interested in conducting research and welcome inquiries from the agency regarding collaboration of education and service.

There are numerous nursing texts on the market that describe the research process in detail. Three particularly helpful ones are Polit and Hungler (1985); Waltz, Strickland, and Lenz (1984); and Wilson and Hutchinson (1986). The research process begins with an overview of the problem and the purpose for the study. It defines a specific problem and, depending upon the nature of the research, lists hypotheses or specific related questions. A review of the literature provides an overview of the research conducted in the past and the underlying theories and concepts that relate to the problem under study. The theoretical framework synthesizes the review of the literature and provides the conceptual leap from the theory base to the study of the problem in the practice setting.

The design of the study is specified and includes the description of the population under study, the basic research instrument, and the methods for data analysis. Permission from an appropriate institutional review board for protection of human subjects' rights is required before proceeding with the study. After the data are collected, analyzed, and interpreted, the findings and implications for application to practice and/or further research are discussed.

There is little research relating to the current home health care nursing field of practice. Thus, the following study of client outcomes in home health care was selected to demonstrate application of the research process as previously outlined and to share the research questions generated. It is hoped that nurses will continue to investigate the problems relating to nursing process and the diagnostic classification systems frameworks as they apply to home health care practice.

## SAMPLE RESEARCH PROJECT: THE MEASUREMENT OF CLIENT OUTCOMES IN HOME HEALTH CARE AGENCIES*

### PURPOSE

The purpose of the project was to develop a reliable and valid tool for measuring the health status of patients receiving nursing care through certified home health agencies. It was proposed that such a tool would

---

* Keating, in press.

increase knowledge concerning the nature and quality of nursing care received by clients within the health care system. According to the literature review, reliable and valid tools for measuring patient-centered outcomes and nursing's accountability to the consumer are needed (Gordon, 1982; Atwood, 1980; Horn, 1980; Kreuger, 1980).

## CONCEPTUAL FRAMEWORK

Part of nursing's uniqueness lies in the classification of client health problems labeled as nursing diagnosis. Since the 1950s, this term has entered the nursing literature, and, after the first meeting of the National Group for the Classification of Nursing Diagnoses, it has become a model for defining nursing (Carpenito, 1983). Several of the classification systems have been discussed in this text (Carpenito, 1983; Gordon, 1982; Kim and Moritz, 1982; and Visiting Nurse Association of Omaha, 1980). Carpenito's (1984) definition for a nursing diagnosis was used for this study:

> Nursing Diagnosis is a statement that describes a health state or an actual or potential altered interaction pattern of an individual, family, group, to life processes (psychological, physiological, socio-cultural, developmental, and spiritual) which legally, the nurse can identify and order the primary interventions to maintain the health state or to reduce, eliminate, or prevent client alterations (p 1418–1419).

The early texts on classification systems did not include specific goals related to the diagnoses to provide the standards of care relating to each of the categories. Carpenito (1983) was one of the first nursing authors to add other components to the nursing diagnosis categories. Included with the diagnoses were definition, etiologic and contributing factors, defining characteristics, focus assessment criteria, nursing goals and principles, and rationale for nursing care. Carpenito defines outcome criteria or client goals as "the expected changes in the status of the client after he has received nursing care" (p 41).

The evaluation tool that was developed and tested for this study was based on Carpenito's (1983) framework for measuring client-centered outcomes. Positive outcome criteria include

1. Improvement in the client health status by increasing client comfort and coping abilities
2. Maintenance of present optimal level of health, optimal levels of coping with significant others, optimal adaptation to deterioration of health status, optimal adaptation to terminal illness
3. Collaboration and satisfaction with health care providers

Negative outcome criteria were complications, disabilities, and unwarranted death. According to Carpenito, outcome criteria should include in their format measurable verbs and specific content and time parameters, and they should be attainable (p 42). The advantage of the nursing diagnosis model for the development of a tool to measure patient outcomes was its wide applicability to nursing practice and its increasing acceptance by the profession as one parameter of practice. The nursing diagnosis model could also be tested as part of the data base that fits into the diagnostic-related groupings (DRGs) categories of the prospective payment method for financing health care.

*PROBLEM STATEMENT BASED ON*
*THE CONCEPTUAL FRAMEWORK*

Based on the review of the literature and the decision to develop an evaluation tool to measure nursing care outcomes, the following research question was formulated:

To what extent can quality of nursing care be measured by an instrument that is derived from specific patient outcomes or goals related to the nursing diagnosis classification of client health problems?

In order to develop an instrument to measure quality of nursing care, the following specific questions relating to the problem statement were developed:

1. To what extent do nursing diagnoses apply to home health care clientele?
2. To what extent are the diagnoses and their outcomes found in agency records?
3. To what extent do the nursing diagnoses relate to medical diagnoses?

*DESIGN OF THE STUDY*

The human subject review boards of the participating agencies granted approval for the research. Audits of client records used code numbers, and at no time were the identities of participants in the study or clients disclosed. The study was conducted in several stages. The first stage addressed the first two specific research questions concerning the relevance of the nursing diagnosis classification system to home health care clientele and their documentation in records. The second stage focused on the major question related to the development of an evaluation tool to measure client outcomes and pilot tested the initial tool and a revised version of the tool in several home health care agencies located in two major geographical areas of the country.

The last stage re-examined the fit of the nursing diagnosis classification system to client health problems recorded, as well as the documentation of medical diagnoses and their relationship to nursing (related question 3). Major statistical procedures included content and description analyses, and for reliability and validity, coefficient alpha, and intra- and interrater reliability rates of agreement between experts.

### METHOD FOR MEASURING RELEVANCE OF NURSING DIAGNOSIS CLASSIFICATION SYSTEM TO HOME HEALTH CARE

Nursing administrators and staff nurses were asked to rate the relevance of the nursing classification system model to their practice. A detailed blueprint with six objectives to measure the reliability and validity of the nursing diagnoses' relevance to home health care was developed. Table 12-1 lists the nursing diagnoses identified by the participants as relevant to their practice.

### METHOD FOR DEVELOPING A TOOL FOR MEASURING PATIENT OUTCOMES

A preliminary tool for measuring client outcomes was developed, and home health care nurses were asked to review it for its relevance to practice. The majority of the staff nurses found the tool relevant to client records and appropriate for collecting data. The tool was pilot tested

**Table 12-1.** *List of Nursing Diagnoses Rated by Experts as Having Relevance to Home Health Care Clientele★*

| | |
|---|---|
| Activity intolerance | Noncompliance |
| Anxiety | Alterations in nutrition: Less than body requirements |
| Alterations in bowel elimination | |
| Alterations in cardiac output | Alterations in nutrition: More than body requirements |
| Alterations in comfort | |
| Impaired verbal communication | Respiratory function, alterations in |
| Coping, ineffective individual | Self-care deficit |
| Coping, ineffective family | Sensory-perceptual alterations |
| Alterations in family processes related to an ill family member | Impairment of skin integrity |
| | Sleep pattern disturbance |
| Decreased fluid intake | Social isolation |
| Fluid volume excess: Edema | Alterations in thought processes |
| Grieving | Alterations in tissue perfusion |
| Alterations in health maintenance | Alterations in pattern of urinary elimination |
| Impaired home maintenance | |
| Impaired physical mobility | |

★ Indicated by listing the 10 most frequently encountered diagnoses and by rating each diagnosis on a scale of 1 to 4 according to frequency of encounter.

through a review (audit) of clients' records in a Visiting Nurse Association (VNA). Three nursing faculty with experience in home health care conducted the audit. Only the nursing diagnoses and their related goals, medical diagnoses, positive and negative outcomes, and time factors were recorded during the initial audit. The recordings were then subjected to analysis for interrater reliability. It was found that the three raters were consistent in their reviews of the records. The range of interrater agreement was from 60% to 80%.

Based on the results, it was decided to edit the tool and conduct an additional pilot study in three types of community-based health care agencies in northern California. The revised tool (Fig. 12-1) was used for record audits in a hospital-based home health agency, a county public health agency, and a combined public health/home health care agency. Twenty-five client records from each agency were randomly selected for audit by three expert nursing faculty. At the time of publication, the inter- and intrarater reliability and validity analyses were not available. Frequencies for types of medical and nursing diagnoses were counted and presented some interesting comparisons of nursing diagnoses with the initial pilot study; differences in diagnoses between types of agencies were also noted.

## DATA ANALYSIS: RELEVANCE OF THE NURSING DIAGNOSIS CATEGORIES TO HOME HEALTH CARE

Seventeen directors of home health agencies and 15 staff nurses in a large VNA in upstate New York participated in the initial pilot study. Since the study was an initial inquiry into the application of the nursing diagnosis model and related outcomes, the reliability and validity studies were norm referenced rather than criterion referenced (Waltz, Strickland, and Lenz, 1984).

The data collected from a scale for rating the relevance of the nursing diagnoses to practice were coded and analyzed using the Statistical Package for the Social Sciences (SPSS; Nie, Hull, Jenkins, Steinbrenner, and Bent, 1975), Subprogram: FREQUENCIES. Table 12-1 lists those diagnoses that were rated by the participants in upstate New York as the most frequently encountered in home health care practice. Table 12-2 lists the most frequently reported nursing diagnoses collected from an audit of client records in northern California using the revised tool for measuring client outcomes.

Several reliability and validity procedures were conducted for the initial pilot study and are planned for the second phase. Reliability measures include the following:

*Internal Consistency*—to measure the consistency of the 39 nursing diagnoses derived from Carpenito's (1983) text. An alpha coefficient of

Tool for Measuring Client Outcomes

| Client Identification No. | Medical Diagnosis | | Nursing Diagnosis | | Goal | | Positive Outcome Goal Met | Negative Outcomes | | | Date Admitted | Date Discharged | Time Lapse (in days) |
|---|---|---|---|---|---|---|---|---|---|---|---|---|---|
| | Code | Title | Code | Title | Code | Title | | Complications | Disabilities | Unwarranted Death | | | |
| | | | | | | | | | | | | | |

Figure 12-1. Tool for measuring client outcomes.

330

**Table 12-2.** List of Medical and Nursing Diagnoses Reported Frequently in Client Records by Type of Community Health Agencies

| Type of Agency | Medical/Health Problem | Related Nursing Diagnoses |
|---|---|---|
| County Health Department | Prenatal care number = 5 | Health maintenance, alterations in<br>Knowledge deficit<br>Noncompliance<br>Parenting, alterations in |
| | Postpartum number = 5 | Communication, impaired<br>Family processes, alterations in<br>Knowledge deficit<br>Parenting, alterations in |
| | Well-baby care number = 4 | Communication, impaired<br>Knowlege deficit<br>Parenting, alterations in |
| | Family planning number = 3 | Health maintenance, alterations in<br>Knowledge deficit<br>Noncompliance<br>Parenting, alterations in |
| Home Health Agency (Hospital and Community-Based) | Cancer number = 10 | Bowel elimination, alteration in<br>Comfort, alterations in<br>Knowledge deficit<br>Mobility, impaired<br>Nutrition, alterations in<br>Respiratory function, alterations in<br>Skin integrity, impairment of |
| | Cardiovascular problems number = 10 | Cardiac output, alterations in<br>Health maintenance, alterations in<br>Nutrition, alterations in<br>Knowledge deficit<br>Respiratory function, alterations in |
| | Orthopedic number = 7 | Comfort, alterations in<br>Bowel elimination, alterations in<br>Health maintenance, alterations in<br>Home maintenance management, impaired<br>Injury, potential for<br>Knowledge deficit<br>Mobility, impaired<br>Nutrition, alterations in<br>Skin integrity, impairment of<br>Urinary elimination, alterations in |

*(continued)*

**Table 12-2.** *List of Medical and Nursing Diagnoses Reported Frequently in Client Records by Type of Community Health Agencies (Continued)*

| Type of Agency | Medical/Health Problem | Related Nursing Diagnoses |
|---|---|---|
| | Cerebral vascular accident number = 6 | Bowel elimination, alterations in Cardiac output, alterations in Mobility, impaired Comfort, alterations in Health maintenance, alterations in Injury, potential for Self-care deficit Thought processes, alterations in |

0.364 was the index of reliability. It is hypothesized that the relatively low coefficient is due to the discriminant nature of the diagnoses within the classification system.

*Interrater reliability*—to measure the consistency of performance across the experts. Coefficient alpha was used for the upstate New York group and is planned for the northern California study. Each of the experts

**Table 12-3.** *Nursing Diagnoses with a High Percentage★ of Agreement Between Two Experts in Community Health Nursing (Number of Cases = 25)*

| Diagnosis | Percentage | Number of Cases |
|---|---|---|
| Anxiety | 75 | 4 |
| Bowel elimination, alterations in | 100 | 5 |
| Cardiac output, alterations in | 92 | 13 |
| Comfort, alteration in | 88 | 8 |
| Communication, impaired | 100 | 2 |
| Family processes, alterations in | 100 | 1 |
| Mobility, impaired physical | 77 | 9 |
| Nutrition, alterations in | 73 | 11 |
| Respiratory function, alterations in | 100 | 4 |
| Self-care deficit | 100 | 13 |
| Skin integrity, impairment of | 83 | 12 |
| Urinary elimination, alteration in patterns of | 100 | 7 |

★ Equal to or greater than 75%

randomly selected three client records and conducted a second audit. Analysis of the reviews found a coefficient alpha of 0.999.

*Content validity*—to determine the relevance of the diagnoses to practice. The nurses judged the classification system and were asked to list any client problems that were omitted, with general comments concerning the purpose of the research.

All statistical procedures were based on Waltz et al (1984) recommendations for reliability and validity studies.

## PILOT STUDY OF NURSING DIAGNOSIS DOCUMENTATION IN CLIENT RECORDS USING THE INITIAL EVALUATION TOOL FOR COLLECTING DATA

Although the directors of nursing and staff nurses in New York reported that nursing diagnoses and their related patient outcomes could be found in client records, the audit using the evaluation tool had mixed results. Nursing diagnoses were located; however, outcomes were more difficult to find. In addition, the tool did not yield all the data anticipated. It was decided by the researcher to return to two of the specific questions of the study: (1) To what extent are the diagnoses and their outcomes found in agency records? (2) To what extent do the nursing diagnoses relate to medical diagnoses? Only medical and nursing diagnoses were sought.

Twenty-five client records were randomly selected and reviewed by two expert community health nurses. Tables 12-3 and 12-4 list the nurs-

**Table 12-4.** *Nursing Diagnoses With Low Percentage of Agreement Between Two Experts in Community Health Nursing (Number of Cases = 25)*

| Diagnosis | Percentage | Number of Cases |
|---|---|---|
| Activity intolerance | 0 | 1 |
| Coping, ineffective | 33 | 3 |
| Fluid volume deficit | 1 | 1 |
| Grieving | 0 | 1 |
| Health maintenance, alteration in | 25 | 4 |
| Injury, potential for | 0 | 2 |
| Ineffective breathing patterns | 0 | 1 |
| Self-concept, disturbance in | 0 | 1 |
| Thought processes, alterations in | 0 | 1 |
| Total | | 9 |

**Table 12-5.** *Nursing Diagnoses Not Listed in Client Records Reviewed by Two Experts in Community Health Nursing*

| | |
|---|---|
| Diversional activity deficit | Powerlessness |
| Fear | Rape trauma syndrome |
| Home maintenance management, impaired | Sensory-perceptual alterations |
| Impaired gas exchange | Sexual dysfunction |
| Ineffective airway clearance | Sleep pattern disturbance |
| Knowledge deficit | Social isolation |
| Noncompliance | Spiritual distress |
| Oral mucous membranes, alterations in | Tissue perfusion, alterations in |
| Parenting, alterations in | Violence, potential for |

**Table 12-6.** *Nursing Diagnoses Frequently Listed in Client Records Regardless of Type of Agency (Northern California, 1986)*

| Diagnoses | Frequency |
|---|---|
| Bowel elimination, alterations in | 9 |
| Cardiac output, alterations in | 6 |
| Comfort, alterations in | 6 |
| Health maintenance, alterations in | 9 |
| Knowledge deficit | 15 |
| Mobility, impaired | 9 |
| Noncompliance | 15 |
| Parenting, alterations in | 12 |
| Respiratory function, alterations in | 8 |
| Skin integrity, impairment of | 5 |
| **Less than 5, but with interrater reliability rate of > 67%:** | |
| Coping, ineffective | 2 |
| Family processes, alterations in | 3 |
| Home maintenace management, impaired | 3 |
| Injury, potential for | 4 |
| Nutrition, alterations in | 3 |
| Ineffective breathing patterns | 1 |
| Self-care deficit | 3 |
| Sensory-perceptual alterations | 4 |
| Thought processes, alterations in | 1 |
| Urinary elimination, alteration in | 2 |

ing diagnoses with high and low rates of agreement between the experts. Table 12-5 lists those nursing diagnoses not found in client records.

Of the 95 nursing diagnoses identified in client records by the experts, 26 were not related to a medical diagnosis. Additionally, there were 27 medical diagnoses listed that were not nursing diagnoses. The overall rate of agreement between the judges in locating client health problems was 73%. Some of the variance was accounted for by judges placing client health problems into different nursing diagnostic categories. Three client records were randomly selected and subjected to intrarater reliability for the two researchers with an overall rate of 0.92.

After the evaluation tool used in upstate New York was revised, three nursing faculty members in northern California conducted audits of 25 client records randomly selected in each of three types of agencies.

**Table 12-7.** *List of Nursing Diagnoses Omitted in Home Health Care Client Records According to Geographic Location and Data*

| Upstate New York 1983 | Northern California 1986 |
|---|---|
| | Activity intolerance |
| | Anxiety |
| Diversional activity deficit | Diversional activity deficit |
| Fear | Fear |
| Home maintenance management, impairment | |
| Impaired gas exchange | Impaired gas exchange |
| Ineffective airway clearance | Ineffective airway clearance |
| Knowledge deficit | |
| Noncompliance | |
| Oral mucous membranes, alterations in | Oral mucous membranes, alterations in |
| Parenting, alterations in | Parenting, alterations in |
| Powerlessness | Powerlessness |
| Rape trauma syndrome | Rape trauma syndrome |
| Sensory-perceptual alterations | |
| Sexual dysfunction | Sexual dysfunction |
| Sleep pattern disturbance | Sleep pattern disturbance |
| Social isolation | Social isolation |
| Spiritual distress | Spiritual distress |
| Tissue perfusion, alterations in | Tissue perfusion, alterations in |
| Violence, potential for | Violence, potential for |

Table 12-6 lists the nursing diagnoses most frequently listed in client records regardless of the type of agency. Table 12-7 compares nursing diagnoses omitted from the records of home health care clients according to geographic location (upstate New York and northern California) and time (1983 and 1986).

### SUMMARY OF FINDINGS

Although the sample size was small and applied to no more than 25 clients for each of four agencies in two locations of the country, more than 27 nursing diagnoses were found in client records and seemed relevant to home health clientele. There appeared to be three categories of client problems amenable to services by home health care providers and documented in client records: nursing diagnoses, collaborative diagnoses (nursing and other health care providers), and medical diagnoses.

Nursing claims to be holistic and concerned about the biopsychosocial needs of the client; however, an audit of the diagnoses recorded in family folders produced a preponderance of problems focused on physiologic needs. The situation probably reflects the imperative to provide services that are reimbursable from major funding sources. A home health care staff nurse was asked why diagnoses such as spiritual distress, anxiety, and sexual dysfunction that seemingly relate to home health care problems do not appear in records. The answer was that nurses do assist clients with these problems, but recording them is not cost-effective.

Based on the preliminary screening of the data, the conceptual model for applying the nursing diagnosis classification system to home health care appears to fit. These findings related to two of the specific questions in the inquiry.

The major research question, "To what extent can quality of nursing care be measured by an instrument that is derived from specific patient outcomes or goals related to the nursing diagnosis classification system of client health problems?" was rated by staff nurses as appropriate to their practice. An audit of client records using the initial tool found that goals for clients were recorded but that they did not consistently relate to specific nursing diagnoses. Flow sheets recording each visit and the client's progress did not document the client's progress toward the goal, but rather recorded the implementation of the nursing care plan. Thus, the flow sheets reflected mean standards rather than end standards.

It is likely that the selection of records of clients currently receiving care rather than those of clients discharged from service was in error. The current clients' records reflected process evaluation. Discharged clients' records might have provided the product evaluation data measuring the positive or negative outcomes of care. The revised tool used in northern California did find goals related to each nursing diagnosis, and a preliminary content analysis of the data found that outcomes were easily identified in terms of positive and negative outcomes. All records selected in the latter study reflected clients who were discharged from service.

## INTERPRETATIONS AND IMPLICATIONS

For this study, the nursing diagnosis classification system applied to clients receiving home health care. There were three types of health care problems: (1) collaborative (with other care providers), (2) medical, and (3) uniquely nursing diagnoses (Carpenito, 1984).

Nursing directors and staff indicated that some of the diagnostic categories were not applicable. The audit verified their statement (see Table 12-7). Further study is indicated, because many categories logically apply to client health situations such as "sexual dysfunction related to loss of a body part" or "spiritual distress related to the loss of a loved one." Other diagnoses probably do not apply as often in home health care agencies, such as "rape trauma syndrome" or "parenting, alterations in." In the northern California study, the addition of a county health department nursing service demonstrated the different types of health problems and nursing diagnoses carried by public health agencies and home health care agencies. Thus, "parenting, alterations in" was commonly found in the public health records.

The evaluation tool from this study needs to be applied to a larger representative sample for further reliability and validity studies. One of the advantages of the tool is the short length of time for collecting data. The preliminary pilot study in New York took each of the two researchers 1½ hours to review 25 client records. The three researchers in the second study in northern California took 2 to 3 hours to review 25 records in each type of agency.

Additional study is indicated to identify the more common categories of nursing diagnoses and their potential for building standards of care. Each nursing diagnosis could be subjected to analysis for its underlying dimensions relative to client, nurse, and health care system characteristics. The three researchers of the study in northern California identified a variety of nursing diagnoses related to medical or health problems that were not verified by the other two researchers. It is possible that these diagnoses need further clarification for etiologic and defining characteristics to prioritize the most relevant diagnosis to the client's condition. The lack of interrater agreement in this instance most likely reflects the infancy of the application of the nursing classification systems and the imperative to build a data base on which to refine the systems. The authors suggest the use of the Diagnostic Clusters for Home Health Care Nursing conceptual model in this text as a possible guide for refining nursing diagnoses, especially as they relate to home care.

## Issues: Meeting the Challenge

### Overview

With the spiraling health care delivery costs in the 1980s and the need to control costs, the federal prospective payment method of financing medical/ health care was conceived and implemented. In a very short period of time, the new financing system had a tremendous impact on the health care system and resulted in increased acuity levels of patients discharged from hospitals. Small home health care agencies were spawned, including hospital-based home care units, specialty services, and nurse registries. These became the "cottage" industries of the home health care system. Many of these agencies merged into large corporations or conglomerates to provide a myriad of home health care services.

Traditional public health agencies faced the dilemma of choosing to add home health care services and/or continuing to provide primary levels of prevention. Owing to the financial realities of reimbursement for tertiary levels of care, many primary and secondary levels of prevention programs received less attention and were eventually lost. The effect of this loss of emphasis in public health has yet to be realized and bears investigation. An interesting aspect to the problem is the increased participation in self-care on the part of the consumer and the role that nursing should play. The rapidity of the change in the health care system, the increasing acuity levels of the client population, the aging population and its related multiple chronic diseases, the emerging roles of paraprofessionals in the health care field, nursing's development and its controversial role as a profession, and the entrepreneurial opportunities are all issues confronting nursing and health care.

### Ethical Dilemmas for Home Health Care Nurses

Home health care nurses are faced with ethical dilemmas relating to placement of clients at the appropriate level of care. Some of the dilemmas include: (1) the right to die at home and when; (2) placement of ill homeless people who have no shelter to which to return; (3) the conflict between the cost of care and the inability to continue services when third-party payments cease; (4) the need for agencies to maintain economically feasible client caseloads; (5) the competitive market among individual providers and agencies; (6) confusing families and clients; and (7) an increasing awareness on the part of the consumer to choose quality home health care mandating professional accountability.

An example of such a dilemma occurs when the client needs antibiotic intravenous therapy at home. The home health care agency is paid by the nurse visit or procedure, not by the hours spent in the home. Looking at the situation from a cost-efficient standpoint, the agency will lose money if the nurse has to spend more hours in the home when she or he could be generating other funds through additional visits. A visit from a nurse based in a registry type of service is more cost-effective, because the agencies are usually paid by the nurse-hours spent rather than by the visit or procedure. The impact on the client who receives services becomes obvious; the client may have to absorb the cost, and, in some instances, quality of care is not necessarily ensured.

All the components of the home health care field provide a social condition in contemporary society calling for action on the part of politicians, government, consumers, and professionals. The home care setting has become a part of the multifaceted health care system that impinges on the wholeness of the family. It intrudes into the physical and emotional home milieu and extracts family resources—financially, physically, emotionally, and socially. Yet it continues to operate in a health care system that provides limited care for the sick at home. Third-party payment, including health insurance, Medicare, and Medicaid, fail to provide the comprehensive health benefits needed to care for the ill at home. Thus, in many instances, the success of home health care is measured according to the wealth or non-wealth of the client, or the self-limiting characteristics of the disease process.

The health care system continues to focus on and provide care for sickness. Although many consumers and far-sighted health care providers recognize the need for health promotion and prevention of disease, the financial system fails to support health-related activities. Resources pour into high technology, which at times emphasizes life support without thought to quality of life. Few resources are invested in creating healthy living environments, health maintenance activities, and support for self-care. The original instructive visiting nurses provided care to the sick and, at the same time, taught home health care and preventive techniques to family members. With a financial system that cannot withstand additional costs, health care providers need to incorporate health-teaching activities that allow families and clients to assume more of their care, thus relieving some of the costs to the system and, at the same time, creating home and family environments conducive to care, recovery, and health promotion.

## Financial and Administrative Issues in Home Health Care

### National Association for Home Care's 1987 Blueprint for Action

The National Association for Home Care's (NAHC) *1987 Blueprint for Action* presents key legislative and regulatory issues that address many of the problems previously discussed. The following list of selected issues from the *Blueprint* summarizes them in relation to home health care nursing.

1.  Oppose Medicare and Medicaid budget cuts by

    · Maintaining calculation of home health cost limits on an aggregate basis, as established by Congress in SOBRA 1986
    · Opposing cost sharing (deductible and co-insurance for home health care by Medicare beneficiaries, which would reduce accessibility to the home health benefit
    · Rejecting Administration proposals for reduction in federal Medicaid expenditures (NAHC, 1987, p 1).

Financial support for comprehensive home health care services for clients is included in these selected issues. NAHC is recommending that home health agencies be allowed to aggregate costs of visits, that is, to balance costs of services that may be more expensive (social work) against lower cost visits (home health aides). On July 5, 1985, the Health Care Financing Administration set new cost limits for home care agencies that disallowed aggregating or averaging out of costs. However, on July 1, 1986, Congress overturned these limits through the Sixth Omnibus Reconciliation Act (SOBRA, P.L. 99–509). SOBRA establishes a percentage of the mean of visit costs (112% to 120%) to restore the ability of agencies to aggregate costs.

The Administration has proposed that Medicare beneficiaries share in the cost of home health services by co-payments for visits. The NAHC is concerned that further cuts in the financing of home care and instituting co-insurance programs place an additional burden on clients who can ill afford to pay for home visits. Of special concern are the frail elderly with limited incomes. It is feared that clients would avoid home care owing to their inability to finance co-payments. The situation could lead to increased client hospitalizations from the lack of home care services, which help to prevent deterioration of the medical condition.

The Administration is also proposing Medicaid reductions by capping federal reimbursement and passing on the costs to the states' Medicaid programs. Such action could prevent many needy clients from receiving home health care.

2.  Clarify the home care benefit by

    · Ensuring reasonable, fair, and appropriate application of the "intermittent care" requirement
    · Ensuring reasonable, fair, and appropriate application of the "homebound" requirement (NAHC, 1987, p 1).

The current definitions for allowable costs in home care as contrasted to "24-hour care" are based on the terms *homebound* and *intermittent*. The definitions are vague and their implementation for reimbursing services are inconsistent. NAHC is recommending that intermittent care be defined as one or more visits per day (as necessary) on a daily basis and up to 90 days of services. Daily visits should be defined as 7 days per week; currently, in some states, they are defined as 3 to 5 days per week.

The term *homebound* is defined as those clients who are able to leave their homes for short, intermittent periods of time for purposes of medical treatment, or other short trips such as a walk, a trip to a store, beauty salon, and so on. NAHC is recommending that *homebound* be expanded in its interpretation. *Homebound* should be defined as "for the client where home health care is the appropriate level of care." It would permit clients to receive home care and yet increase their mobility by allowing flexibility in the reasons for leaving home for short periods of time.

3. Reform reimbursement by

   · Introducing prospective payment system for home health care that would provide predictable payment for services while decreasing administrative burdens on providers
   · Providing additional Medicare reimbursement for high-technology services (NAHC, 1987, p 1).

The NAHC is recommending a prospective payment method for financing home health care similar to that implemented in hospitals. It is believed that the system would allow home health agencies to develop predictive and reasonable budgets. It would also help to reduce the administrative costs that currently accompany the retrospective reimbursement system. NAHC is encouraging the inclusion of home health services into the recently passed catastrophic illness coverage for Medicare beneficiaries. Services would include care for both acute and chronic illnesses, such as Alzheimer's disease, in the home and would provide a broader spectrum of home health services in lieu of more expensive hospitalizations or institutionalizations.

4. Make the home care benefit more available to populations in need by

   · Authorizing a program of pediatric home care to support fragile children and their families
   · Including respite care in the Medicare hospice benefit
   · Financing hospice benefits for children
   · Authorizing coverage of nutritional services and IV therapy as part of the Medicare home care benefit
   · Financing a humane system of care for the patient with acquired immunodeficiency syndrome (AIDS; NAHC, 1987, p 1).

These issues relate to increasing home health care services for client groups with special needs. The present health care financial system does not reimburse home care services for fragile infants and children who thus remain hospitalized for longer periods of time than necessary. It disallows IV therapy, nutritionist services, and respite care for the primary care provider. These are essential services for maintaining clients in their homes and avoiding higher cost health care services and providing a caring environment for the ill family member. In-home respite services would provide rest and comfort for both the client and family and/or support systems. This facilitates the maintenance of the client at home rather than transferring the person to an institutional setting for care.

The AIDS epidemic has created a population of gravely ill young people who, many times, prefer to remain at home for supportive care and to die at home. Most of these clients do not have adequate health care insurance or have used up all their benefits. The health care system does not have the resources to support the acute care that they require. Home care provides a cost-effective and humane option of care. The concern for these special-need client groups is the lack of support for comprehensive services. Home care services for these clients could prove to be cost-effective by decreasing length of stay in the hospital, preventing re-admission, and providing care in a humanistic environment that promotes recovery, provides comfort, and supports the client and family and/or significant other structures.

5.  Improve quality of care by

    ·   Enacting legislation creating minimal standards for all home care programs receiving federal funds
    ·   Promoting state licensure programs that establish standards for administrators, professionals, and paraprofessionals (NAHC, 1987, p 1).

NAHC reports that 15 states have no licensure or accreditation regulations for home health agencies. To ensure quality of services, NAHC believes that Congress should enact legislation requiring standards for all Medicare- and Medicaid-financed programs. Standards should include regulation of individual care providers and administrators, training of home health aides and homemakers, and supervision of health care providers to ensure quality of care. NAHC recommends accreditation by such organizations as the National League for Nursing, the Joint Commission on Accreditation of Hospitals, and the National Home Care Association and through Medicare regulations.

Embedded in the quality assurance issues are NAHC's concerns about elder abuse. NAHC reports that whereas most elder abuse occurs by family members, some providers have abused clients in their care. NAHC strongly recommends that Congress enact legislation that will institute programs to identify, treat, and prevent cases of elder abuse.

## Political Action: Implications for Nursing

Political action on the part of nurses is indicated through involvement with national and local health policies and legislation (Mason and Talbott, 1985). Nurses must bring the attention of the public and lawmakers to the present and future health care needs of the population. The demographics of today's

American society imply increasing demands on an already overburdened health care system.

Demographics include a mobile, transient, and aging population. Senator Bill Bradley (Caring, 1985, p 4) states that by the year 2000, the over-85 population will be 60% larger than it is today. More than 15 million older Americans will suffer chronic disease, limiting their daily activities, an increase of 50% over 1980 statistics. Currently, the major third-party payment systems (Medicare and private health insurance) do not provide adequate coverage for home health care or long-term care to meet the needs of the chronically ill.

## Research and Program Development: Implications for the Future

The shrinking size of the American family owing to fewer children, divorce, more women in the work force, and mobility has an effect on the support systems available for providing home health care to family members. Limited family size creates a need for respite care for the family member who is expected to become the major care provider for the ill member at home. Home care appears to be more cost-effective than institutional care in terms of health care dollars. The intrinsic benefits to the client and family, including the sense of client self-sufficiency, self-worth, and self-esteem have not been measured. They provide excellent research questions for nurses in home health care to demonstrate the worth of nursing services.

Multiple issues of concern to home health care nurses call for their involvement in program development to meet the needs of the aggregate client system. Examples of problems include nurse-managed home health care services and nursing centers, recreational and health promotion services for the elderly to prevent or slow the advance of chronic illnesses, volunteer programs to visit the elderly at home, adult day-care centers and nursing homes without walls, and integration of population age groups (e.g., day care for children and for senior citizens).

Clients with chronic disease and expensive illnesses requiring high technology and those who choose to die at home need support systems from society and the health care system to provide them with quality care. There is a need to create solvent financial support systems for clients. Home health care coverage as part of health insurance benefits should be mandated. Tax deductions for home health costs and adult day care should be part of the tax structure.

Computerization is a part of the current health care delivery system and will expand in its application in the future. Systems will be developed for assessing, diagnosing, and treating client health problems in the home by communicating between systems in the home, agency, and medical centers. Patient- and family health–teaching computerized programs exist and will be developed in the future. Instructional videotapes for home use to teach and reinforce procedures will become commonplace. An excellent resource for existing computer-assisted health care education is found in *Bolwell's Software Directory* (1986).

There is a need for quality assurance programs for the agencies who provide care. Highly skilled technicians are needed in home health care. Nursing must take the responsibility for ensuring quality staff and services (Griffith, 1986). Nursing must provide adequate supervision of paraprofessional staff and must guard against a predominance of low-level, poorly prepared health care providers who threaten the well-being of the clients.

Professional nurses must become more knowledgeable and competent in the field in order to create the clinical specialty of home health care for today's health care system. Home health care nurses need to conduct research and collaborate with each other (acute care and community-based professionals) to meet the needs of the consumers of home health care and their families.

## Conclusions

### Practice

Home health care nurses are the pioneers of a new frontier of health care. They need to be visionary, highly skilled in "caring" strategies, advocates for clients, and risk takers. The nurse remains the pivotal figure in providing optimal care for the client of home health care services. Nursing must assume responsibility for equal access, adequate services, and quality care for clients in a financially restrictive health care system. To accomplish these tasks, nurses must become involved in political activist roles in home health care program planning, policymaking, and legislation.

### Education

Staff development programs and continuing education for nurses will continue to provide home health care knowledge and skills necessary for nurses to provide services from community- and hospital-based home care agencies. Home videotapes for teaching and reinforcing techniques and skills are examples of learning opportunities for professional, paraprofessional, and family home health care providers. Collaboration between nursing service and education can provide the resources and personnel for creating continuing education programs appropriate to the needs of nurses who are providing services in a constantly changing home health care system.

Education in both the undergraduate and graduate curricula will undergo changes to incorporate home health care into the theory base and practice of nursing. Baccalaureate programs continue to produce generalists through curricula that include the introduction of theory and practice in specialities that should include home health care. The programs will not produce specialists in the field but, with collaboration from home health care service, can expect to prepare graduates who function at beginning levels of home care practice under the mentorship of an experienced nurse or through planned internships.

Baccalaureate programs may choose to integrate home health care concepts and clinical skills into acute care settings, such as adult, child, and gerontologic nursing, or community-based settings, such as community/ public health, mental health, and home health care nursing. At the senior level, some schools of nursing may offer areas of concentration or preceptorship clinical models in home health care. Since a great percentage of nursing practice will take place in the home or community setting in the near future, it is imperative that nursing education and service collaborate for the preparation of beginning level practitioners in home health care.

Home health care nursing tracks for clinical specialists, administrators/ managers, or staff developers/client educators are being developed at the master's level. Research in home health care will provide new knowledge and opportunities for doctoral study and dissertation topics for high-level nurse scholars.

## Research

Theoretical frameworks and conceptual models such as the Diagnostic Clusters Model proposed by the authors are needed as paradigms for home health care nursing. The frameworks will serve to demonstrate the uniqueness of nursing services in home care, the cost-effectiveness of home-based nursing services, and the quality of services through improved client and family outcomes. Nursing research will provide a sound base for the practice of home health care nursing, and replication of studies will validate or refute findings, ultimately leading to improved health care services for clients. With research findings to validate its significance and contribution to quality client services, nursing will demonstrate its leadership role in home health care.

## References

Atwood JR: A research perspective. Nursing Research 29(2):105–108, 1980
Bolwell C: Software Directory. April, 1986. Saratoga, CA, DISKOVERY Computer Assisted Healthcare Education, 1986
Carpenito LJ: Nursing Diagnosis Application to Clinical Practice. Philadelphia, JB Lippincott, 1983
Carpenito LJ: Is the problem a nursing diagnosis? American Journal of Nursing 11:1418–1419, 1984

Gordon M: Manual of Nursing Diagnosis. New York, McGraw-Hill, 1982

Griffith DG: Building key ingredients to assure quality in home health care. Nursing and Health Care 7(6):300–302, 1986

Horn BJ: Establishing valid and reliable criteria: A researcher's perspective. Nursing Research 29(2):88–90, 1980

Keating S: Measurement of client outcomes in home health agencies. In The Measurement of Clinical and Education Nursing Outcomes. New York, Springer Publishing, (in press)

Kim MJ, Moritz S: Classification of Nursing Diagnoses: Proceedings of the Third and Fourth National Conferences. New York, McGraw-Hill, 1982

Krueger JC: Establishing priorities for evaluation and evaluation research: A nursing perspective. Nursing Research 29(2):115–118, 1980

Legislative feature. Caring 4(4):4–37, 1985

Manfredi C: Reliability and validity of the Phaneuf nursing audit. Western Journal of Nursing Research 8(2):168–180, 1986

Mason D, Talbott S: Political Action Handbook for Nurses. Menlo Park, CA, Addison-Wesley Publishing Co, 1985

National Association for Home Care: 1987 Blueprint for Action. Developed by NAHC Government Affairs Committee and Approved by NAHC Board of Directors, 1987

Nie NH, Hull CH, Jenkins JG, Steinbrenner K, Bent DH: Statistical Package for the Social Sciences, 2nd ed. New York, McGraw-Hill, 1975

Phaneuf MC: Quality assurance: A nursing view. Hospitals 47:62–68, 1973

Polit DF, Hungler BP: Essentials of Nursing Research. Philadelphia, JB Lippincott, 1985

Visiting Nurse Association of Omaha: A Classification Scheme for Client Problems in Community Health Nursing. US Dept of Commerce, National Technical Information Service, DHHS Publica. No HRA 80–16, June, 1980

Waltz CF, Strickland OL, Lenz ER: Measurement in Nursing Research. Philadelphia, FA Davis, 1984

Ward MJ, Lindeman CA: Western Council on Higher Education for Nursing. Western Interstate Commission for Higher Education. Instruments for Measuring Nurse Practice and Other Health Care Variables, vols 1 and 2. Washington, US Dept of Health, Education anad Welfare, 1978

Wilson HS, Hutchinson SA: Applying Research in Nursing. Menlo Park, CA, Addison-Wesley Publishing Co, 1986

# Community Assessment Model for Home Health Care

## Description of the Community

### Horizontal Patterns

I. Boundaries—Geopolitical Lines
II. Population Characteristics
  A. Vital Statistics: Total Population
    1. Age groups
    2. Birth- and death rates
    3. Immigration and emigration statistics
  B. Demographics
    1. Socioeconomic factors
      a. Mean income
      b. Major sources of income
      c. Major industries and commerce
    2. Major religious preferences
    3. Major cultural/ethnic representations
    4. Educational level characteristics
    5. Common family structures
  C. Health Statistics
    1. Leading mortality rates
    2. Leading morbidity rates
    3. Health care utilization patterns
      a. Private physicians
      b. Ambulatory care
      c. Long-term care
      d. Acute care

       e.  Home health care
       f.  Clinics and outpatient facilities
    4.  Financial support patterns for health care services
       a.  Private fees
       b.  Philanthropic
       c.  Insurance (Medicare, Blue Cross, Blue Shield, etc.)
       d.  Government support (Medicaid, Women Infants Children, Supplementary Security Income, etc.)

III.  Community Resources
    A.  Health Agencies
       1.  Hospitals
       2.  Long-term facilities
       3.  Health-related facilities
       4.  Home health agencies (for-profit and nonprofit)
       5.  Health departments
       6.  Combined health agencies
       7.  Ambulatory facilities
       8.  Private physicians and other health care providers
    B.  Health Care Providers
       1.  Numbers and types
       2.  Qualifications
       3.  Ratios to clients and needs

## Vertical Patterns

  I.  Type of Community Within County, State, and National Contexts (rural, urban, suburban, predominant political processes, type of government)
  II.  Population Characteristics—Comparisons With State and National Data (e.g., age groups, socioeconomic status, birth- and death rates)
III.  Health Care Resources From State and National Levels
    A.  Types of Agencies
    B.  Patterns of Health Care Services Utilization
    C.  Financial Support for Health Care Agencies, Client Care, Support Services and Equipment, and Health Care Providers

# Classification of Functional Patterns and Nursing Diagnoses

| Functional Pattern | Diagnosis |
|---|---|
| 1. Health perception— health management | *Altered growth and development<br>Health maintenance, alterations in<br>Potential for injury<br>Noncompliance |
| 2. Nutritional—metabolic | Fluid volume deficit<br>Fluid volume excess<br>*Hyperthermia<br>*Hypothermia<br>*Ineffective thermoregulation<br>*Infection, potential for<br>Nutrition, alterations in, less than body requirements<br>Nutrition, alterations in, more than body requirements<br>Oral mucous membrane, alterations in<br>*Potential alteration in body temperature<br>Skin integrity, impairment in<br>*Impaired swallowing |
| 3. Elimination | Bowel elimination, alterations in: constipation<br>Bowel elimination, alterations in: diarrhea<br>Bowel elimination, alterations in: incontinence<br>*Functional incontinence<br>*Reflex incontinence |

| Functional Pattern | Diagnosis |
|---|---|
| | *Stress incontinence |
| | *Total incontinence |
| | *Urge incontinence |
| | Urinary elimination, alterations in, patterns of |
| | *Urinary retention |
| 4. Activity—Exercise | Activity intolerance |
| | Airway clearance, ineffective |
| | Breathing patterns, ineffective |
| | Cardiac output, alterations in: decreased |
| | Diversional activity deficit |
| | Gas exchange, impaired |
| | Home maintenance management: impaired |
| | Mobility, impaired physical |
| | Respiratory function, alterations in |
| | *Impaired tissue integrity |
| | *Post-trauma syndrome |
| | Self-care deficit: |
| |     Total |
| |     Feeding |
| |     Bathing/hygiene |
| |     Dressing/grooming |
| 5. Sleep—Rest | *Sleep—Pattern disturbance |
| 6. Cognitive—Perceptual | *Altered comfort: chronic pain |
| | Comfort, alterations in, pain |
| | Impaired adjustment |
| | Knowledge deficit |
| | Sensory–Perceptual alterations: |
| |     Visual |
| |     Auditory |
| |     Kinesthetic |
| |     Gustatory |
| |     Tactile |
| |     Olfactory |
| | Thought processes: alterations in |
| 7. Self-perception | Anxiety |
| | Fear |
| | *Hopelessness |
| | Powerlessness |
| | Self-concept, disturbance in |
| 8. Role—Relationship | Communication, impaired verbal |
| | Family processes, alterations in |

| Functional Pattern | Diagnosis |
|---|---|
|  | Grieving (specify) |
|  | ★Unilateral neglect |
|  | Parenting, alterations in |
|  | ★Social interactions, impaired |
|  | Social isolation |
|  | Violence, potential for |
| 9. Sexuality—Reproductive | Rape–trauma syndrome |
|  | Sexual dysfunction |
|  | ★Altered sexuality patterns |
| 10. Coping—Stress tolerance | Coping, ineffective individual |
|  | Coping, ineffective family |
| 11. Value—Belief | Spiritual distress |

★ From *New Diagnoses Accepted by NANDA* (1986)
Diagnoses are grouped according to *Gordon's Functional Health Patterns* [1982] and *New Diagnoses Accepted by NANDA* [1986]. The authors of this text have classified them by functional patterns.)

# Diagnostic Divisions and Nursing Diagnoses as Developed by Doenges and Moorhouse (1985)

| Diagnostic Division | Nursing Diagnosis |
|---|---|
| 1. Activity/rest | Activity intolerance<br>Activity intolerance, potential<br>Divisional activity, deficit<br>Sleep pattern disturbance |
| 2. Circulation | Cardiac output, alteration in: decreased<br>Tissue perfusion, alteration in |
| 3. Elimination | Bowel elimination, alteration in constipation<br>Bowel elimination, alteration in diarrhea<br>Bowel elimination, alteration in incontinence<br>Urinary elimination, alteration in, patterns of |
| 4. Emotional reactions | Anxiety<br>Coping, ineffective individual<br>Fear<br>Grieving, anticipatory<br>Grieving, dysfunctional<br>Powerlessness<br>Rape-trauma syndrome<br>Self-concept, disturbance in: body image; self-esteem; role performance; personal identity |

| Diagnostic Division | Nursing Diagnosis |
|---|---|
| | Social isolation |
| | Spiritual distress |
| | Violence, potential for |
| 5. Family pattern alterations | Coping, family: potential for growth |
| | Coping, ineffective family: compromised |
| | Coping, ineffective family: disabling |
| | Family process, alteration in |
| | Parenting, alteration in: actual or potential |
| 6. Food/fluid | Fluid volume deficit, potential |
| | Nutrition, alteration in: less than body requirements |
| | Nutrition, alteration in: more than body requirements |
| | Nutrition, alteration in: potential for more than body requirements |
| | Oral mucous membranes, alteration in |
| 7. Hygiene | Self-care deficit (specify level: feeding, bathing/hygiene, dressing/grooming, toileting) |
| 8. Neurologic | Communication, impaired: verbal |
| | Sensory–perceptual, alteration in |
| | Thought processes, alteration in |
| 9. Pain | Comfort, alteration in: pain (acute and chronic) |
| 10. Safety | Injury, potential for |
| | Mobility, impaired physical |
| | Skin integrity, impairment of: actual |
| | Skin integrity, impairment of: potential |
| | Sexual dysfunction |
| 11. Teaching/learning | Health maintenance, alteration in |
| | Home maintenance management, impaired |
| | Knowledge deficit (specify) {Learning need [specify]} |
| | Noncompliance (specify) {Compliance [specify]} |
| 12. Ventilation | Airway clearance, ineffective |
| | Breathing pattern, ineffective |
| | Gas exchange, impaired |

# Classification Scheme for Client Problems in Community Health Nursing Developed by the Visiting Nurse Association of Omaha (Simmons, 1980)

Problems are listed as follows: Domain, problem label, modifier, sign or symptom.

## Environmental

*Income: Deficit*

    Low/no income
    High medical expenses not covered by insurance
    Expresses/demonstrates difficulty understanding money management
    Able to buy only necessities (e.g., food, clothing)

*Sanitation: Deficit*

    Soiled living area
    Inadequate/improper food storage/disposal
    Insects/rodents present
    Foul odor
    Inadequate water supply
    Inadequate sewage disposal

## Safety Hazards: Residence

> Structurally unsound
> Inadequate heat
> Steep stairs
> Obstructed exits/entries
> Cluttered living space
> Unsafe storage of dangerous objects/substances
> Unsafe mats and throw rugs
> Lacks needed safety devices
> Lead base paint present
> Unsafe gas/electrical appliances

## Safety Hazards: Neighborhood

> High crime rate
> High pollution level (e.g., noise, waste)
> Uncontrolled animals
> High traffic area

# Psychosocial

## Communication with Community Resources: Impairment

> Unfamiliar with procedures for obtaining services (e.g., education, health care, transportation, food, day care, recreation, furniture, clothing, religion)
> Difficulty understanding roles of service providers
> Unable to communicate concerns to care provider
> Expresses dissatisfaction with service provided
> Language barrier

## Isolation: Social

> Lacks contact with family/friends
> Alone most of time
> Uses health care provider for social contact
> Minimal outside stimulation/leisure time activities

## Behavioral Pattern: Impairment

> Demonstrates inappropriate suspicion
> Demonstrates inappropriate manipulation

Exhibits compulsive behavior
Demonstrates passive-aggressive behavior

## *Role Change: Impairment*

Reversal of traditional male/female roles
Reversal of dependent/independent roles
Assumes new role with loss of previous role
Assumes additional role(s)

## *Interpersonal Conflict*

Expresses disillusionment with relationship
Lacks shared activities
Incongruent values/goals
Poor interpersonal communication
Expresses prolonged, unrelieved stress

## *Grief*

Exhibits shock and disbelief
Exhibits denial
Exhibits anger
Exhibits bargaining
Family/individual in conflicting stages of grief process
Exhibits nonacceptance

## *Confusion*

Diminished attention span
Disoriented to time/place/person
Forgetful
Inability to do simple calculations
Inability to concentrate

## *Depression*

Downcast/sad/tearful
Expresses feelings of hopelessness/worthlessness
Loss of interest/involvement in activity
Excessive inward focus
Flat affect (e.g., monotone speech, limited body language)
Expresses wish to die
Attempts suicide
Fails to meet personal needs

*Anxiety*

Expresses feelings of apprehension
Irritable
Undefined fear(s)
Much purposeless activity
Inappropriate concern over minor things
Tremors
Narrow perception focus to scattering of attention

*Human Sexuality: Impairment*

Fails to recognize consequences of sexual behavior
Relates difficulty expressing intimacy
Sexual identity confusion

*Parenting: Impairment*

Provides restrictive environment
Handles child with difficulty
Expresses dissatisfaction with parenting role
Communicates inappropriately with child
Uses excessive/inadequate/inconsistent control
Conveys expectations incongruent with child's level of growth and
    development
Lacks skills for caretaking (e.g., feeding, bathing, elimination)
Inappropriate health care for minor injuries/accidents

*Neglect: Child/Adult*

Primary caretaker inappropriately relinquishes responsibilities
Fails to recognize psychosocial needs of child/adult
Poor personal/environmental hygiene
Child/adult left alone inappropriately
Child/adult lacks necessary supervision
Child/adult lacks appropriate stimulation/care

*Abuse: Child/Adult*

Harsh discipline
Welts/bruises observed/reported
Injury with questionable explanation
Verbal attacks

Child/adult exhibits fearful behavior
Physical violence
Scapegoating
Child/adult constantly receives negative messages
Sexual violence

## Growth and Developmental Lag

Abnormal results of developmental screening tests (improvised/ standardized)
Slow gain in weight/height/head circumference in relation to growth curve
Behavior inappropriate for age

# Physiological

## Hearing: Impairment

Unable to hear normal speech tones
Limited/abnormal response to sound
Favors one ear for listening
Abnormal results of hearing screening test (improvised/standardized)

## Vision: Impairment

Difficulty/inability to see small print/callibrations (e.g., syringes, thermometer)
Difficulty/inability to see distant objects
Difficulty/inability to see close objects
Abnormal results of vision screening test (improvised/standardized)
Limited/abnormal response to visual stimuli
Squinting/blinking/tearing/blurring
Color blindness

## Speech and Language: Impairment

Lacks ability to speak
Demonstrates inability to understand
Relies heavily on nonverbal communication
Uses inappropriate sentence structure
Demonstrates poor enunciation or clarity
Uses words inappropriately

## Dentition: Impairment

Missing/broken teeth
Decayed teeth
Sore gums
Ill-fitting dentures

## Respiration: Impairment

Abnormal breath patterns (e.g., shortness of breath, dyspnea)
Cough
Cyanosis (with or without activity)
Abnormal sputum
Noisy respirations
Rhinorrhea
Abnormal breath sounds

## Circulation: Impairment

Edema
Cramping/pain in extremities
Decreased pulse
Discoloration of skin/cyanosis
Temperature change in affected area
Varicosities
Syncopal episodes
Abnormal blood pressure reading
Pulse deficit

## Circulation: Impairment (continued)

Irregular heart rate
Excessively rapid/slow heart rate
Reports anginal pain
Abnormal heart sounds

## Neuro-Musculo-Skeletal Function: Impairment

Limited range of motion (e.g., contractures)
Poor coordination
Gait/ambulation disturbance
Decreased muscle strength/muscle tightness
Inability to manage activities of daily living
Tremors

## Digestive Function: Impairment

Nausea/vomiting
Difficulty chewing/swallowing
Indigestion/heartburn
Anorexia
Anemia
Abnormal weight loss

## Reproductive Function: Family Planning

Inappropriate/insufficient knowledge of family planning method(s)
Inaccurate/inconsistent use of family planning methods(s)
Dissatisfied with present family planning method

## Reproductive Function: Pregnancy

Inability to cope with changing body
Lifestyle incongruent with physiologic change
Minor discomfort
Fear of delivery procedure
Inability to cope with present body needs

## Reproductive Function: Impairment

Unusual/abnormal discharge
Abnormal menstrual patterns
Unusual changes in breasts
Unusual changes in testicles/penis
Dyspareunia (e.g., painful intercourse)

## Bowel Function: Impairment

Diarrhea
Constipation
Pain with defecation
Minimal bowel sounds
Blood in stools
Abnormal color
Reports cramping/abnormal discomfort
Increased frequency of stools
Incontinence of stools

## *Urinary Function: Impairment*

Incontinent of urine
Urgency/frequency
Burning/painful urination
Inability to empty bladder
Nocturia
Polyuria
Hematuria

## *Integument: Impairment*

Lesion (e.g., wound, burn, incision)
Rash
Hypertrophy of nails
Excessive oily
Inflammation
Drainage

## *Pain*

Statement of client
Elevated pulse/respiration/blood pressure
Movement compensation
Restless behavior
Facial grimaces
Pale or sweating

## *Consciousness: Impairment*

Lacks response to normal stimuli (e.g., touch, noise)

## **Health Behaviors**

## *Nutrition: Impairment*

Weight 10% more or less than average
Lacks/excess established standards for daily caloric intake
Improper feeding schedule for age
Emaciated/obese

## *Sleep and Rest Patterns: Impairment*

Sleep/rest pattern interferes with family lifestyle
Wakes frequently during night

Somnabulism (e.g., walks in sleep)
Insomnia
Nightmares
Insufficient sleep/rest for age/physical condition

## Physical Activity: Impairment

Sedentary lifestyle
Lacks regular exercise routine
Type/amount of exercise inappropriate for age/physical condition

## Personal Hygiene: Deficit

Dirty clothing
Dirty skin

## Personal Hygiene (continued)

Body odor
Matted/unclean hair
Unclean teeth
Halitosis

## Substance: Misuse

Abuses nonprescription drugs (e.g., medication, alcohol, nicotene)
Unable to perform normal routine
Reflex disturbance
Demonstrates change in behavior

## Therapeutic Regime Noncompliance: Medical/Dental Supervision

Fails to obtain routine medical/dental evaluation
Fails to seek care for symptoms requiring medical/dental evaluation
Fails to return as requested by physician/dentist
Lacks consistent source of medical/dental care
Medical/dental supervision sought by client but prescribed regime appears inadequate to meet client needs

## Therapeutic Regime Noncompliance: Prescribed Treatment Plan

Fails to perform treatment as prescribed
Fails to obtain needed equipment

*Therapeutic Regime Noncompliance:*
*Prescribed Medication*

> Deviates from prescribed dosage
> Lacks system for taking medication
> Medication improperly stored
> Fails to obtain refills appropriately
> Fails to obtain immunizations

*Therapeutic Regime Noncompliance:*
*Prescribed Diet*

> Inability to integrate dietary prescription into balanced nutritional
>   pattern
> Does not adhere to diet as prescribed

*Technical Procedure: Deficit*

> Unable to demonstrate/relate procedure adequately
> Requires nursing skills
> Unable to perform procedure without assistance
> Unable to operate special equipment correctly

*Appendix* | **E**

# Assessment Guidelines for Family Profile of Home Health Care Clients

## A. Subjective Data (Health History)

1. *Identifying Data:*

    Family Name:
    Address:
    Directions:
    Phone #'s:

    *Primary Care Provider(s):*
    Name:
    Address:
    Phone:

    *Insurance or Financing of Health Care:*

    | | |
    |---|---|
    | Type: | Coverage: |
    | Title: | Number: |
    | Contact person: | |

    *Informant:*
    Family members or significant others in home:
    Birthdates:
    Soc. Sec. #'s:

## 2. *Physiologic Data:*

*Health of Family Members:*

Name:                          Age:          Role in family:
Overall health status: (eventually complete health histories on all
                  family members)

*Home Health Care Client:*

Date cf referral:
Source of referral:
Name:                          Age:          Role in family:
Overall health status:
Medical diagnosis(es):
Chief complaint/analysis of symptom:
Prescribed therapeutic regimens:

## 3. *Psychological Data:*

Major cultural and language influences:

*Family Dynamics:*

| Members | Role | Primary Function | Interaction with Other Members |
|---------|------|------------------|--------------------------------|

*Impact of Illness on Family*

Home health care: major provider:
Child care: major provider:
Occupational demands:
House maintenance:
Leisure time activities:
Spiritual needs:
Grieving process:
Health–illness knowledge level:
Anxiety and/or fear expressions:
Dietary practices:
Nutritional needs:

## 4. *Sociologic Data*

Family economics:
Major income provider(s):   Name:
                   Occupation:
                   Work hours:

Other resources:          Insurance:
                                 Financial aid:
Major expenditures:     Housing:
                                 Food:
                                 Clothing:
                                 Health care:
Overall economic status of family:

*Potential Resources for Additional Aid:*
Family:
Community agencies:
Social services:

*Home Environment:*

Type of housing
Rent or own:
Number of floors and rooms:
Number of occupants:
Facilities:

*Neighborhood Resources:*

Neighbors involvement:
Outdoor access:
Transportation facilities:
Nearby stores and types:
Meals-on-Wheels:
Church/organizations, locations:
Quality of environment: climate, air, water, sewage, garbage,
                             sidewalks, streets, lighting
Milieu:

*Community Resources:*

Location of health care agencies and providers:
Social services:
Transportation:
Communication:
Educational opportunities:
Recreational opportunities:
Church/socializing institutions:
Industry:
Commerce:
Government:
Politics:
Law enforcement:
Emergency services:

### B.  Objective Data (Physical Examinations of Client and Family Members: Home Facilities)

1.  *Physical Examination*

    *Client:* Initial complete examination, continued monitoring of chief complaint(s)

    *Family Members:* Eventual complete baseline examinations

2.  *Home Facilities:*

    Location of client's room and access to: bathroom facilities, water, socialization with others

    Storage area for equipment protected from possible contamination or loss

    Home sterilization facilities (stove, oven, and pans)

    Location of safe storage of medications

    Condition of floors, stairs, and furnishings for mobility of client

    Special installations: appliances, handrails, ramps, raised toilet seats, commode, shower chair, hospital bed, assistive devices, wheel chairs, lounge chairs, etc.

    Preparation of food: refrigeration, stove, sink, basic stock items

    Method of waste removal

### C.  Assessment: Nursing Diagnostic Cluster

   Person:

   Environment:

   Specific Nursing Diagnoses and Related Client-Centered Goals:

### D.  Initial Plan of Care:


_____

Signature


_____

Date

# *Checklist for Selection of Vendors*

Vendor Name: _____

Contact Person: _____

Address: _____

Phone: _____

Hours: _____

| Criteria | Yes | No | Comments |
|---|---|---|---|
| 1. Geographic location/ accessibility | ____ | ____ | _____ |
| 2. Operating hours | ____ | ____ | _____ |
| 3. Set-up and delivery | ____ | ____ | _____ |
| 4. Financial billing/charging | ____ | ____ | _____ |
| 5. Maintenance and repair of equipment | ____ | ____ | _____ |
| 6. Back-up system | ____ | ____ | _____ |
| 7. Compatibility of equipment | ____ | ____ | _____ |
| 8. Inventory and condition of equipment | ____ | ____ | _____ |
| 9. Nurse's role/availability | ____ | ____ | _____ |

| Criteria | Yes | No | Comments |
|---|---|---|---|
| 10. Comparative costs with other vendors | ___ | ___ | _____ |
| 11. Total services vs other vendors | ___ | ___ | _____ |
| 12. Communication | ___ | ___ | _____ |

Overall Evaluation: Excellent ___    Good ___    Fair ___    Poor ___

Recommend: Yes ___    No ___

_____

Evaluator

_____

Date

# Home Environment Assessment Guide

## General Information

Family Name: _____ Date _____

Address: _____

_____

Phone: _____

Directions: _____

_____

Type of living quarters: Single room __ Apartment __ Home __

If a room or apartment: Floor: _____

Rent: __ Own: __

Method for gaining access into home: Front door __ Back door __

Other __ Elevator __ Stairs __

Family prefers that nurse call ahead: __ Ring bell __ Knock __

A. Outside access has adequate: Room for entry __ Lighting __

Facilities for handicapped or needed equipment and appliances _____

_____

Environmental conditions can be controlled (ice, mud, etc.) _____

_____

Security measures/personnel _____

_____

B. Surrounding grounds provide opportunities for change of scene, recreation, exercise. Neighborhood is safe and secure. Sidewalks, shopping,
and public transportation are available. Describe briefly:

_____

_____

_____

C. Living quarters have adequate utilities:

Telephone ___ Heat ___ Lighting ___ Garbage disposal ___

Hot and cold water from safe supply ___ Sewage disposal ___

Food storage and preparation ___ Bathing facilities ___

Furniture ___ Sleeping room ___

Study and leisure time facilities _____

Other:

_____

_____

D. The ill client's room or care providing site has space for:

   1. Equipment and supplies_____

   2. Storage facilities _____

   3. Ambulation and mobility _____

   4. Privacy _____

                     adequate:

   5. Access to water and disposal of wastes _____

   6. Lighting _____

Summary of assessment data: _____

_____

_____

## Diagnostic Cluster: Environment: Safety Patterns

Problem list of actual or potential environmental hazards:
1.
2. . . . etc.

Nursing Diagnoses: Coping, ineffective, family
                      Family processes, alterations in
                      Health maintenance, alterations in
                      Home maintenance management, impaired
                      Infection, potential for
                      Injury, potential for
                      Knowledge deficit
                      Mobility, impaired, physical
                      Self-care deficit, total or partial

related to:
1.
2. . . . etc.

Long-term Goals (outcomes): 1.
                                 2. . . . etc.

Short-Term Goals (objectives) for each long-term goal
1. Specific outcome desired
2. Measurable action verb
3. Extent of expectations
4. By whom
5. Time frame

Nursing Care Plan
1. What is to be done
2. By whom
3. When and how often
4. Where
5. Method(s)
6. Documentation

Evaluation
Progress as measured by meeting objectives:

Outcome as measured by meeting long-term goal(s):

Diagnosis #: Resolved on Date _____

Not resolved: Reasons _____

_____

Signed _____ , RN

_____

Client/Family Member

# AIDS Information Sources, Programs, and Legal Resources

## Information Sources and Programs— Northern California

AIDS Health Project (Mental Health)
333 Valencia Street, 4th Floor
San Francisco, CA 94103
(415) 626–6637

AIDS Interfaith Network
890 Hayes Street
San Francisco, CA 94117
(415) 928–HOPE

American Association of Physicians for Human Rights
P.O. Box 14366
San Francisco, CA 94114
(415) 558–9353
(415) 673–3189

California Nurses Association
AIDS Activities
1855 Folsom Street, Room 670
San Francisco, CA 94103
(415) 864–4141

Jewish Emergency Assistance Network (JEAN)
(415) 567–8860
(415) 788–3630

National Association of People with AIDS
519 Castro #46
San Francisco, CA 94114
(415) 553–2509

Pacific Center AIDS Project
400 40th Street, #200
Oakland, CA 94609
(415) 420–8181

San Francisco AIDS Foundation
Includes Women's Project
333 Valencia Street, 4th Floor
San Francisco, CA 94103
(415) 863–2437
(800) FOR–AIDS (Northern California outside San Francisco)
(415) 864–6606 TTY/TDD for the hearing-impaired

Shanti Project
890 Hayes Street
San Francisco, CA 94117
(415) 558–9644

## *Information Sources and Programs—Southern California*

AIDS Project Los Angeles
1362 Santa Monica Boulevard
Los Angeles, CA 90046
(213) 876–AIDS

San Diego AIDS Project
Includes Mothers of AIDS Patients (MAP)
P.O. Box 89049
San Diego, CA 92138
(619) 543–0300
(619) 234–3432

## *Information Sources and Programs—Midwest*

National Coalition of Gay Sexually Transmitted Disease Services
% Mark Behar
P.O. Box 239
Milwaukee, WI 53201
(414) 277–7671

## Legal Resources

Bay Area Lawyers for Individual Freedom (BALIF)
(415) 982–9211

Lambda Legal Defense and Education Fund
132 W. 43rd Street, Fifth Floor
New York, NY 10036
(212) 944–9488

National AIDS Network
1012 14th Street, N.W., Suite 601
Washington, DC 20005
(202) 347–0390

National Association of People with AIDS
P.O. Box 65472
Washington, DC 20035
(202) 483–7979

National Lesbian and Gay Health Foundation
P.O. Box 65472
Washington, DC 20035
(202) 797–3708

## Information Sources and Programs—New York

Gay Men's Health Crisis
P.O. Box 274
132 West 24th Street
New York, NY 10011
(212) 807–6655

Hispanic AIDS Forum
% APRED
853 Broadway, Suite 2007
New York, NY 10003
(212) 870–1902
(212) 870–1864

National Council of Churches
AIDS Task Force and Minority Task Force on AIDS
475 Riverside Drive, Room 572
New York, NY 10115
(212) 870–2421

National Gay Task Force
80 Fifth Avenue, Suite 1601

New York, NY 10011
(212) 807–6016
(800) 221–7044
National Hemophilia Foundation
Soho Building
110 Greene Street, Room 406
New York, NY 10012
(212) 219–8180

## Information Hotlines (toll free)

United States Public Health Service AIDS Hotline
(800) 342–AIDS
(404) 329–3534 (Atlanta)
United States Centers for Disease Control
(800) 447–AIDS
National Gay Task Force
AIDS Information Hotline
(800) 211–7044
(212) 529–1604 (New York State)

## Information Sources and Programs—England and Europe

The Terrence Higgins Trust
BM A.I.D.S., London WC1N 3XX
01–833 2971

## Information Sources and Programs—United States Government

United States Public Health Service
Public Affairs Office
Hubert H. Humphrey Building
Room 725–H
200 Independence Avenue, S.W.
Washington, DC 20201
(202) 245–6867
National Institute of Allergy and Infectious Diseases
Office of Research Reporting and Public Response
(301) 496–5717

# Information Sources and Programs—Washington, DC

American Red Cross AIDS Education Office
1730 D Street, N.W.
Washington, DC 20006
(202) 639–3223

AIDS Action Council
729 Eighth Street, S.E.
Suite 200
Washington, DC 20003
(202) 547–3101

# Index

Page numbers in *italics* refer to figures; page numbers followed by *t* indicate tables.